Mayo Clinic Atlas of Regional Anesthesia and Ultrasound-Guided Nerve Blockade

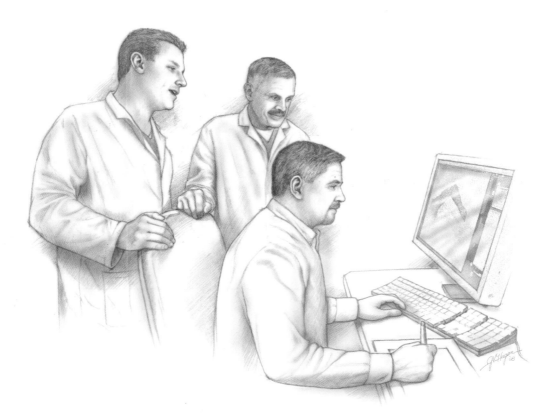

Dr. James R. Hebl (left), Dr. Robert L. Lennon (center), and Mr. John V. Hagen (right), the medical illustrator, conferring about one of the many drawings in this book.

Mayo Clinic Atlas of Regional Anesthesia and Ultrasound-Guided Nerve Blockade

Editors

James R. Hebl, M.D.
Robert L. Lennon, D.O.

Associate Editors
Adam K. Jacob, M.D.
Hugh M. Smith, M.D., Ph.D.

Illustrator
John V. Hagen

MAYO CLINIC SCIENTIFIC PRESS   OXFORD UNIVERSITY PRESS

Oxford University Press

Oxford University Press, Inc., publishes works that further
Oxford University's objective of excellence
in research, scholarship, and education.

Oxford New York
Auckland Cape Town Dar es Salaam Hong Kong Karachi
Kuala Lumpur Madrid Melbourne Mexico City Nairobi
New Delhi Shanghai Taipei Toronto

With offices in
Argentina Austria Brazil Chile Czech Republic France Greece
Guatemala Hungary Italy Japan Poland Portugal Singapore
South Korea Switzerland Thailand Turkey Ukraine Vietnam

Published by Oxford University Press, Inc.
198 Madison Avenue, New York, New York 10016
www.oup.com

Oxford is a registered trademark of Oxford University Press

Library of Congress Cataloging-in-Publication Data

Mayo Clinic atlas of regional anesthesia and ultrasound-guided nerve blockade / edited by James
R. Hebl, Robert L. Lennon.
    p. ; cm.
  Includes bibliographical references and index.
  ISBN 978-0-19-974303-2
  1. Conduction anesthesia--Atlases. 2. Nerve block--Atlases. 3. Operative ultrasonography--
Atlases. I. Hebl, James R. II. Lennon, Robert L. III. Mayo Foundation for Medical Education
and Research. IV. Title: Atlas of regional anesthesia and ultrasound-guided nerve blockade.
  [DNLM: 1. Anesthesia, Conduction--methods--Atlases. 2. Nerve Block--methods--Atlases.
3. Ultrasonography--methods--Atlases. WO 517 M473 2010]
  RD84.M39 2010
  617.9'60223--dc22

                                                                      2009042450

9 8 7 6 5 4 3 2 1

Printed in China
on acid-free paper

We undertook this project to enhance the well-being of our patients, to strengthen the education of our residents and fellows, and to stimulate dialogue in regional anesthesia among our colleagues both inside and outside our institution. It is our belief that advancing the art and science of regional anesthesia will occur only after achieving these goals.

With deep gratitude, we dedicate this book to our families. Their encouragement, love, and support make all things possible.

To my wife, Heather, and our children, Zachary, Matthew, and Gabriela.

J. Hebl

To my wife, Kit, and our family, Rob and Courtney, Becky and Bill and their daughter, Katie.

R. Lennon

FOREWORD

In 1981, I moved to Seattle, Washington, for a 1-year fellowship in regional anesthesia at Virginia Mason Clinic. Although the geographic setting was spectacular, it was the novel approach to patient management that impressed and ultimately convinced me that peripheral nerve blockade was more than a challenging technical skill with questionable clinical applicability. At that time, very few anesthesia departments had the expertise to utilize regional anesthesia routinely within the surgical suite. But at Virginia Mason Clinic, the surgeons demanded regional anesthesia for their patients. For this reason, patients *expected* to have neural blockade incorporated into their anesthetic experience. As a result, a group of senior anesthesiologists—all having excellent technical skills, an unflagging work ethic, and strong convictions about the benefits of neural blockade—provided a superior service to these patients. In fact, they had convinced their surgical colleagues through a combination of patient satisfaction and evidence-based publications that regional anesthesia was superior to general anesthesia alone. The result was an environment well suited to clinical studies, resident teaching, patient satisfaction, and excellent rapport between anesthesia and surgery colleagues. I rejoined Mayo Clinic in 1982 with the goal of creating a similar regional-anesthesia–friendly environment. This was accomplished with the help of dedicated colleagues, a strong relationship with the orthopedic surgeons, and an ultimate shared goal of improved patient care.

The past 2 decades have seen a renaissance in regional anesthesia—particularly peripheral nerve blockade. This has been fueled by several factors, including an emphasis on perioperative pain management, the appearance of evidence-based investigations within the literature, improvements in equipment, and widespread educational offerings. However, perhaps the most important change affecting this practice during the past decade has been the advancement of technology. The application of ultrasound to assist in the identification and localization of neural structures—and the accurate and safe injection of local anesthetic—has been an exciting and potentially revolutionary addition to the practice of neural blockade.

The *Mayo Clinic Atlas of Regional Anesthesia and Ultrasound-Guided Nerve Blockade*, edited by Drs. James R. Hebl and Robert L. Lennon, is the result of a highly innovative practice developed by a dedicated group of regional anesthesiologists at Mayo Clinic. These individuals, coming from a rich legacy of neural blockade, have embraced new technology and present it in a format that is novel and immediately useful to clinicians. The use of ultrasound in the practice of regional anesthesia exemplifies the rapid application of cutting-edge technology into clinical practice. Whether ultrasound technology revolutionizes the practice of neural blockade or simply becomes a useful tool for specific applications, this text helps define and clarify the technique and, as such, will be an invaluable addition to the library of academicians and clinicians alike.

Denise J. Wedel, M.D.
Consultant, Department of Anesthesiology, Mayo Clinic, Rochester, Minnesota;
Professor of Anesthesiology, College of Medicine, Mayo Clinic;
Past-President, American Society of Regional Anesthesia and Pain Medicine

PREFACE

"Regional anesthesia has come to stay."

This was the prediction of William J. Mayo, M.D., in his foreword to Gaston Labat's book, *Regional Anesthesia: Its Technic and Clinical Application*, in 1922. Now, more than 85 years later, this quotation has taken on new meaning in the field of regional anesthesia and pain medicine. The subspecialty of regional anesthesia has seen tremendous growth and interest during the past decade. These have been driven by multiple factors, including an aging patient population, evidence-based publications demonstrating the clinical benefits of regional anesthetic techniques, a greater demand for orthopedic (e.g., joint replacement) surgery, and advancements in endoscopic techniques, biocompatible materials, imaging equipment, and computer-guided technologies. In fact, the American Academy of Orthopaedic Surgeons and the National Center for Health Statistics estimate that more than 8.2 million orthopedic procedures are performed annually—nearly 30% of all major surgical interventions. Many of the patients having these procedures will benefit from regional anesthetic techniques during the perioperative period.

The primary goal of this regional anesthesia text and atlas is to promote the art and science of regional anesthesia and acute pain management. The text is *not* intended to be a comprehensive or exhaustive review of regional anesthesia but rather a practical guide for residents-in-training and clinicians who hope to expand their knowledge and gain greater familiarity with regional anesthestic techniques. Furthermore, the text emphasizes the importance of a detailed knowledge of applied anatomy to safely and successfully perform regional anesthetic techniques. In 1922, Labat noted that, "The practice of regional anesthesia is an art. It requires special knowledge of anatomy, skill in the performance of its various procedures, experience in the method of handling patients, and gentleness in the execution of surgical procedures." We hope that the vivid illustrations and artistic excellence of John V. Hagen in this atlas further emphasize this point and provide clinicians with the anatomical foundations necessary to understand the concepts essential to regional anesthesia.

A secondary goal of this text and atlas is to provide an overview of the emerging field of ultrasound-guided regional anesthesia. Recently, the use of ultrasound has received tremendous interest as technologic improvements enhance the image quality of neurovascular structures. Furthermore, clinicians have begun to recognize the potential benefits of the technique, including direct visualization of neural and vascular structures, rapid and reliable identification of both normal and variant anatomy, confirmation of circumferential spread of local anesthetic around neural targets, and the placement of perineural catheters under direct vision. The benefits and future applications of ultrasound-guided technology as it applies to regional anesthesia and acute pain medicine are just beginning to emerge. Future studies will delineate where and how this technology may further promote and advance the art and science of regional anesthesia.

Clearly, most anesthesiologists have had little formal training in ultrasonography or its application to regional anesthesia. In an attempt to introduce this new technology to residents-in-training and clinicians interested in expanding their clinical expertise, we have dedicated an entire section (Section III) of this text and atlas to the fundamental principles of ultrasound-guided regional anesthesia. Section III (Chapters 6-8) reviews the basic principles and concepts of ultrasonography, describes the sonoanatomy and appearance of neural structures, and provides clinical pearls on how to acquire the technical proficiency necessary to perform ultrasound-guided regional anesthetic techniques. In addition, detailed information on patient-provider orientation, ultrasound probe positioning, needle insertion site, and pearls to enhance image acquisition are provided throughout Section IV ("Upper Extremity Peripheral Nerve Block Techniques") and Section V ("Lower Extremity Peripheral Nerve Block Techniques"). Finally, each ultrasound image is accompanied by an anatomical illustration that corresponds precisely to the sonographic image. This method of pairing an ultrasound image with a corresponding anatomical illustration facilitates the learning of sonoanatomy and neurovascular pattern recognition and has been extremely useful and well received within our residency and fellowship programs.

The practice of regional anesthesia is experiencing renewed interest and widespread application. Advancements in peripheral techniques, neural localization, block success, and overall safety have improved intraoperative anesthesia, perioperative pain management, patient satisfaction, and surgical outcomes. The art and science of regional anesthesia has come to stay—a visionary sentiment as true today as it was nearly a century ago.

James R. Hebl, M.D.
Robert L. Lennon, D.O.

ACKNOWLEDGMENTS

Bradly J. Narr, M.D., and Mark A. Warner, M.D., have been the driving force and inspiration for this book. Drs. Narr (Chair, Mayo Clinic Department of Anesthesiology, 2005-present) and Warner (Chair, Mayo Clinic Department of Anesthesiology, 1999-2005) have provided us with the necessary time, resources, and sustaining encouragement to bring this atlas to completion. We are grateful to both of them for their dedication and commitment to the advancement of medical education.

We extend our appreciation and gratitude to the members of the Section of Orthopedic Anesthesia for their chapter authorship and enduring support and encouragement. This project would not have been possible without their thoughtful and valuable contributions.

To Duane K. Rorie, M.D., Ph.D., for addressing our many questions and concerns with his wealth of anatomical and regional anesthesia knowledge and for his meticulous anatomical dissections and guidance in the laboratory.

To John V. Hagen, for his dedication and skillful execution of the original artwork. Our hope is to educate clinicians and residents-in-training on the art and science of regional anesthesia through John's masterful illustrations.

To Stephen N. Boyd and Joan Beck, who created much of the original artwork for the textbook *Mayo Clinic Analgesic Pathway: Peripheral Nerve Blockade for Major Orthopedic Surgery* (Lennon RL and Horlocker TT, editors). Several of the illustrations, most in Section V, are modifications or variations of this original work.

To Parker C. Smith for his assistance in the acquisition of ultrasound images.

To the editorial staff: Roberta Schwartz, Production Editor; LeAnn Stee, Editor; Traci Post, Scientific Publications Specialist; Jane M. Craig, Editorial Assistant; Kenna L. Atherton, Copy Editor/Proofreader; and Ryan Ledebuhr, designer. This project would not have been possible without their professional contribution and dedication to the advancement of medical science.

TABLE OF CONTENTS

CONTRIBUTORS

Douglas R. Bacon, M.D., M.A.
Consultant, Department of Anesthesiology*
Professor of Anesthesiology and of
History of Medicine†

David E. Byer, M.D.
Consultant, Department of Anesthesiology*
Assistant Professor of Anesthesiology†

Paula A. Craigo, M.D.
Consultant, Department of Anesthesiology*
Assistant Professor of Anesthesiology†

John A. Dilger, M.D.
Consultant, Department of Anesthesiology*
Assistant Professor of Anesthesiology†

Christopher M. Duncan, M.D.
Consultant, Department of Anesthesiology*
Instructor in Anesthesiology†

Edward D. Frie, M.D.
Consultant, Department of Anesthesiology*
Instructor in Anesthesiology†

James R. Hebl, M.D.
Consultant, Department of Anesthesiology*
Associate Professor of Anesthesiology†

Adam K. Jacob, M.D.
Consultant, Department of Anesthesiology*
Assistant Professor of Anesthesiology†

Thomas J. Jurrens, M.D.
Clinical Associate, Department of Anesthesiology*

Michelle A. O. Kinney, M.D.
Consultant, Department of Anesthesiology*
Assistant Professor of Anesthesiology†

Sandra L. Kopp, M.D.
Consultant, Department of Anesthesiology*
Assistant Professor of Anesthesiology†

Robert L. Lennon, D.O.
Supplemental Consultant,
Department of Anesthesiology*
Associate Professor of Anesthesiology†

Carlos B. Mantilla, M.D., Ph.D.
Consultant, Department of Anesthesiology*
Associate Professor of Anesthesiology
and of Physiology†

Steven R. Rettke, M.D.
Consultant, Department of Anesthesiology*
Professor of Anesthesiology†

Kenneth P. Scott, M.D.
Consultant, Department of Anesthesiology*
Instructor in Anesthesiology†

Hugh M. Smith, M.D., Ph.D.
Consultant, Department of Anesthesiology*
Assistant Professor of Anesthesiology†

Laurence C. Torsher, M.D.
Consultant, Department of Anesthesiology*
Assistant Professor of Anesthesiology
and of Medical Education†

Mark A. Warner, M.D.
Consultant, Department of Anesthesiology*
Professor of Anesthesiology†

Jack L. Wilson, M.D.
Consultant, Department of Anesthesiology*
Assistant Professor of Anesthesiology†

Kimberly P. Wynd, M.B., B.Ch.
Regional Anesthesia Fellow,
Department of Anesthesiology,
Mayo School of Graduate Medical Education†

Mayo Clinic, Rochester, Minnesota.
†*College of Medicine, Mayo Clinic.*

MEMBERS OF THE SECTION OF
ORTHOPEDIC ANESTHESIA

James R. Hebl, M.D., Section Head

Douglas R. Bacon, M.D., M.A.
David E. Byer, M.D.
Paula A. Craigo, M.D.
John A. Dilger, M.D.
Christopher M. Duncan, M.D.
Edward D. Frie, M.D.
Terese T. Horlocker, M.D.*
Adam K. Jacob, M.D.
Thomas J. Jurrens, M.D.
Michelle A. O. Kinney, M.D.
Sandra L. Kopp, M.D.
Robert L. Lennon, D.O.*
Carlos B. Mantilla, M.D., Ph.D.
Steven R. Rettke, M.D.*
Duane K. Rorie, M.D., Ph.D.*†
Kenneth P. Scott, M.D.
Rungson Sittipong, M.D.†
Hugh M. Smith, M.D., Ph.D.
Laurence C. Torsher, M.D.
Jack L. Wilson, M.D.

Previous Section Head
†*Emeritus Member*

SECTION

I

Principles of Peripheral Nerve Blockade

1

Regional Anesthesia: Past, Present, and Future

John A. Dilger, M.D.

Carlos B. Mantilla, M.D., Ph.D.

Douglas R. Bacon, M.D., M.A.

A Historical Perspective

Regional anesthesia has been an important part of medical practice for more than a century. In fact, experts have identified Egyptian pictographs dating back to 3000 BC showing a physician compressing a nerve in the antecubital fossa while an operation is being performed on the hand. Yet, it would not be until the latter half of the 19th century that regional anesthesia became possible. In 1884, Carl Koller, M.D. (1857-1944; Austrian ophthalmologist), showed that a solution of cocaine could anesthetize the eye and function as a local anesthetic. Koller first reported his findings at the Congress of Ophthalmology in Heidelberg, Germany. Within a year of that report, more than 100 papers were published on various cocaine-based regional anesthetic techniques. The careers of William J. Mayo, M.D. (1861-1939), and Charles H. Mayo, M.D. (1865-1939), founders of Mayo Clinic in Rochester, Minnesota, further illustrate the importance of Koller's discovery. They used local infiltration anesthesia during surgical procedures from the inception of Saint Marys Hospital in September 1889. The operative reports from C. H. Mayo between 1890 and 1892 indicate that local anesthesia was used in 9% of cases.

William Halsted, M.D. (1852-1922; Chair, Department of Surgery, Johns Hopkins Hospital), took an approach different from that of the Mayo brothers. Halsted used cocaine as local infiltration as he dissected down toward major nerve trunks. He then injected cocaine around them, performing regional blockade under direct vision. In many ways, this technique foreshadowed the ultrasound technology used today. By the turn of the 20th century, local anesthesia was used in approximately 7% of surgical procedures performed at Saint Marys Hospital by Mayo Clinic surgeons.

Despite the medical benefits of cocaine, there were also significant concerns about its use. Halsted became addicted to the drug through self-experimentation while trying to understand the most efficacious way to use the solution. Furthermore, regional blockade with cocaine was often not uniformly dense, and 13 fatalities were reported in the literature within the first 7 years of its use. Because of these concerns, physicians began searching for alternatives to cocaine. In 1905, Alfred Einhorn (1856-1917; German chemist) synthesized procaine. The drug was soon found to be a safer and more reliable alternative to cocaine. This newly discovered local anesthetic forever changed the practice of regional anesthesia. In 1908, August Bier, M.D. (1861-1949; German surgeon, known as the Father of Spinal Anesthesia), introduced intravenous local anesthesia at a surgical meeting in Berlin. Despite its initial acceptance, the Bier block technique was soon abandoned because it was both difficult to perform and resulted in the immediate return of pain after tourniquet deflation.

In 1911, Diedrich Kulenkampff, M.D. (German surgeon), continued the German-based research efforts in regional anesthesia and used surface anatomy to locate the brachial plexus. He found that there was a fascial sheath that confined the local anesthetic to the area surrounding

the nerves. Kulenkampff described the first supraclavicular technique of brachial plexus blockade. He inserted a needle above the first rib and produced a paresthesia before injecting local anesthetic. In 1919, Karl Mulley published an article that described the interscalene approach to the brachial plexus. Using surface anatomy formed by the sternocleidomastoid muscle, the scalene muscles, and the clavicle, Mulley elicited a paresthesia for neural localization before injecting local anesthetic.

In 1920, C. H. Mayo traveled to Paris, France, to visit his surgical colleague, Victor Pauchet, M.D. (1869-1936), and to observe new surgical techniques. Pauchet had mastered the German techniques of transcutaneous regional anesthetic blockade. Pauchet's pupil, Gaston Labat, M.D. (1876-1934), was finishing his training with Pauchet and provided the anesthesia while Mayo and Pauchet operated. Mayo was so impressed with these regional techniques that he recruited Labat to Mayo Clinic. As part of his employment, Labat was to teach regional anesthesia to the surgeons in practice at Mayo Clinic and to write a book describing percutaneous regional anesthesia (Figure 1).

By October 1, 1920, Labat had begun his work in Rochester, Minnesota, where he would stay for a year. The book, which was richly illustrated by Mayo Clinic artists (Figures 2 through 8, with portions of the original figure legends), was published after Labat accepted a position as a regional anesthetist at Bellevue Hospital in New York City. Largely a translation of Pauchet's *L'Anesthesie Regionale* with a new section on the regional anesthetist as a specialist, Labat's book, *Regional Anesthesia: Its Technic and Clinical Application*, was a medical bestseller well into the 20th century. Before leaving Mayo Clinic, Labat instructed William Meeker, M.D., in the techniques of regional anesthesia. In 1924, just before his departure from Mayo Clinic, Meeker taught John Lundy, M.D. (1894-1973), Labat's techniques. Recruited to chair the Section on Regional Anesthesia (which by the end of the decade was the Section on Anesthesia), Lundy was responsible for all anesthetics, supplemental oxygen therapy, and blood transfusions at Mayo Clinic. By 1931, approximately 30% of all anesthetics given at

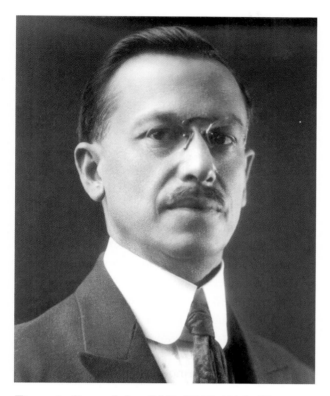

Figure 1. Gaston Labat, M.D. (1876-1934). (From Physicians of the Mayo Clinic and Mayo Foundation. St. Paul [MN]: Bruce; c1923.)

Mayo Clinic involved a regional technique—a practice that continues today.

In Paris in the early 1920s, a new technique for blocking the brachial plexus from an axillary approach was introduced. M. Reding, M.D., studying the anatomy of the axilla, discovered that the nerves of the plexus surround the artery in a fascial sheath. Thus, using the artery as a landmark, Reding found that the fascial compartment could be filled with local anesthetic to result in brachial plexus blockade. Reding blocked the musculocutaneous nerve, which lay outside the sheath, by infiltrating the coracobrachialis muscle. Interestingly, this technique was never described in Labat's classic text.

The Labat tradition of percutaneous regional anesthesia gradually spread across the United States. The clinical success of regional anesthesia at both Mayo Clinic and Bellevue Hospital in New York further propagated this

interest. Thus, C. H. Mayo's recognition of the benefits of regional anesthesia helped its use spread from the Midwest to the East Coast and, eventually, across the nation. The techniques provide patients with exceptional intraoperative and postoperative analgesia while avoiding many of the side effects commonly associated with general anesthesia.

Nerve Localization Techniques

Percutaneous regional anesthesia is successful only when local anesthetic can be accurately and reproducibly placed in the vicinity of nerves. Since the inception of regional anesthetic techniques, various localization methods have been developed and used successfully. These include paresthesia-seeking techniques, peripheral nerve stimulation, stimulating catheters, and direct visualization with ultrasound-guided technology. Ultrasound guidance may represent the 21st century's version of Halsted's anatomical dissection down to the brachial plexus.

The use of patient-reported paresthesias to guide local anesthetic injection has a long and successful tradition in regional anesthesia as a result of the simplicity of the technique. Other than a needle, no special equipment is required. Importantly, paresthesia-seeking techniques require an intimate knowledge of neuroanatomy and a cooperative patient. Minimal sedation is recommended to allow appropriate and useful patient feedback. Traditionally, it has been assumed that needle-to-nerve contact produces the paresthesia. However, paresthesias can also arise from contact with the needle shaft or traction on nearby tissues. Although paresthesia-seeking techniques are sometimes painful to patients, clinical studies have not shown a significant increase in neurologic complications after their use. When paresthesia techniques are used for blocks involving separate peripheral nerves (e.g., axillary blockade), multiple injection sites or stimuli are recommended to facilitate successful blockade.

Paresthesia technique—the long-preferred method of regional anesthesiologists—was slowly replaced during the 1980s as peripheral nerve stimulation began to emerge.

During its development, peripheral nerve stimulation was thought to provide superior localization of neural structures compared with blind paresthesia-seeking techniques. Peripheral nerve stimulators transmit a small electric current through a stimulating needle that, when in proximity to neural structures, causes depolarization and muscle contraction. The mechanics of nerve stimulation are based on several important principles. First, true nerve stimulation results from the activation and depolarization of A-α motor fibers. A-α fibers require less current for depolarization than A-δ or C pain fibers. Therefore, painful paresthesias are avoided during muscle contraction. Second, the choice of electrodes during stimulation is important. The negative terminal (cathode) should be attached to the needle, and the positive terminal (anode) attached to the patient. Depolarization occurs as the negative terminal allows current to flow from the needle to adjacent neural structures. If the terminals are reversed, hyperpolarization occurs as current flows away from the needle. Finally, the nerve stimulator must be designed to allow adjustment of several key features and to confirm the presence (or absence) of a complete circuit. Adjustable features may include current output, stimulation frequency, and pulse duration.

The most common feature that is routinely adjusted during each regional technique is the stimulating current. High-current outputs (>1.5 mA) are more likely to stimulate neural structures across tissue planes. However, this may result in unnecessary forceful or even painful motor contractions. With the exception of the needle tip, most modern stimulating needles are coated with a thin layer of insulation. This produces a spherelike area of current density at the distal needle tip, which results in a more discrete field of stimulation. Once the appropriate motor response is identified, the current is gradually decreased as the needle is advanced toward the nerve. Although there is no optimal current at which a block will be reliably successful, most experts agree that a current of 0.5 mA or less with preservation of a motor response is acceptable for the delivery of local anesthetic or placement of a catheter. However, the ability to blindly stimulate a peripheral nerve should *never* supersede a detailed knowledge of the relevant anatomy and pertinent superficial landmarks. Therefore, the anatomical expertise acquired during the early part of the 20th century continues to be a cornerstone of regional anesthesia practice today.

Continuous peripheral nerve blocks have been used with increasing frequency during the 21st century for the management of moderate to severe postoperative pain. Perineural catheters have been shown to provide extended site-specific postoperative analgesia, reduce opioid-related side effects, improve patient satisfaction, accelerate rehabilitation and functional recovery, and shorten the duration of hospitalization compared with intravenous opioid-based analgesic techniques. However, the success of continuous peripheral nerve catheters depends on the accurate and reliable placement of perineural catheters adjacent to neural structures. Perineural catheters may be placed using stimulating or nonstimulating techniques. Proponents of stimulating catheter techniques report a more accurate placement of catheters adjacent to neural targets. The electrophysiologic principles associated with stimulating catheters are similar to those of single-injection techniques. Stimulating catheters concentrate their energy in a spherelike area of current density at the catheter tip in a manner similar to that of stimulating needles. Once an appropriate motor response is elicited using a stimulating needle, the current is transferred to the stimulating catheter. The catheter is then advanced while maintaining the same motor response. This technique ensures that the catheter remains close to the neural target for administration of local anesthetic.

Ultrasound-guided regional anesthesia is a rapidly evolving technique for the identification and localization of neural structures. Ultrasound technology may improve block success by allowing clinicians to directly visualize the deposition of local anesthetic around neural targets. Technologic improvements in ultrasound equipment have resulted in a dramatic improvement in image quality, which makes recognition of nerves and nerve patterns accessible to anyone willing to learn the art of sonographic interpretation. Ultrasonography is ideally suited to regional anesthetic techniques for upper extremity surgery because the brachial plexus is sufficiently superficial to allow optimal imaging. In addition, ultrasound technology provides a greater understanding of neuroanatomy, which can facilitate the teaching of existing nerve block techniques and development of new approaches.

Importance of Peripheral Nerve Blockade

An important legacy of pioneering physicians Carl Koller, Gaston Labat, and William Halsted is the ability to provide surgical levels of anesthesia using peripheral nerve block techniques. Today, regional blocks are increasingly popular alternatives to general anesthesia for surgery and postoperative analgesia. The superior analgesia and avoidance of general anesthesia and its associated complications have made peripheral techniques appealing to both patients and clinicians. Additional advantages include reducing opioid consumption and minimizing opioid-related side effects such as nausea, vomiting, pruritus, and somnolence. Moreover, the use of regional techniques minimizes or eliminates recovery room stays, facilitates rehabilitation, and may shorten hospitalization. A multimodal analgesic regimen that incorporates regional anesthetic techniques and oral analgesics can maximize these benefits and improve surgical outcomes.

Regional anesthesia is a dynamic and evolving subspecialty of anesthesia practice. Peripheral nerve blockade is clinically applicable to a wide spectrum of anatomical regions and incorporates a variety of technical approaches, specialized equipment, local anesthetics, and adjuvants. Performed as either single-injection or continuous catheter techniques, peripheral nerve blockade can provide both postoperative analgesia and surgical anesthesia. Providers have the ability to customize the regional anesthetic technique to the patient, to the unique surgical procedure, and to his or her technical strengths.

Implications of Peripheral Nerve Blockade

In contemporary medical practice, regional anesthetic techniques have expanding socioeconomic and clinical implications. For example, studies evaluating patient satisfaction have found that perioperative analgesia and the avoidance of nausea and vomiting are consistently two of the highest concerns among patients. In an increasingly competitive medical environment, patient satisfaction and improved anesthetic and surgical outcomes will have a considerable impact on where and how patients choose to receive their medical care. In addition, when directly compared with general anesthesia, regional techniques are more cost-effective because of accelerated recovery and rehabilitation and shortened hospital stay. Regional techniques also allow surgeons to perform increasingly invasive and more complex procedures on an outpatient basis— a trend that may help contain increasing medical costs. Furthermore, these techniques and their associated benefits are allowing surgical procedures to be performed on elderly patients whose comorbidities may have previously precluded them from being surgical candidates.

Recent developments in local anesthetic delivery systems have the potential to further improve peripheral techniques. Technologic advancements such as microspheres, microemulsions, and nanoparticles have been investigated for their potential to prolong sensory blockade after a single injection. Current limitations of these advancements include safe and consistent drug delivery, unpredictable drug plasma levels, and local anesthetic neurotoxicity.

Summary

The practice of regional anesthesia is experiencing renewed interest and widespread application. Advancements in peripheral techniques, neural localization, block success, and overall safety have improved perioperative pain management, patient satisfaction, surgical outcomes, and health-related quality of life. Despite recent progress, future research should focus on appropriately designed prospective, randomized, controlled trials that further evaluate novel therapeutics, drug delivery systems, and the economic impact of regional anesthesia. The notable efforts of both historical and contemporary practitioners have secured a bright and promising future for regional anesthesia. In 1922, William J. Mayo, M.D., predicted that "Regional anesthesia is here to stay." This visionary sentiment is as true today as it was nearly a century ago.

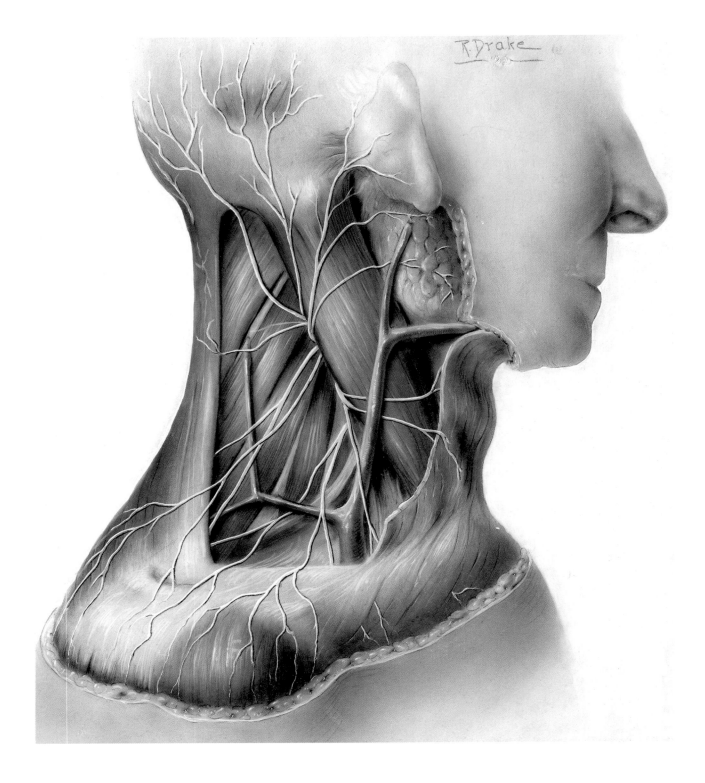

Figure 2. Superficial branches of the cervical plexus at their emergence on the posterior margin of the sternocleido-mastoid muscle. (From Labat G. Regional anesthesia: its technic and clinical application. Philadelphia and London: W. B. Saunders; c1922.)

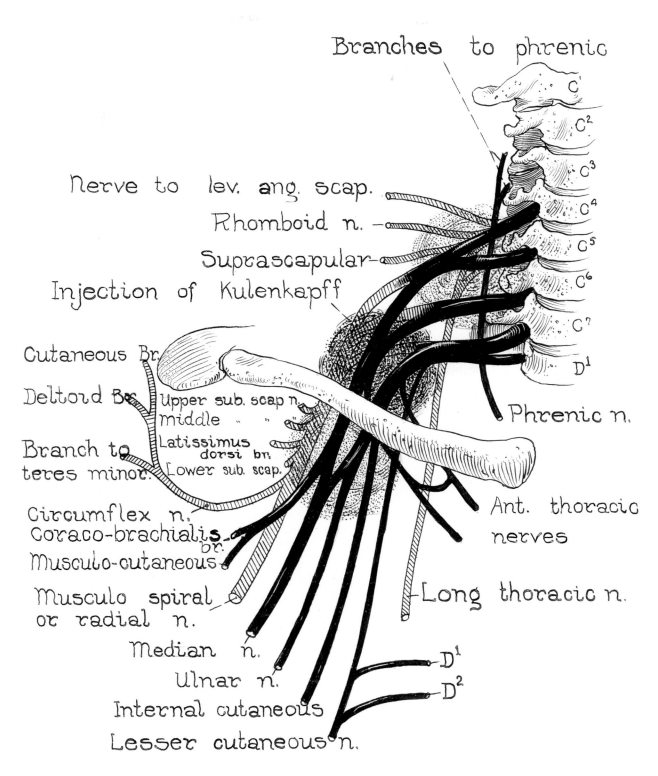

Figure 3. Diagrammatic illustration of the brachial plexus, showing the supraclavicular and infraclavicular branches of the plexus. (From Labat G. Regional anesthesia: its technic and clinical application. Philadelphia and London: W. B. Saunders; c1922.)

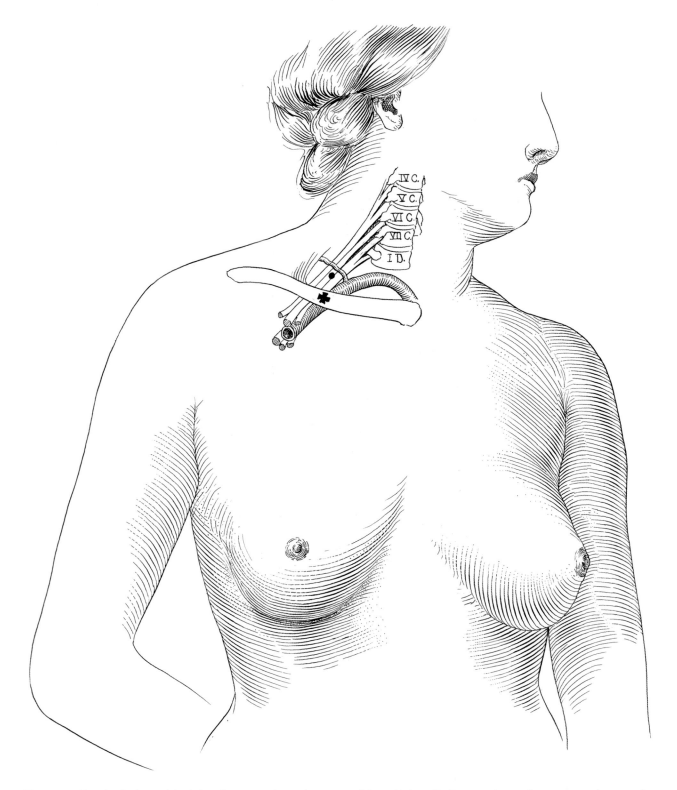

Figure 4. Brachial plexus block by the supraclavicular route. (From Labat G. Regional anesthesia: its technic and clinical application. Philadelphia and London: W. B. Saunders; c1922.)

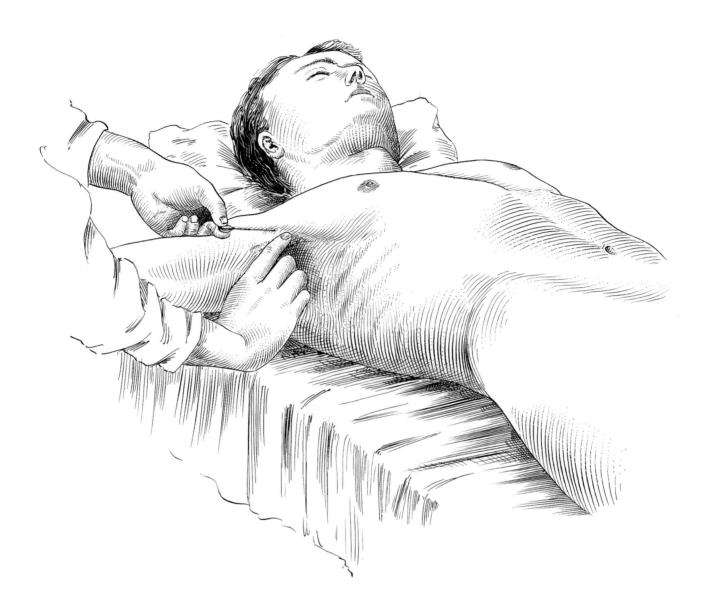

Figure 5. Brachial plexus block by the axillary route. (From Labat G. Regional anesthesia: its technic and clinical application. Philadelphia and London: W. B. Saunders; c1922.)

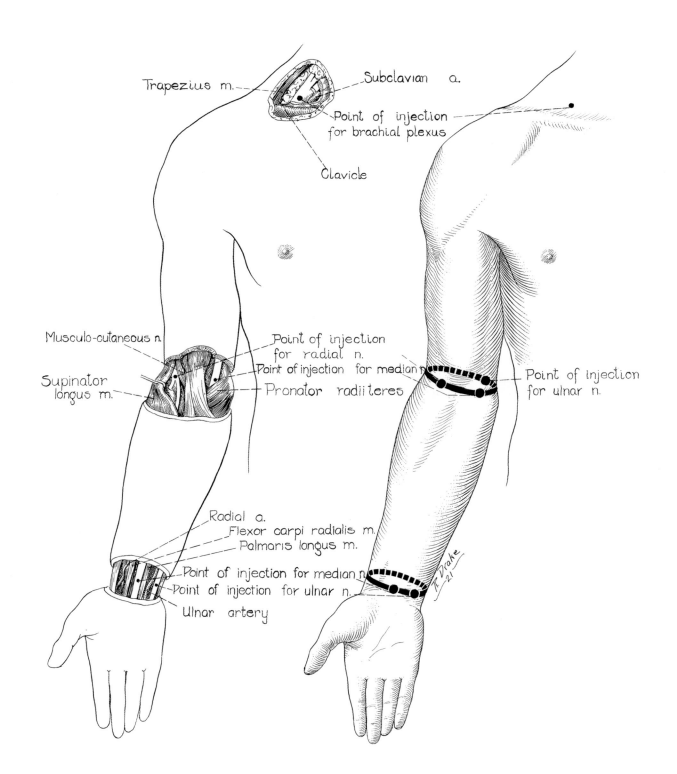

Figure 6. Synoptic illustration of the blocking of the brachial plexus and its branches. (From Labat G. Regional anesthesia: its technic and clinical application. Philadelphia and London: W. B. Saunders; c1922.)

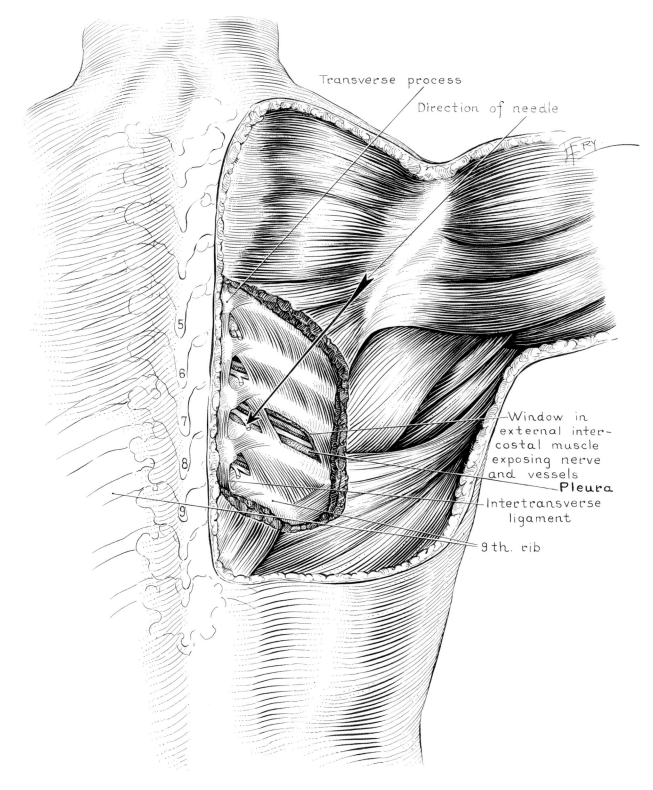

Figure 7. Paravertebral dorsal block. (From Labat G. Regional anesthesia: its technic and clinical application. Philadelphia and London: W. B. Saunders; c1922.)

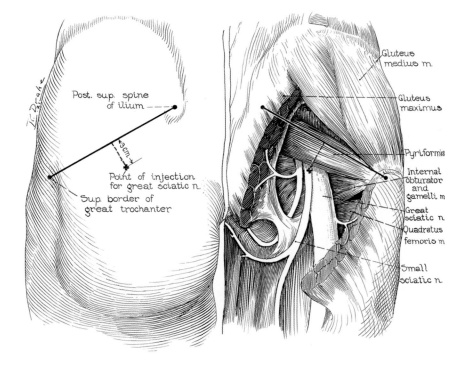

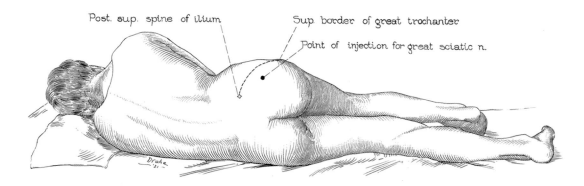

Figure 8. Sciatic nerve block. (From Labat G. Regional anesthesia: its technic and clinical application. Philadelphia and London: W. B. Saunders; c1922.)

Suggested Reading

Bacon DR. Regional anesthesia and chronic pain therapy: a history. In: Brown DL, editor. Regional anesthesia and analgesia. Philadelphia: W. B. Saunders; c1996. p. 10-22.

Brown DL, Winnie AP. Biography of Louis Gaston Labat, M.D. Reg Anesth. 1992 Sep-Oct;17(5):249-62.

Côté AV, Vachon CA, Horlocker TT, Bacon DR. From Victor Pauchet to Gaston Labat: the transformation of regional anesthesia from a surgeon's practice to the physician anesthesiologist. Anesth Analg. 2003 Apr;96(4):1193-200.

De Andrés J, Sala-Blanch X. Peripheral nerve stimulation in the practice of brachial plexus anesthesia: a review. Reg Anesth Pain Med. 2001 Sep-Oct;26(5):478-83.

Ford DJ, Pither C, Raj PP. Comparison of insulated and uninsulated needles for locating peripheral nerves with a peripheral nerve stimulator. Anesth Analg. 1984 Oct;63(10):925-8.

Goerig M, Agarwal K, Schulte am Esch J. The versatile August Bier (1861-1949), father of spinal anesthesia. J Clin Anesth. 2000 Nov;12(7):561-9.

Halsted WS. Practical comments on the use and abuse of cocaine: suggested by its invariably successful employment in more than a thousand minor surgical operations. N York M J. 1885;42:294.

Horlocker TT. Peripheral nerve blocks: regional anesthesia for the new millennium. Reg Anesth Pain Med. 1998 May-Jun;23(3):237-40.

Horlocker TT, Wedel DJ. Ultrasound-guided regional anesthesia: in search of the holy grail. Anesth Analg. 2007 May;104(5):1009-11.

Ilfeld BM, Enneking FK. Continuous peripheral nerve blocks at home: a review. Anesth Analg. 2005 Jun;100(6):1822-33.

Koller C. Personal reminiscences of first use of cocain as local anesthetic in eye surgery. Anesth & Analg. 1928;7:9-11.

Kopp SL, Horlocker TT, Bacon DR. The contribution of John Lundy in the development of peripheral and neuraxial nerve blocks at the Mayo Clinic: 1925-1940. Reg Anesth Pain Med. 2002 May-Jun;27(3):322-6.

Kulenkampff D. [Anesthesia of the brachial plexus]. Zentralbl f Chir. 1911;38:1337-40. German.

Liu SS, Strodtbeck WM, Richman JM, Wu CL. A comparison of regional versus general anesthesia for ambulatory anesthesia: a meta-analysis of randomized controlled trials. Anesth Analg. 2005 Dec;101(6): 1634-42.

Liu SS, Wu CL. The effect of analgesic technique on postoperative patient-reported outcomes including analgesia: a systematic review. Anesth Analg. 2007 Sep;105(3):789-808.

Marhofer P, Chan VW. Ultrasound-guided regional anesthesia: current concepts and future trends. Anesth Analg. 2007 May;104(5):1265-9.

Morin AM, Eberhart LH, Behnke HK, Wagner S, Koch T, Wolf U, et al. Does femoral nerve catheter placement with stimulating catheters improve effective placement? A randomized, controlled, and observer-blinded trial. Anesth Analg. 2005 May;100(5):1503-10.

Mulley K. [A modification of Kulenkampff's brachial block technic in order to avoid pleural injury.] Beitr Klin Chir. 1919;114:666-80. German.

Pham-Dang C, Kick O, Collet T, Gouin F, Pinaud M. Continuous peripheral nerve blocks with stimulating catheters. Reg Anesth Pain Med. 2003 Mar-Apr;28(2):83-8.

Pulido JN, Bacon DR, Rettke SR. Gaston Labat and John Lundy: friends and pioneer regional anesthesiologists sharing a Mayo Clinic connection. Reg Anesth Pain Med. 2004 Sep-Oct;29(5):489-93.

Reding M. [A new method of regional anesthesia of the upper extremity.] Presse Med. 1921;29:294-6. French.

Rodgers A, Walker N, Schug S, McKee A, Kehlet H, van Zundert A, et al. Reduction of postoperative mortality and morbidity with epidural or spinal anaesthesia: results from overview of randomised trials. BMJ. 2000 Dec 16;321(7275):1493.

Salinas FV, Neal JM, Sueda LA, Kopacz DJ, Liu SS. Prospective comparison of continuous femoral nerve block with nonstimulating catheter placement versus stimulating catheter-guided perineural placement in volunteers. Reg Anesth Pain Med. 2004 May-Jun;29(3):212-20.

Smith HM, Bacon DR. The history of anesthesia. In: Barash PG, Cullen BF, Stoelting RK, editors. Clinical anesthesia. 5th ed. Philadelphia: Lippincott Williams & Wilkins; c2006. p. 3-26.

Urmey WF, Stanton J. Inability to consistently elicit a motor response following sensory paresthesia during interscalene block administration. Anesthesiology. 2002 Mar;96(3):552-4.

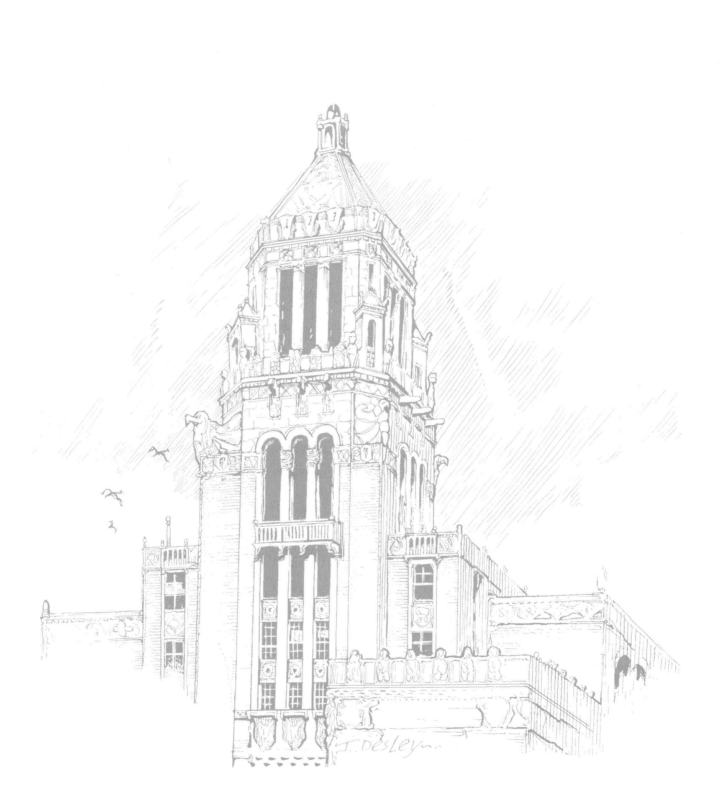

CHAPTER

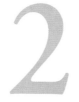

Pharmacology of Neural Blockade

Christopher M. Duncan, M.D.

Paula A. Craigo, M.D.

Local anesthetics have been used for more than a century to provide anesthesia for patients undergoing invasive surgical procedures. In 1884, William Halsted, M.D., was the first to inject cocaine around a sensory nerve under direct vision to provide surgical anesthesia. Since that time, local anesthetics and their adjuvants have played an important role in providing anesthesia and perioperative analgesia for upper and lower extremity surgery. The wide spectrum of local anesthetics available today allow clinicians to tailor the use of regional anesthesia and peripheral nerve blockade to address procedural requirements, patient comfort, and safety issues. Adjuvant medications that may enhance the clinical effects of local anesthetics are also available.

Mechanism of Action

Local anesthetics act by inhibiting sodium influx through voltage-gated sodium channels within neuronal cell membranes. The inhibition of sodium influx prevents an action potential from being generated and blocks overall signal conduction. The site of receptor blockade is thought to be on the cytoplasmic side of the sodium channel. Therefore, local anesthetics must first pass through the neuronal membrane before binding to the receptor at the cytoplasmic site. Local anesthetics that can easily translocate across a lipid bilayer (i.e., lipid-soluble compounds) are able to bind more quickly to receptor sites than lipid-insoluble drugs. Furthermore, local anesthetics bind more readily to sodium channel receptors that are in an "open" state. Therefore, neurons that fire in rapid succession tend to have a faster onset of conduction blockade when exposed to local anesthetics.

Clinical Features

Potency

The potency of a local anesthetic, or the ability of a drug to produce a desired effect, is primarily associated with lipid solubility. Local anesthetics that are highly lipophilic tend to penetrate neuronal membranes more easily, resulting in a higher degree of conduction blockade with less drug. Therefore, local anesthetics that are highly lipophilic (e.g., bupivacaine) are more potent than those with a lower degree of lipid solubility (e.g., chloroprocaine).

Onset

Onset of action is largely dependent on the pK_a of the local anesthetic and the total dose administered. Nonionized forms of local anesthetics are able to pass through lipid bilayers more readily than ionized compounds. Therefore, the ability to penetrate neural tissue is favored by local anesthetics with pK_a levels near physiologic pH (i.e., higher concentrations of non-ionized drug). The result is a faster onset of conduction blockade for agents such as lidocaine (pK_a 7.8) and mepivacaine (pK_a 7.7).

Duration

The duration of a local anesthetic is primarily associated with plasma protein binding (α_1-acid glycoprotein). Local anesthetics with a strong affinity for protein (e.g., bupivacaine) have a longer duration of action than agents

with weaker protein affinity (e.g., lidocaine). Recently, liposomal encapsulation of local anesthetics has been shown to substantially extend the duration of anesthesia and analgesia.

Dose

Local anesthetics commonly used for peripheral nerve blockade are listed in Table 1. Maximal doses for local anesthetics are recommended by drug manufacturers and are not supported by evidence-based investigations. In general, the lowest effective dose and concentration should be used to minimize the risk of systemic and neural toxicity.

The dose of local anesthetic should be individualized and based on the site of injection, patient age and weight, and preexisting medical conditions that could affect the pharmacology and toxicity of a local anesthetic (Table 2). Because of the potential for accumulation of local anesthetic, these considerations are believed to be most critical when large doses of local anesthetics are injected. In addition, these considerations must be taken

Table 1.   Common Local Anesthetics and Recommended Maximal Doses

Local anesthetic	Maximal dose, mg
Lidocaine	300
With epinephrine	500
Mepivacaine	400
With epinephrine	550
Bupivacaine	175
With epinephrine	225
Continuous infusion	400/24 h
Ropivacaine	225
With epinephrine	225
Continuous infusion	800/24 h

Modified from Lennon RL, Horlocker TT, editors. Mayo Clinic analgesic pathway: peripheral nerve blockade for major orthopedic surgery. Rochester (MN): Mayo Clinic Scientific Press and Boca Raton (FL): Taylor & Francis; c2006.

into account when repeated blocks are performed or during continuous infusions of local anesthetics.

Metabolism

Local anesthetics are classified as either amino esters or amides. The two compounds differ in both the site and the mechanism of metabolism. Amino esters are metabolized by pseudocholinesterase-mediated ester hydrolysis. Ester hydrolysis is very rapid, with the resultant water-soluble metabolites being secreted in the urine. One metabolite of importance, para-aminobenzoic acid (PABA), has been associated with allergic reactions. In contrast, amino amides are metabolized by microsomal enzymes in the liver. The rate of metabolism depends on the specific agent, but it is much slower than ester hydrolysis. Decreased hepatic function or reduced liver blood flow (i.e., congestive heart failure) will reduce the metabolic rate and predispose patients to systemic toxicity. Currently, nearly all upper and lower extremity nerve blocks are performed with amino amide local anesthetics.

Toxicity

Although complications from peripheral nerve blockade are infrequent, the use of local anesthetics is not without risk. The administration of these drugs, often in high volumes, may result in untoward and potentially toxic local and systemic effects.

Local Toxicity

Evidence has suggested that local anesthetics can cause microstructural changes in nerve and muscle tissue after local administration. In rare cases, these changes are substantial enough to produce clinically relevant neuromuscular deficits. The dose of local anesthetic and additives such as epinephrine may increase the risk of both neurotoxicity and myotoxicity.

Systemic Toxicity

The conduction of electric impulses occurs in a similar manner within both the central and peripheral nervous systems and the myocardium (cardiac conduction system). Because the effects of local anesthetics are not specific to peripheral nerves, severe and potentially fatal side effects may occur within the central nervous system and myocardium. Systemic toxicity occurs after the intravascular uptake (either direct or indirect) of local anesthetic. In general, the brachial plexus has relatively limited vascular uptake compared with that of other sites of local anesthetic injection (e.g., caudal, intercostal). Therefore, most systemic complications associated with brachial plexus blockade occur during inadvertent intravascular injection.

Signs and symptoms of systemic toxicity develop progressively. Initial features include excitatory central nervous system symptoms (e.g., tinnitus, perioral numbness), followed by inhibitory central nervous system events (e.g., sedation, loss of consciousness), electrocardiographic

Table 2. Patient-Related Factors Affecting the Pharmacology of a Local Anesthetic	
Factor	**Dose modification**
Age	
<4 months	Reduce dose by 15%
>70 years	Reduce dose by 10%-20%
Renal dysfunction	Reduce dose by 10%-20%, including continuous infusions
Hepatic dysfunction	Reduce dose by 10%-20%, more with continuous infusions
Congestive heart failure	Reduce dose by 10%-20%, including continuous infusions
Pregnancy	Reduce concentration because of increased sensitivity to local anesthetics

Modified from Lennon RL, Horlocker TT, editors. Mayo Clinic analgesic pathway: peripheral nerve blockade for major orthopedic surgery. Rochester (MN): Mayo Clinic Scientific Press and Boca Raton (FL): Taylor & Francis; c2006.

abnormalities, and ultimately cardiac arrest. Changes seem to correlate with increasing plasma levels of the drug, acute increases being more detrimental than gradual increases. When multiple local anesthetics are used simultaneously, drug levels and adverse effects tend to be additive.

Treatment

If a patient develops signs or symptoms of local anesthetic toxicity, the injection or administration (i.e., continuous infusion) of additional local anesthetic should be immediately discontinued. The treatment of local anesthetic toxic reactions is similar to the management of other medical emergencies and focuses on ensuring adequate airway, breathing, and circulation. Ensuring adequate oxygenation and ventilation is paramount to avoid progressive acidosis. If a patient experiences a seizure, general tonic-clonic activity can be terminated with a small dose of thiopental, propofol, or benzodiazepine without causing cardiovascular compromise. In the case of cardiac toxicity, the primary treatment is supportive care until the local anesthetic is sufficiently cleared and a perfusing rhythm and hemodynamic stability are restored. The intense protein-binding properties of bupivacaine may require prolonged resuscitative efforts, including the initiation or use of cardiopulmonary bypass. Recent evidence suggests that intravenous lipid emulsion therapy may be an effective antidote to local anesthetic-induced cardiac toxicity.

Adjuvant Medications

The word *adjuvant* comes from the Latin *ad-* to, *juvare-* to help. Several adjuvants, or additives, have been described for use in peripheral nerve blockade to extend or enhance the clinical effects of local anesthetics.

Epinephrine

Epinephrine is the most commonly used adjuvant during peripheral nerve blockade. Its sympathomimetic activity serves dual purposes when added to local anesthetics. First, the onset of chronotropy and systemic vasoconstriction allows for the early detection of intravascular injection or absorption. Second, its vasoconstrictive properties

decrease the vascular uptake of local anesthetic, resulting in lower peak plasma levels, prolonged contact between the nerve and local anesthetic, and extended duration of neuronal blockade.

When epinephrine is used as an adjuvant, doses range from 1.7 to 5 mcg/mL of local anesthetic (1:600,000 to 1:200,000, respectively). Its benefit is dose-dependent up to a concentration of 5 mcg/mL. At a higher concentration, side effects may increase without improving the quality or duration of the block. Commercially prepared solutions with epinephrine have a lower pH than those in which it is freshly added; a lower pH results in a higher percentage of ionized drug molecules. Because these ionized molecules do not readily cross the neural membrane, the onset of local anesthetic action is delayed after injection. The addition of epinephrine to local anesthetics with intrinsic vasoconstrictive properties, such as ropivacaine, may not increase block duration but can still facilitate the detection of intravascular injection or systemic uptake.

The use of epinephrine is not without risk and should be avoided during distal peripheral and digital nerve blocks of the upper and lower extremities. Vasoconstriction may reduce neuronal blood flow and predispose neural tissue to ischemic injury. This may be a particular concern in patients with preexisting microangiopathy or neuropathy. Lower concentrations of epinephrine (1.7-2.5 mcg/mL) are known to have little effect on nerve blood flow and should be considered a reasonable alternative in high-risk patients. In addition, tachycardia resulting from the intravascular injection or systemic uptake of epinephrine may precipitate cardiac ischemia in vulnerable patients. Concerns regarding neural or cardiac ischemia must be balanced with the need to detect intravascular injection. In general, because large doses of local anesthetics are administered during peripheral nerve blockade, the benefits of adding epinephrine may outweigh the potential risks.

Clonidine

Clonidine is an α_2-receptor agonist that may prolong the duration of anesthesia and analgesia after peripheral nerve blockade. Although its exact mechanism is unclear, clonidine seems to exert a beneficial effect when administered *either* locally or systemically. However, the effect is most likely peripherally mediated and dose-dependent. Clonidine seems most effective when added to intermediate-acting local anesthetics (e.g., mepivacaine), consistently prolonging the time to the first request for postoperative analgesia. When coupled to long-acting local anesthetics (e.g., bupivacaine), its benefit is less clear. Commonly reported side effects of bradycardia, hypotension, and sedation are unlikely to occur at doses used during peripheral nerve blockade (1-1.5 mcg/kg).

Other Adjuvants

The use of alternative adjuvant medications such as tramadol, opioids, verapamil, neostigmine, and hyaluronidase has been reported in the literature. However, none of these agents seem to provide substantial benefit or clear improvement in the quality or duration of peripheral nerve blocks.

Suggested Reading

Auroy Y, Narchi P, Messiah A, Litt L, Rouvier B, Samii K. Serious complications related to regional anesthesia: results of a prospective survey in France. Anesthesiology. 1997 Sep;87(3):479-86.

Faccenda KA, Finucane BT. Complications of regional anaesthesia: incidence and prevention. Drug Saf. 2001;24(6):413-42.

Korevaar WC, Burney RG, Moore PA. Convulsions during stellate ganglion block: a case report. Anesth Analg. 1979 Jul-Aug;58(4):329-30.

Neal JM, Hebl JR, Gerancher JC, Hogan QH. Brachial plexus anesthesia: essentials of our current understanding. Reg Anesth Pain Med. 2002 Jul-Aug;27(4):402-28. Erratum in: Reg Anesth Pain Med. 2002 Nov-Dec;27(6):625.

Rosenberg PH, Veering BT, Urmey WF. Maximum recommended doses of local anesthetics: a multifactorial concept. Reg Anesth Pain Med 2004 Nov-Dec;29(6):564-75.

Rosenblatt MA, Abel M, Fischer GW, Itzkovich CJ, Eisenkraft JB. Successful use of a 20% lipid emulsion to resuscitate a patient after a presumed bupivacaine-related cardiac arrest. Anesthesiology. 2006 Jul;105(1):217-8.

Singelyn FJ, Gouverneur JM, Robert A. A minimum dose of clonidine added to mepivacaine prolongs the duration of anesthesia and analgesia after axillary brachial plexus block. Anesth Analg. 1996 Nov;83(5):1046-50.

CHAPTER

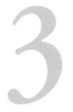

Complications of Peripheral Nerve Blockade

James R. Hebl, M.D.

The use of peripheral nerve blockade for periop-erative anesthesia and analgesia has increased dra-matically during the past several years. The reasons for this increased use may include not only the potential benefits of peripheral nerve blockade (Table 1) but also the avoidance of complications commonly associated with more traditional neu-raxial techniques. These include concerns about perioperative anticoagulation, infectious risks and complications, unwanted hemodynamic instability

(sympathectomy), and delayed hospital dismissal during outpatient surgery.

However, peripheral techniques may be associated with their own unique set of complications and con-cerns. Complications are beginning to be reported at a higher frequency as changes in clinical practice (e.g., aggressive perioperative anticoagulation, new regional techniques, continuous catheters) and the popularity of these blocks continue to evolve. The majority of

Table 1.	Potential Benefits of Peripheral Nerve Blockade

Superior postoperative analgesia
Improved rehabilitative efforts (due to analgesia)
Decreased perioperative nausea and vomiting
Faster emergence and recovery
Earlier mobilization (unilateral blockade)
Less cognitive impairment (avoiding opioids)
Faster eligibility for dismissal
Shorter hospital stay
Extended benefits from continuous catheter
  techniques

these complications can be classified as neurologic complications (i.e., peripheral nerve injuries and systemic local anesthetic toxicity), hemorrhagic or vascular injuries, infectious complications, or complications associated with extended peripheral nerve blockade (i.e., continuous catheter techniques).

Neurologic Complications and Regional Anesthesia

Perioperative nerve injuries have long been recognized as a potential complication of regional anesthesia. In 1914, Neuhof described a musculospiral nerve palsy (i.e., a radial neuropathy) after brachial plexus anesthesia which could not be attributed to the original injury. Subsequently, Woolley and Vandam reviewed the available literature and found several cases of persistent neurologic symptoms after brachial plexus blockade. They reported frequencies of nerve injury ranging from 0.1% to 5.6% and speculated that many of the injuries may be attributed to mechanical trauma or local anesthetic toxicity. Woolley and Vandam recommended that "an atraumatic technic with the use of small gauge needles and avoidance of hematoma formation" be the primary goal. Furthermore, they suggested that the patient be "carefully prepared with sedatives so that the experience of nerve injection is not disagreeable and recollection of the procedure too vivid."

Incidence and Etiology of Neurologic Complications

The incidence and characteristics of serious complications related to regional anesthesia were reviewed by Auroy and colleagues in a large prospective survey conducted in France. A total of 103,730 regional anesthetic procedures, including 71,053 neuraxial anesthetics, 21,278 peripheral nerve blocks, and 11,229 intravenous regional anesthetics, were performed over a 5-month period. Neurologic complications related to regional anesthetic techniques occurred in 34 (0.03%) patients. These represented 26% of all complications related to regional anesthesia. Of the 34 neurologic complications, 24 (70%) occurred during spinal anesthesia, 6 (18%) during epidural anesthesia, and 4 (12%) during peripheral nerve blockade. Additional complications that occurred during peripheral nerve blockade included cardiac arrest (0.01%), death (0.005%), seizures (0.08%), and radiculopathy (0.02%). All neurologic complications occurred within 48 hours of surgery and resolved within 3 months in 85% of patients. In 12 of 19 (63%) cases of radiculopathy after spinal anesthesia and in *all* cases of radiculopathy after epidural or peripheral nerve blockade, needle placement was associated with either a paresthesia during needle insertion or pain on injection. In all cases, the postoperative radiculopathy had the same topography as the associated paresthesia.

In a follow-up investigation, Auroy and colleagues examined an additional 158,083 regional anesthetic procedures—including 50,223 peripheral nerve blocks—performed during a 10-month period. The overall incidence of serious complications related to regional anesthesia (all techniques) was approximately 4 in 10,000 (0.04%) (Table 2). Interestingly, when they specifically examined the risk associated with peripheral nerve blockade, they found an identical incidence of 4 in 10,000 (0.04%). However, a considerably higher percentage of complications was noted with the posterior lumbar plexus block compared with other peripheral techniques (Table 3).

Auroy and colleagues also found that the incidence of cardiac arrest and neurologic complications was substantially higher after spinal anesthesia than after other types

Table 2.   Serious Complications Related to Regional Anesthesia*

Technique	Cardiac arrest	Respiratory failure	Death	Seizure	Neurologic injury
Spinal (n=41,251)	10 (2.4)	2 (0.5)	3 (0.7)	1 (0.2)	14 (3.4)
Epidural (n=35,379)	0	3 (0.8)	0	3 (0.8)	0
Peripheral block (n=50,223)	1 (0.2)	2 (0.4)	1 (0.2)	6 (1.2)	12 (2.4)
IV regional block (n=4,448)	0	0	0	0	0
Peribulbar block (n=17,071)	0	0	0	0	0
Total regional block (N=158,083†)	11 (0.7)	7 (0.4)	4 (0.3)	10 (0.6)	26 (1.6)

*Data presented are number of complications and the estimated (n/10,000), where applicable.

†The entries above do not include 9,711 other types of blocks.

Data from Auroy Y, Benhamou D, Bargues L, Ecoffey C, Falissard B, Mercier F, et al. Major complications of regional anesthesia in France: the SOS Regional Anesthesia Hotline Service. Anesthesiology, 2002 Nov;97(5):1274-80.

of regional anesthesia (Table 2). This finding was also reported in their initial publication. Neurologic complications attributed specifically to the regional technique occurred in 26 (0.02%) patients; recovery was complete within 6 months in 16 of the 26 patients. Of the 12 patients who experienced a neurologic complication after peripheral nerve blockade, 7 had a persistent complication for more than 6 months. In addition, 9 of the 12 regional blocks were performed with the use of a peripheral nerve stimulator.

On the basis of these findings, the authors concluded that needle trauma and local anesthetic neurotoxicity were the primary causes of most neurologic complications.

Table 3.   Serious Complications Related to Peripheral Nerve Blockade*

Technique	Cardiac arrest	Respiratory failure	Death	Seizure	Neurologic injury
Interscalene block (n=3,459)	0	0	0	0	1 (2.9)
Supraclavicular block (n=1,899)	0	0	0	1 (5.3)	0
Axillary block (n=11,024)	0	0	0	1 (0.9)	2 (1.8)
Midhumeral block (n=7,402)	0	0	0	1 (1.4)	1 (1.4)
Posterior lumbar plexus block (n=394)	1 (25.4)	2 (50.8)	1 (25.4)	1 (25.4)	0
Femoral block (n=10,309)	0	0	0	0	3 (3)
Sciatic nerve block (n=8,507)	0	0	0	2 (2.4)	2 (2.4)
Popliteal nerve block (n=952)	0	0	0	0	3 (32)
Total peripheral nerve blocks (N=50,223)	1 (0.2)	2 (0.4)	1 (0.2)	6 (1.2)	12 (2.4)

*Data presented are number of complications and the estimated (n/10,000), where applicable.

Data from Auroy Y, Benhamou D, Bargues L, Ecoffey C, Falissard B, Mercier F, et al. Major complications of regional anesthesia in France: the SOS Regional Anesthesia Hotline Service. Anesthesiology, 2002 Nov;97(5):1274-80.

Furthermore, although these studies found that the incidence of severe anesthesia-related complications is extremely low, they also showed that serious complications may occur in the presence of experienced anesthesiologists. This finding suggests that continued vigilance in patients undergoing regional anesthesia is not only warranted but also critical to minimize perioperative nerve injuries.

Closed Claims Analysis

Cheney and colleagues examined the American Society of Anesthesiologists Closed Claims database to further delineate the role of nerve damage in malpractice claims filed against anesthesia-care providers. Of the 4,183 claims reviewed, 670 (16%) were for anesthesia-related nerve injury. The most frequent sites of injury were the ulnar nerve (28%), brachial plexus (20%), lumbosacral nerve roots (16%), and spinal cord (13%); the remaining claims (22%) were for additional mononeuropathies. Overall, regional anesthesia was more frequently associated with nerve damage claims than general anesthesia. The only exception was ulnar nerve injuries, which were predominantly associated with general anesthesia (85%).

Regional anesthetic techniques (axillary, interscalene, and supraclavicular blockade) were attributed specifically to 16% of all brachial plexus injuries, in which 31% of patients experienced a paresthesia either during needle placement or with injection of local anesthetic. In contrast, 30% of ulnar nerve injuries were attributed to regional anesthetic techniques in which a mechanism of injury was explicitly stated. Interestingly, none of these claims involved the elicitation of a paresthesia. In these cases, the onset of symptoms occurred immediately within the postoperative period in 21% of patients and was delayed from 1 to 28 days postoperatively (median, 3 days) in 62% of cases. Neurologic deficits that arise within the first 24 hours postoperatively may represent extraneural or intraneural hematoma, intraneural edema, or a lesion involving a sufficient number of nerve fibers to allow immediate diagnosis. In contrast, delayed neurologic findings, in which symptoms develop several days or even weeks postoperatively, may represent an alternative cause such as a tissue reaction or scar formation leading to

degeneration of nerve fibers. However, the available data do not allow determination of whether this reaction is due to mechanical trauma, local anesthetic neurotoxicity, or a combination of both.

In a more recent review of the Closed Claims database, Lee and colleagues specifically examined serious injuries associated with regional anesthesia that occurred during the period 1980-1999. During that time, a total of 1,005 regional anesthesia claims were identified, of which 368 (37%) were obstetric-related claims and 637 (63%) nonobstetric claims. All obstetric claims were related to complications associated with neuraxial anesthesia or analgesia. In contrast, of the 637 nonobstetric claims, 134 (21%) were related specifically to complications occurring during peripheral nerve blockade. Axillary blocks were used in most of the peripheral blocks (44%), followed by intravenous regional anesthesia (21%), interscalene blocks (19%), and supraclavicular blocks (7%). The damaging event was related to the block technique in more than 50% of cases. Overall, temporary or permanent peripheral nerve injury occurred in 79 (59%) of 134 peripheral nerve claims. Upper extremity techniques were more commonly associated with peripheral nerve claims than lower extremity techniques. Additional complications occurring during peripheral nerve blockade included death or brain damage (13%), pneumothorax (10%), emotional distress (2%), inflammatory skin reactions (2%), and miscellaneous (14%).

Perioperative Nerve Injury

Several basic science and clinical investigations have examined peripheral nerve injury in an attempt to identify risk factors commonly associated with postoperative neurologic dysfunction. As a result of this work, a multitude of patient, surgical, and anesthetic risk factors have been identified that may contribute to perioperative nerve injury (Table 4).

Patient Risk Factors

Patient risk factors commonly associated with perioperative nerve injury include male sex, increasing age, extremes of body habitus, and preexisting diabetes

Table 4. Potential Risk Factors Contributing to Perioperative Nerve Injury

Patient risk factors

Preexisting neurologic disorders	Increasing age	Preexisting diabetes mellitus
Male sex	Extremes of body habitus	

Surgical risk factors

Surgical trauma or stretch	Perioperative inflammation	Cast compression or irritation
Tourniquet ischemia	Postoperative infection or abscess	Patient positioning
Vascular compromise	Hematoma formation	

Anesthetic risk factors

Local anesthetic toxicity	Needle- or catheter-induced mechanical trauma
Perineural edema	Ischemic injury (vasoconstrictors)

mellitus. However, patients with preexisting neurologic deficits also may be at increased risk. The presence of chronic, underlying neural compromise due to mechanical (e.g., compression), ischemic (e.g., peripheral vascular disease), toxic (e.g., cisplatin chemotherapy), or metabolic (e.g., diabetes) derangements may theoretically place these patients at increased risk of further neurologic injury. Upton and McComas were the first to describe the *double-crush phenomenon*, which suggests that patients with preexisting neural compromise may be more susceptible to injury at another site when exposed to a secondary insult (Figure 1). Secondary insults may include various concomitant patient, surgical, or anesthetic risk factors. Osterman emphasized not only that two low-grade insults along a peripheral nerve trunk are worse than a single site but also that the damage of the dual injury far exceeds the expected additive damage caused by each isolated insult. It may be further postulated that the secondary insult need not be along the peripheral nerve trunk itself but rather at any point along the neural transmission pathway. Therefore, the performance of neuraxial—and peripheral—techniques in patients with preexisting neurologic disorders may theoretically place them at increased risk of a double-crush phenomenon.

Surgical Risk Factors

Surgical risk factors include direct intraoperative trauma or stretch, vascular compromise, perioperative infection, hematoma formation, prolonged tourniquet ischemia, or improperly applied casts or dressings. Horlocker and colleagues examined the cause of perioperative nerve injury in 607 patients undergoing 1,614 blocks for upper extremity surgery. Surgical variables were believed to be the cause in 55 of 62 (88.7%) neurologic complications identified. Direct surgical trauma or stretch occurred in 40 (73%) cases, inflammation or infection in 6 (11%) cases, hematoma or vascular compromise in 4 (7%) cases, cast irritation in 3 (5%) cases, and tourniquet ischemia in 2 (4%) cases. Interestingly, all complications involving motor deficits had a surgical cause. Fourteen patients (25%) required subsequent surgical intervention to restore nerve function.

Anesthetic Risk Factors

Regional anesthetic factors that may contribute directly or indirectly to perioperative nerve injury include needle- or catheter-induced mechanical trauma, ischemic nerve injury due to vasoconstrictors or neural edema, and chemical injury from direct local anesthetic neurotoxicity. Several authors have investigated the role of mechanical trauma,

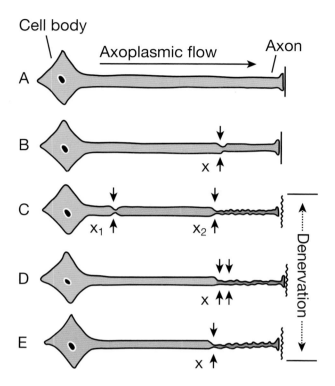

Cell body

Axoplasmic flow

Axon

Figure 1. Neural lesions resulting in denervation. Axoplasmic flow is indicated by the degree of shading. Complete loss of axoplasmic flow results in denervation (C, D, and E). A, Normal neuron. B, Mild neuronal injury at a single site (x) is insufficient to cause denervation distal to the insult. C, Mild neuronal injury at two separate sites (x_1 and x_2) may cause distal denervation (i.e., double crush). D, Severe neuronal injury at a single site (x) may also cause distal denervation. E, Axon with a diffuse, preexisting underlying disease process (e.g., toxic, metabolic, ischemic) may have impaired axonal flow throughout the neuron, which may or may not be symptomatic but predisposes the axon to distal denervation after a single minor neural insult at x (i.e., double crush).

including the role of needle gauge, type, and bevel configuration on peripheral nerve injury. The disruption of perineural tissue around nerve fascicles compromises the blood-nerve barrier and results in the herniation of endoneurial contents (i.e., myelinated nerve fibers) into the perineural space. However, needle-to-nerve contact by itself—in the absence of local anesthetic injection—rarely produces clinical or functional abnormalities.

Rather, it is the combined effect of needle penetration and injection of local anesthetic into the neural fascicle that likely causes axonal degeneration and subsequent neurologic injury.

Neural ischemia from local anesthetic additives or perineural edema may also contribute to perioperative nerve deficits. Epinephrine is a common local anesthetic adjuvant used to prolong neural blockade, identify intravascular injection, and reduce the systemic uptake of local anesthetic. However, its use may contribute to neural compromise by amplifying the vasoconstrictive effects of local anesthetics and reducing nerve blood flow in epineurial vessels sensitive to the adrenergic effects of epinephrine. The risk of adverse events from neural ischemia may be of greatest concern in patients with preexisting neural compromise.

Finally, clinical experience has shown that the use of local anesthetics is overwhelmingly safe when they are administered correctly and in the recommended concentrations. However, when local anesthetic concentrations are inappropriately high, exposure times are prolonged (i.e., continuous infusions, repeated block techniques, epinephrine use), or injections are intraneural, severe degenerative changes may occur within neural fibers which lead to long-lasting neurologic sequelae. For example, several investigations have shown the acute toxic effects of local anesthetics within animal models. In general, most outcome studies have found that the neurotoxic effects are concentration-dependent, with the highest concentrations of local anesthetics inducing the most severe nerve injury. Furthermore, the order of potency of local anesthetics causing nerve injury is associated with the degree of motor nerve conduction blockade. Therefore, many experts have concluded that local anesthetic toxicity may directly parallel anesthetic potency.

Hemorrhagic Complications and Peripheral Nerve Blockade

Hemorrhagic complications are rare but potentially devastating complications of peripheral nerve blockade. They have been reported with various techniques, including interscalene, supraclavicular, infraclavicular, axillary, intercostal, femoral, ilioinguinal, posterior lumbar plexus, and lumbar sympathetic blockade. Patients at greatest risk may include those receiving hemostasis-altering medications such as low-molecular-weight heparin (LMWH), antiplatelet aggregation medications, or antithrombolytic therapy. However, relatively few data exist on the risk of hemorrhagic complications within these patient populations after peripheral nerve blockade.

In general, localized bruising and tenderness are exceedingly common after peripheral techniques, with frequencies as high as 8% to 23% being reported. However, true hemorrhagic complications are relatively uncommon. For example, reported frequencies of hematoma formation during brachial plexus blockade range from 0.2% to 3%. In most circumstances, hematomas are small, unrecognized, and clinically inconsequential. However, there have been reports of severe hemorrhagic complications and of serious neurologic impairment after hematoma formation.

Single-Injection Techniques

Stan and colleagues examined the neurologic and vascular complications in 1,000 consecutive patients undergoing transarterial axillary brachial plexus blockade. Reported vascular complications included transient arterial vasospasm in 10 (1%) patients, unintentional intravascular injection in 2 (0.2%) patients, and small (0-2 cm) hematoma formation in 2 (0.2%) patients. None of these complications resulted in perioperative morbidity, nor did they require intervention other than close observation. In contrast, Ben-David and Stahl report a case of radial nerve dysfunction associated with a large axillary hematoma in a patient after a single-dose transarterial axillary block. Laboratory investigation found normal prothrombin and partial thromboplastin times. The patient was observed for hematoma expansion and treated conservatively with arm elevation, splinting, and passive physiotherapy to maintain range of motion. Neurologic function gradually improved during the next several weeks and returned to normal 6 months postoperatively with no evidence of residual neurologic deficit.

Continuous Catheter Techniques

Hematoma formation has also been described with the use of continuous catheter techniques. Ekatodramis and colleagues reported two cases of prolonged Horner syndrome due to a neck hematoma after continuous interscalene blockade. In both cases, an expanding neck hematoma developed between the prevertebral and anterior scalene muscles within 24 to 72 hours of catheter placement. Both techniques were reportedly uneventful and atraumatic. Presenting symptoms included visual disturbances and painful swelling along the lateral aspect of the neck. Characteristic features of Horner syndrome (myosis, ptosis, enophthalmia, and anhidrosis) were identified on the side ipsilateral to the block in both patients. Interestingly, symptoms persisted in both cases for more than 6 months and achieved near complete resolution by 1 year. Ultrasonography and magnetic resonance imaging of the neck showed that the brachial plexus was free from compression in both patients. The authors concluded that prevertebral hematomas compressed and injured preganglionic cervical sympathetic fibers, resulting in an extended Horner syndrome. The spontaneous resolution of symptoms over 1 year indicates the time required for complete regeneration of nerve fibers.

As these cases show, hematoma formation should be considered in the differential diagnosis of any patient with neurologic impairment after peripheral nerve blockade. Surgical decompression and hematoma evacuation may become necessary if 1) the hematoma continues to expand, 2) progressive neurologic deterioration occurs, 3) neural dysfunction does not improve despite resolution of the hematoma, or 4) there is evidence of vascular or lymphatic obstruction. In select cases in which these criteria are not met, observation and conservative management may be appropriate.

Unlike the known risks of spinal hematoma arising from concomitant anticoagulation and neuraxial anesthesia, the risk for peripheral nerve blockade is not clearly defined, nor are guidelines available. Although the consensus statements on neuraxial anesthesia and anticoagulation published by the American Society of Regional Anesthesia and Pain Medicine may be applied to any regional technique, a more liberal application may consider the compressibility of the needle insertion site and the vascular structures at risk. Accordingly, the use of peripheral techniques in patients with coagulopathy should be based on a careful risk-benefit analysis, and they should be performed with caution. This caution is particularly important if the block is to be performed in a region where an expanding hematoma could compress the airway (e.g., interscalene) or go unrecognized for several hours or days in a noncompressible site (e.g., lumbar plexus).

Bleeding into a nerve sheath does not represent the same catastrophe, in terms of severity and significance of neural compromise, as bleeding into the spinal canal. Cardiac catheterization involves the placement of a large cannula in a femoral or brachial vessel with subsequent anticoagulation, yet neurologic dysfunction is rare. Indeed, single-dose and continuous peripheral blocks may be suitable alternatives to neuraxial techniques in a patient who has had anticoagulation. Communication between clinicians involved in the perioperative management of patients receiving anticoagulants for thromboprophylaxis is essential to decrease the risk of serious hemorrhagic complications. Patients should be closely monitored perioperatively for early signs of neural compression such as pain, numbness, or weakness. A delay in diagnosis and intervention may lead to irreversible neural ischemia.

Infectious Complications and Peripheral Nerve Blockade

Infection can complicate any regional anesthetic technique. The infectious source may be exogenous (e.g., contaminated equipment or medication) or endogenous (e.g., a bacterial source in the patient seeding to the remote site of needle or catheter insertion). Although infection at the site of needle insertion is an absolute contraindication to regional anesthesia, common sense dictates that encroaching cellulitis, lymphangitis, or erythema may also preclude a regional anesthetic technique.

Indwelling catheters may increase the risk of an infectious complication. A review of the literature shows that infectious complication rates range from 0% to 3.2% for both upper and lower extremity catheters (Table 5). Gaumann and colleagues reported a 27% colonization rate for indwelling axillary catheters that had remained in situ an average of 3.7±0.7 days. However, no signs of local or systemic infection were noted in any patient. Similarly, Bergman and colleagues reported a single (0.2%) superficial axillary infection in 405 consecutive continuous axillary catheters. Interestingly, the patient was being treated for reflex sympathetic dystrophy and did not receive the standard 2 days of antibiotic therapy commonly administered to surgical patients.

The infectious risk of femoral nerve catheters was evaluated by Cuvillon and colleagues in 211 consecutive patients undergoing perineural catheter placement. Patients received standardized postoperative analgesic and antibiotic therapy. After 48 hours, each catheter was removed and semiquantitative bacteriologic culture studies were performed. Bacterial colonization had occurred on 57% of the catheters, with *Staphylococcus epidermidis* being the most frequent microorganism. Of the catheters colonized, 53% were colonized with a single organism. Neither cellulitis nor abscess occurred. Three (1.4%) transitory bacteremias were likely related to catheter use. Patients presented with increased temperatures and symptoms of bacteremia at both 24 and 48 hours. Both blood and femoral catheter cultures were positive for the same organisms. Symptoms of bacteremia and the fever dissipated on removal of the catheter and without the addition of antibiotic therapy. No serious long-term infectious complications were noted in any patient.

Currently, there are no definitive recommendations regarding continuous catheter use and routine antibiotic prophylaxis. Signs and symptoms of local or systemic infections should be treated with catheter removal and parenteral antibiotics. Retained catheter fragments may also be a source of infection. Bergman and colleagues described an axillary abscess necessitating surgical intervention in a patient with a fractured catheter. There were no neurologic sequelae.

					Infectious
Reference	**Sample size (N)**	**Catheter type**	**Duration of catheter use**	**Antibiotic administration**	**complication rate, %**
Cuvillon (2001) *Anesthesia & Analgesia*	211	Femoral	48 h	Yes	1.5
Bergman (2003) *Anesthesia & Analgesia*	405	Axillary	55 h	Yes	0.2
Borgeat (2003) *Anesthesiology*	700	Interscalene	4 days	Yes	0.8
Borgeat (2004) *Regional Anesthesia*	237	Popliteal	60 h	Unknown	0
Capdevila (2005) *Anesthesiology*	1,416	Upper and lower extremity	56 h	Variable	0.07
Buckenmaier (2006) *British Journal of Anaesthesia*	305	Upper and lower extremity	10 days	Yes	0.7
Borgeat (2006) *Anesthesia & Analgesia*	1,001	Popliteal	48 h	Yes	0
Neuburger (2007) *Acta Anaesthesiologica Scandinavica*	2,285	Upper and lower extremity	4 days	Yes (97%)	3.2
Wiegel (2007) *Anesthesia & Analgesia*	1,398	Upper and lower extremity	4-6 days	Yes	0.2

Table 5. Infectious Complications of Peripheral Nerve Catheters

Complications of Continuous Peripheral Nerve Catheters

The incidence and characteristics of complications associated with continuous peripheral nerve catheters were recently examined by Capdevila and colleagues in a large, multicenter European trial. The authors prospectively studied 1,416 patients scheduled to undergo major orthopedic surgery and continuous peripheral nerve blockade to assess the risk of neurologic, hemorrhagic, infectious, and technical complications. During the investigation, 394 (28%) minor adverse events were noted. Most of these events (n=253; 64%) were technical complications associated with the catheter or infusion device. Accidental withdrawal of catheters, kinked or inadvertently displaced catheters, catheter leakage, and technical complications with the infusion device occurred most commonly.

Twelve (0.84%) serious adverse events directly related to the catheter technique were noted (Table 6). All events resolved without sequelae.

Among the 969 (68%) catheters submitted for culture studies, 278 (28.7%) had positive bacterial colonization (growth of at least 1 microorganism on quantitative culture). The majority of these cases (n=242, 87%) were colonized by a single organism. The bacterial species most commonly identified was *Staphylococcus epidermidis* (61%). Forty-two (3%) patients had evidence of a localized inflammatory reaction (erythema, tenderness, induration) at the site of catheter insertion. In these patients, 44.2% of catheters were colonized, whereas 18.6% of catheters were colonized in patients without signs or symptoms of localized inflammation (P=.001). One psoas

Table 6.   Serious Adverse Events Associated With Continuous Peripheral Nerve Blockade

Adverse event	ISB (n=256)	AXB (n=126)	PCB (n=20)	Femoral (n=683)	Fascial (n=94)	Sciatic (n=32)	Popliteal (n=167)	Distal (n=38)
Neuropathy	0	0	0	3 (0.4%)	0	0	0	0
Acute respiratory failure	2 (0.8%)	0	0	0	0	0	0	0
Laryngeal nerve paralysis	2 (0.8%)	0	0	0	0	0	0	0
Severe hypotension	0	0	3 (15%)	0	0	0	0	0
Systemic local anesthetic toxicity	0	1 (0.08%)	0	0	0	0	0	1 (2.5%)
Abscess	0	0	0	1 (0.14%)	0	0	0	0

AXB, axillary block; Distal, distal peripheral catheters; ISB, interscalene block; PCB, psoas compartment block.
Modified from Capdevila X, Pirat P, Bringuier S, Gaertner E, Singelyn F, Bernard N, et al; French Study Group on Continuous Peripheral Nerve Blocks. Continuous peripheral nerve blocks in hospital wards after orthopedic surgery: a multicenter prospective analysis of the quality of postoperative analgesia and complications in 1,416 patients. Anesthesiology. 2005 Nov;103(5):1035-45. Used with permission.

muscle abscess was noted in a diabetic patient undergoing total knee arthroplasty with a continuous femoral nerve catheter. No bacteremia was found, and the patient recovered fully with targeted antibiotic therapy. No hemorrhagic complications were noted during the study. Independent risk factors for neurologic and infectious complications are listed in Table 7.

Summary
Neurologic, hemorrhagic, and infectious complications have been reported after peripheral nerve blockade. Of these complications, peripheral nerve injury may be the most catastrophic perioperative complication. Patient, surgical, and anesthetic risk factors have all been identified as potential causes, and multiple factors commonly play a role. The double-crush phenomenon suggests that patients with several concomitant risk factors may be at greatest risk for development of postoperative neurologic complications. A comprehensive understanding of the complexities of perioperative nerve injury is critical to rapidly assess patients, identify potential causes, and intervene when appropriate immediately postoperatively. Successful long-term management is highly dependent on realistic patient and physician expectations and on an individualized, multidisciplinary therapeutic approach.

Suggested Reading
Auroy Y, Narchi P, Messiah A, Litt L, Rouvier B, Samii K. Serious complications related to regional anesthesia: results of a prospective survey in France. Anesthesiology. 1997 Sep;87(3):479-86.

Auroy Y, Benhamou D, Bargues L, Ecoffey C, Falissard B, Mercier FJ, et al. Major complications of regional anesthesia in France: the SOS Regional

Table 7.   Risk Factors for Neurologic and Infectious Complications After Continuous Peripheral Nerve Blockade

Adverse event	Risk factor	Odds ratio (95% CI)	*P* value
Neurologic	Intensive care unit stay	9.8 (2.02-38.5)	0.004
	Patient age <40 y	3.9 (1.6-9.8)	0.006
	Bupivacaine infusion	2.7 (1.06-6.8)	0.02
Infectious	Intensive care unit stay	5.07 (0.33-18.1)	0.004
	Catheter duration >48 h	4.61 (1.57-15.9)	0.008
	Male sex	2.1 (1.07-4.1)	0.008
	No antibiotic prophylaxis	1.92 (1.03-3.9)	0.01

CI, confidence interval.

Modified from Capdevila X, Pirat P, Bringuier S, Gaertner E, Singelyn F, Bernard N, et al; French Study Group on Continuous Peripheral Nerve Blocks. Continuous peripheral nerve blocks in hospital wards after orthopedic surgery: a multicenter prospective analysis of the quality of postoperative analgesia and complications in 1,416 patients. Anesthesiology. 2005 Nov;103(5):1035-45. Used with permission.

Anesthesia Hotline Service. Anesthesiology. 2002 Nov;97(5):1274-80. Erratum in: Anesthesiology. 2003 Feb;98(2):595.

Ben-David B, Stahl S. Axillary block complicated by hematoma and radial nerve injury. Reg Anesth Pain Med. 1999 May-Jun;24(3):264-6.

Bergman BD, Hebl JR, Kent J, Horlocker TT. Neurologic complications of 405 consecutive continuous axillary catheters. Anesth Analg. 2003 Jan;96(1):247-52.

Capdevila X, Pirat P, Bringuier S, Gaertner E, Singelyn F, Bernard N, et al; French Study Group on Continuous Peripheral Nerve Blocks. Continuous peripheral nerve blocks in hospital wards after orthopedic surgery: a multicenter prospective analysis of the quality of postoperative analgesia and complications in 1,416 patients. Anesthesiology. 2005 Nov;103(5):1035-45.

Cheney FW, Domino KB, Caplan RA, Posner KL. Nerve injury associated with anesthesia: a closed claims analysis. Anesthesiology. 1999 Apr;90(4):1062-9.

Cuvillon P, Ripart J, Lalourcey L, Veyrat E, L'Hermite J, Boisson C, et al. The continuous femoral nerve block catheter for postoperative analgesia: bacterial colonization, infectious rate and adverse effects. Anesth Analg. 2001 Oct;93(4):1045-9.

Ekatodramis G, Macaire P, Borgeat A. Prolonged Horner syndrome due to neck hematoma after continuous interscalene block. Anesthesiology. 2001 Sep;95(3)801-3.

Enneking FK, Benzon H. Oral anticoagulants and regional anesthesia: a perspective. Reg Anesth Pain Med 1998 Nov-Dec;23(6 Suppl 2):140-5.

Gaumann DM, Lennon RL, Wedel DJ. Continuous axillary block for postoperative pain management. Reg Anesth. 1988;13(2):77-82.

Horlocker TT, Kufner RP, Bishop AT, Maxson PM, Schroeder DR. The risk of persistent paresthesia is not increased with repeated axillary block. Anesth Analg. 1999 Feb;88(2):382-7.

Horlocker TT, Wedel DJ. Neuraxial block and low-molecular-weight heparin: balancing perioperative analgesia and thromboprophylaxis. Reg Anesth Pain Med. 1998 Nov-Dec;23(6 Suppl 2):164-77.

Lee LA, Posner KL, Domino KB, Caplan RA, Cheney FW. Injuries associated with regional anesthesia in the 1980s and 1990s: a closed claims analysis. Anesthesiology. 2004 Jul;101(1):143-52.

Liu SS, Mulroy MF. Neuraxial anesthesia and analgesia in the presence of standard heparin. Reg Anesth Pain Med. 1998 Nov-Dec;23(6 Suppl 2):157-63.

Löfström B, Wennberg A, Wién L. Late disturbances in nerve function after block with local anaesthetic agents: an electroneurographic study. Acta Anaesthesiol Scand. 1996;10(2):111-22.

Myers RR, Heckman HM. Effects of local anesthesia on nerve blood flow: studies using lidocaine with and without epinephrine. Anesthesiology. 1989 Nov;71(5): 757-62.

Neal JM, Hebl JR, Gerancher JC, Hogan QH. Brachial plexus anesthesia: essentials of our current understanding. Reg Anesth Pain Med. 2002 Jul-Aug;27(4):402-28. Erratum in: Reg Anesth Pain Med 2002 Nov-Dec;27(6):625.

Neuhof H. Supraclavicular anesthetization of the brachial plexus: a case of collapse following its administration. JAMA. 1914;62:1629-31.

Osterman AL. The double crush syndrome. Orthop Clin North Am. 1988 Jan;19(1):147-55.

Rosenquist RW, Brown DL. Neuraxial bleeding: fibrinolytics/thrombolytics. Reg Anesth Pain Med. 1998 Nov-Dec;23(6 Suppl 2):152-6.

Selander D, Brattsand R, Lundborg G, Nordborg C, Olsson Y. Local anesthetics: importance of mode of application; concentration and adrenaline for the appearance of nerve lesions. An experimental study of axonal degeneration and barrier damage after intrafascicular injection or topical application of bupivacaine (Marcain). Acta Anaesthesiol Scand. 1979 Apr;23(2):127-36.

Stan TC, Krantz MA, Solomon DL, Poulos JG, Chaouki K. The incidence of neurovascular complications following axillary brachial plexus block using a transarterial approach: a prospective study of 1,000 consecutive patients. Reg Anesth. 1995 Nov-Dec;20(6):486-92.

Upton AR, McComas AJ. The double crush in nerve entrapment syndromes. Lancet. 1973 Aug 18;2(7825): 359-62.

Woolley EJ, Vandam LD. Neurological sequelae of brachial plexus nerve block. Ann Surg. 1959 Jan;149(1):53-60.

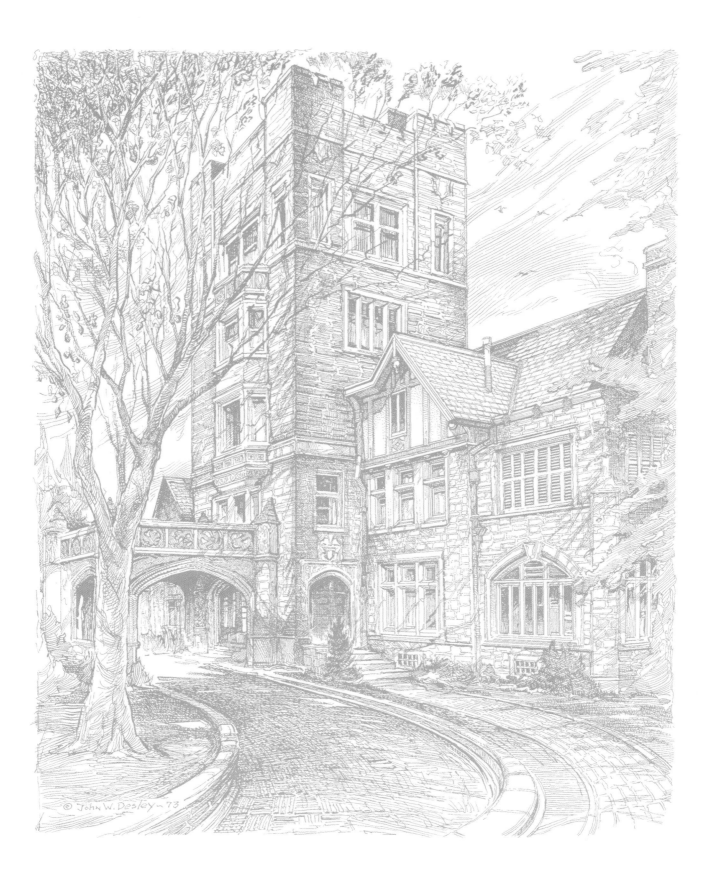

© John W. Dosley – 73

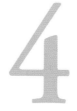

Perioperative Positioning Injuries

Mark A. Warner, M.D.

Patients undergoing upper and lower extremity surgical procedures face unique positioning challenges that may place them at risk for development of various perioperative complications. Central and peripheral neuropathies, compartment syndromes, and soft tissue injuries are just a few of the position-related injuries that may occur. In addition, many patients undergoing upper extremity procedures (e.g., shoulder or upper arm surgery) are placed in head-elevated or semirecumbent positions that may be associated with hemodynamic challenges such as hypotension and peripheral venous pooling. Much of the information available on these potentially devastating perioperative complications is limited to anecdotal case reports and limited case series. Therefore, it is difficult to assess the overall frequency at which these events occur.

Preoperative Considerations

A basic principle that may allow clinicians to avoid many neurologic and soft tissue–related positioning problems is to never exceed ranges of motion that patients cannot comfortably tolerate while awake. Many patients undergoing upper extremity surgical procedures are either elderly or have orthopedic or rheumatic disorders that limit the range of motion in one or more of their joints. Importantly, these joint limitations often involve the head and neck. Some patients have body shapes and sizes (e.g., obesity) that add another level of complexity to safely positioning them. It is always advisable to consider the planned intraoperative position—particularly when it involves a position that may stretch or compress peripheral nerves or soft tissue. Patients should be examined preoperatively to determine specific anatomical or pathologic conditions that may preclude them from being placed in the planned intraoperative position.

Several general positioning issues should be assessed in all patients. However, for patients undergoing upper extremity surgery, additional concerns need to be taken into consideration.

Shoulder Procedures and the Lawn-Chair Position
Shoulder procedures are often performed with patients in a head-elevated position with the operating table configured to resemble a lawn chair. With this position, it is critically important to assess patients for their ability to tolerate cervical rotation, flexion, and extension. Although cervical movement should be minimized as much as possible, some patients (e.g., those with rheumatic disorders) are unable to tolerate even a modest degree of cervical manipulation. Prolonged or permanent neurologic injury of both the ipsilateral and the contralateral upper extremities has been reported after prolonged cervical flexion, extension, or rotation in patients with preexisting cervical radiculopathies. Obesity, or more specifically a body habitus with a protuberant abdomen, is also an important consideration when positioning patients. The lawn-chair position has been associated with increased intra-abdominal pressure and difficulty with ventilation in short, obese patients. The degree of upper torso inclination typically used in lawn-chair positions may not be well tolerated by patients within this group. Under these circumstances,

surgeons should be notified that they may need to modify or adjust the operative position accordingly.

Shoulder Procedures and the Lateral Position
It may be difficult for patients undergoing shoulder procedures to fully recline laterally. For example, some patients may have significant pain and discomfort in the contralateral shoulder. Therefore, modifications to the lateral position, such as placing rolls or blankets between the downward aspect of the chest and the operating table to reduce pressure on the contralateral shoulder, may be necessary during surgical positioning. Mattress alterations may also be useful, including the use of gaps in the mattress that allow the contralateral shoulder to rest without carrying the weight of the upper torso. Regardless, the ability of patients to rest comfortably laterally should be assessed preoperatively and plans modified to adapt to any patient-specific limitations.

Upper Extremity Procedures and the Supine Position
In many supine positions, the arm and forearm are positioned in extension onto an arm board or lateral table extension. This position may be impossible for patients with osteoarthritis, bone spurs, or other bony deformities that prevent full extension of the forearm at the elbow. Furthermore, some patients may have limited range of motion due to restrictive or inflexible soft tissue or scarring. These patients may be particularly susceptible to median neuropathies if the elbow is fully extended during general or regional anesthesia. For example, men between 20 and 40 years old who have exceptionally large biceps (e.g., weight lifters) are limited in their ability to fully extend their forearms at the elbow. Under these circumstances, forceful full extension of the elbow after induction of anesthesia has resulted in postoperative median nerve injury. The cause is not fully understood, but the median nerve may contract in length over time as the elbow's range of motion becomes more restricted. Forceful extension of a contracted nerve may cause a temporary stretch beyond its normal resting length. In mammalian nerves, stretch of more than 5% of their resting length can cause acute ischemic injury and permanent disability if sustained for prolonged periods.

Intraoperative Considerations

Although most patients tolerate short periods of positioning that may make them uncomfortable while awake, there are no clear recommendations regarding the duration that these positions can be sustained without resulting in transient or permanent nerve injury or soft tissue complications. Therefore, avoidance of anesthetized positions that are not tolerable to patients while awake is recommended. Careful preoperative assessment of the patient and direct communication between the anesthesia and surgical teams is critically important when formulating an intraoperative positioning plan that is out of the ordinary. Alternatives to standard intraoperative positions should be developed and discussed preoperatively because it may be difficult to make creative adjustments and build consensus after anesthesia is induced and positioning begins.

Each unique position or variant of a position used for upper extremity surgery needs careful attention to avoid potential neural compromise and soft tissue compression. Several specific issues must be considered.

Shoulder Procedures and the Lawn-Chair Position

Patients undergoing general anesthesia and having definitive airway management (i.e., endotracheal tube or laryngeal mask airway) should have the airway fully supported both during and after surgical positioning. When the patient is maneuvered into a lawn-chair position, attention should be focused on the head and neck to avoid excessive cervical rotation, flexion, or extension. Cervical positions that are not well tolerated by the awake patient may result in severe neurologic injury if sustained at angles beyond that which is considered comfortable by the patient. The head, if secured or stabilized, should not support the weight of the upper torso at any time. The contralateral upper extremity should be positioned within a range of motion deemed comfortable by the patient while awake. In general, elbows should be flexed less than 90° to avoid intrinsic pressure on the ulnar nerve within the cubital tunnel. Studies have shown that elbow flexion of more than 90° may produce high intrinsic pressures under the cubital tunnel retinaculum (Figure 1). The retinaculum

is the proximally thickened tissue of the fascia that joins the medial epicondylar and olecranon heads of the flexor carpi ulnaris. Elbow flexion to more than 90° causes the retinaculum to stretch and compress the ulnar nerve as it passes beneath and between the medial epicondyle and olecranon processes (Figure 2).

Similarly, arms should be abducted less than 90° to avoid stretch of the brachial plexus as it enters and passes through the axilla (Figure 3). Stretch of the nerve tissue within the axilla is further compromised if the cervical spine is also rotated to the contralateral side. Finally, the degree of head elevation (i.e., inclination) may need to be reduced for patients who have large abdomens and in whom ventilation is difficult.

Shoulder Procedures and the Lateral Position

Most modern operating tables have thick, well-cushioned mattress pads. When these pads are used, there are no data to suggest that rolls or padding placed under the chest wall of laterally positioned patients (i.e., axillary rolls) reduces the frequency of neurologic complications or increased compartment pressures within the dependent upper extremity. However, these pads need to be carefully positioned on the table and periodically assessed to ensure that they do not dislodge or advance into the dependent axilla, where they may cause neurovascular compression.

Pads or rolls placed under the dependent chest wall may be beneficial in a select group of anesthetized patients. Adult patients at the extremes of body mass index (i.e., extremely thin or massively obese) seem to have an increased risk for development of compartment syndrome of the dependent extremity when undergoing general anesthesia or deep sedation in the lateral position. During care of these patients, dependent pads or rolls may help reduce pressure on the downward shoulder or decrease compartment pressures within the contralateral upper extremity. Alternatives to chest pads or rolls include a modified lateral position (i.e., semilateral positions) or mattress modifications to accommodate patient limitations.

When an arm board is used to support the nondependent upper extremity during surgical procedures, the

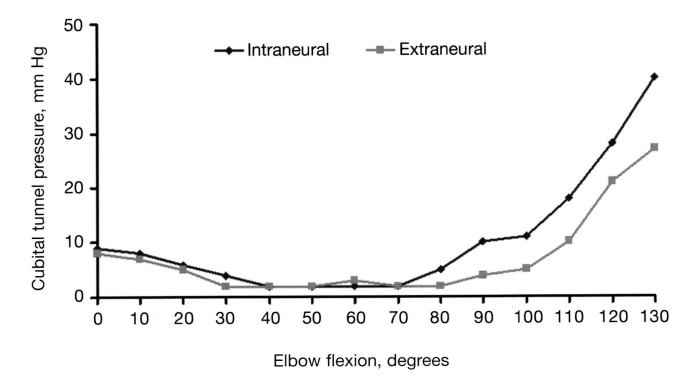

Figure 1. Relationship between degrees of elbow flexion and cubital tunnel pressures. (Modified from Gelberman RH, Yamaguchi K, Hollstein SB, Winn SS, Heidenreich FP Jr, Bindra RR, et al. Changes in interstitial pressure and cross-sectional area of the cubital tunnel and of the ulnar nerve with flexion of the elbow: an experimental study in human cadavera. J Bone Joint Surg Am. 1998 Apr;80(4):492-501. Used with permission.)

support should be well padded and the extremity carefully positioned to avoid points of increased pressure on neurovascular structures (Figure 4).

Upper Extremity Procedures and the Supine Position
Patients with limited extension of the forearm at the elbow may require forearm or hand support intraoperatively. Arms should not be abducted to more than 90° for prolonged periods to avoid stretch of the brachial plexus as it enters and passes through the axilla (Figure 3). In addition, table attachments used to hold equipment, bars, or other supports must not cause points of soft tissue compression. Several case reports and medicolegal cases have been described in which

support bars attached to the operating table have caused clinically significant radial neuropathies postoperatively (Figure 5). Finally, a segment of patients undergoing upper extremity surgery may have prolonged procedure times and benefit from meticulous attention to general body positioning. For example, patients undergoing digit reimplantation (duration >10 hours) have the potential for development of soft tissue compression injuries. In these cases, it may be advisable to periodically alter patient positions to relieve or prevent prolonged soft tissue compression. Modest changes in lower extremity positions, movement of the contralateral arm, and head rotation may help avoid soft tissue ischemia, compartment syndrome, and even alopecia.

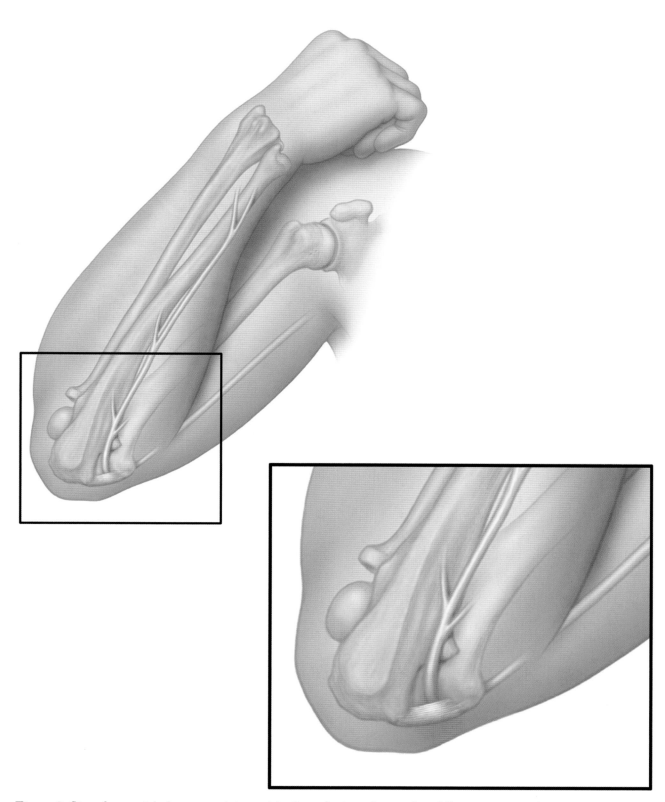

Figure 2. Site of potential ulnar nerve injury with elbow flexion of more than 90°.

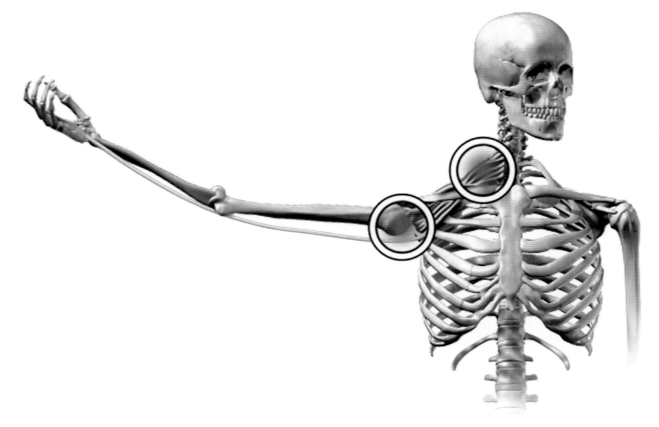

Figure 3. Sites of potential brachial plexus injury with arm abduction and head rotation.

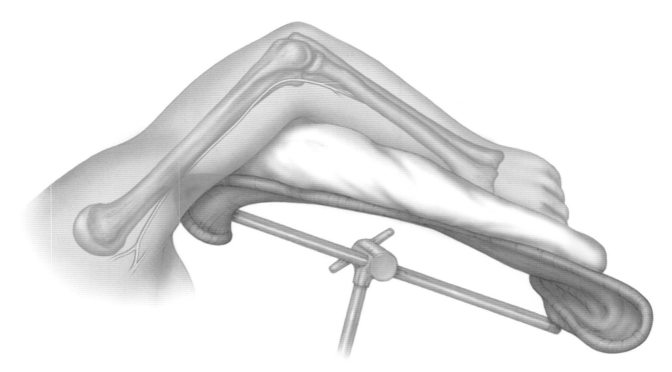

Figure 4. Site of potential nerve injury during intraoperative lateral positioning.

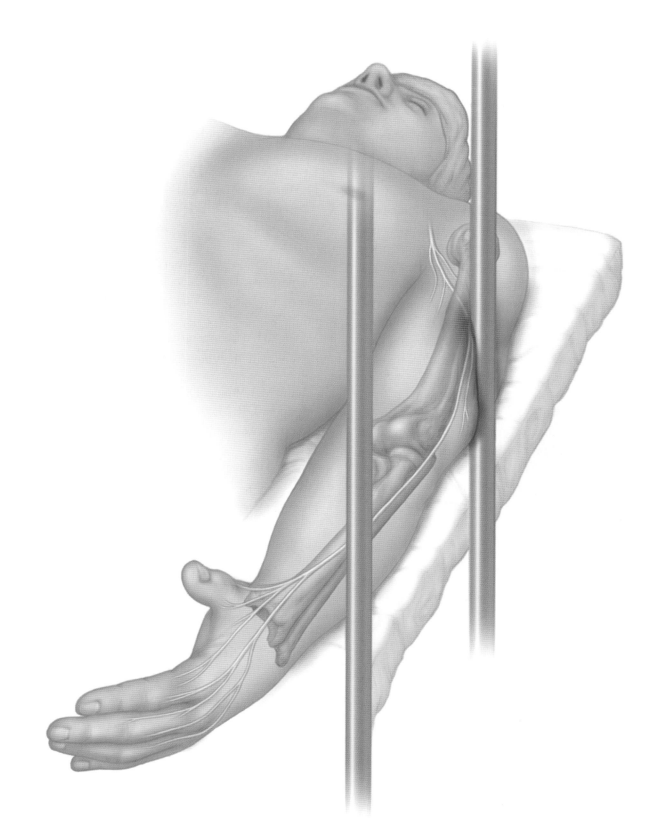

Figure 5. Site of potential radial nerve injury during supine intraoperative positioning.

Summary

The perioperative positioning of patients undergoing upper and lower extremity surgical procedures is an important component of safe patient care. Many of the issues related to patient positioning that are overlooked during the perioperative period can be easily identified during the preoperative evaluation process. A detailed preoperative assessment can provide many of the clues necessary to develop an integrated plan for the intraoperative positioning of patients with potential limitations. Patient positions that minimize the risk of perioperative nerve injury, compartment syndrome, or other soft tissue problems and have a minimal impact on patient hemodynamics and ventilation should be the primary focus of the surgical and anesthesia care teams. In general, the most valuable principle to adhere to is, "Would the planned intraoperative position be comfortably tolerated by the patient while awake?"

Suggested Reading

Practice advisory for the prevention of perioperative peripheral neuropathies: a report by the American Society of Anesthesiologists Task Force on Prevention of Perioperative Peripheral Neuropathies. Anesthesiology. 2000 Apr;92(4):1168-82.

Gelberman RH, Yamaguchi K, Hollstein SB, Winn SS, Heidenreich FP Jr, Bindra RR, et al. Changes in interstitial pressure and cross-sectional area of the cubital tunnel and of the ulnar nerve with flexion of the elbow: an experimental study in human cadavera. J Bone Joint Surg Am. 1998 Apr;80(4):492-501.

Lawson NW, Meyer DJ Jr. Lateral positions. In: Martin JT, Warner MA, editors. Positioning in anesthesia and surgery. 3rd ed. Philadelphia: WB Saunders; c1997. p. 127-52.

Milde LN. The head-elevated positions. In: Martin JT, Warner MA, editors. Positioning in anesthesia and surgery. 3rd ed. Philadelphia: WB Saunders; c1997. p. 71-94.

Warner MA. Perioperative neuropathies. Mayo Clin Proc. 1998 Jun;73(6):567-74.

Warner MA, Warner DO, Matsumoto JY, Harper CM, Schroeder DR, Maxson PM. Ulnar neuropathy in surgical patients. Anesthesiology. 1999 Jan;90(1):54-9.

Warner ME, LaMaster LM, Thoeming AK, Marienau ME, Warner MA. Compartment syndrome in surgical patients. Anesthesiology. 2001 Apr;94(4):705-8.

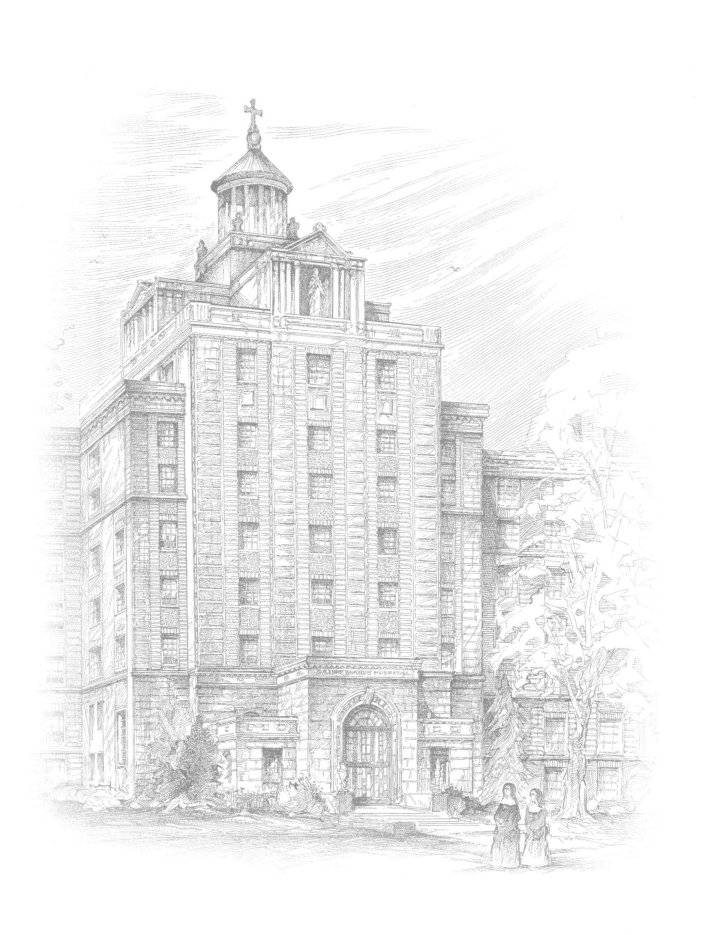

SECTION

II

Anatomy and Regional Anesthesia

CHAPTER

5

Anatomical Considerations for Peripheral Nerve Blockade

James R. Hebl, M.D.

Nomenclature for Anatomical Positioning

Regional anesthesia is the practice of applied anatomy that requires a detailed knowledge of body structures and their relationship to one another. An understanding of the nomenclature used to describe anatomical location(s) and related movement(s) is essential to effectively teach—and learn—regional anesthetic techniques. All descriptions of the human body are based on the assumption that the patient is standing in a normal anatomical position. In this position, the patient is standing upright with the head in the neutral position, arms at the sides, and palms facing forward (Figure 1).

To fully understand proper anatomical orientation, clinicians must be able to recognize the plane from which a specimen is depicted or viewed. There are four primary anatomical planes (Figures 2 and 3):

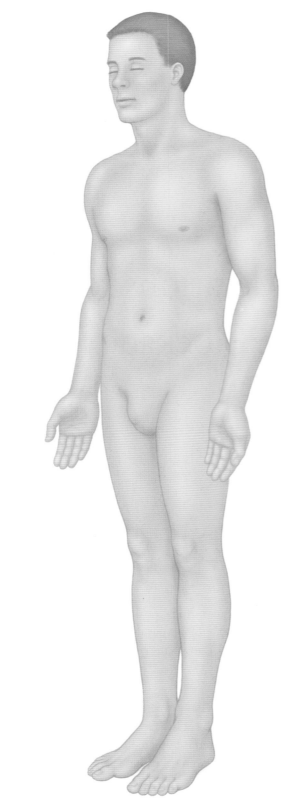

Figure 1. Normal anatomical position.

- *Median sagittal*: Vertical plane passing through the center of the body and dividing it into equal right and left halves
- *Paramedian*: Vertical plane to the right or left of midline and parallel to the median sagittal plane
- *Coronal*: Vertical plane passing through the body perpendicular to the median plane(s)
- *Transverse*: Horizontal plane perpendicular to both the median and the coronal planes

A fundamental knowledge of surface orientation and anatomical movements is essential to effectively communicate and understand the location of anatomical structures relative to one another. Nomenclature for basic surface orientations includes the following (Figures 4 and 5):

- *Anterior (ventral)*: front of the body
- *Posterior (dorsal)*: back of the body
- *Cephalad (superior, rostral)*: toward the upper end (head) of the body
- *Caudad (inferior)*: toward the lower end (feet) of the body
- *Palmar, dorsal*: used to refer to the anterior and posterior aspects of the hand
- *Plantar, dorsal*: used to refer to the sole and the top of the foot
- *Supine*: lying with the posterior surface down
- *Prone*: lying with the anterior surface down
- *Proximal*: a location or movement toward the origin of a limb (near the trunk)
- *Distal*: a location or movement away from the origin of a limb (away from the trunk)
- *Medial*: a location or movement toward the midline of the body or an extremity
- *Lateral*: a location or movement away from the midline of the body or an extremity

Nomenclature for basic body movements of the upper and lower extremity includes the following (Figures 6-11):

- *Flexion*: movement in the sagittal plane in the anterior direction; generally describes the anterior movement of a joint

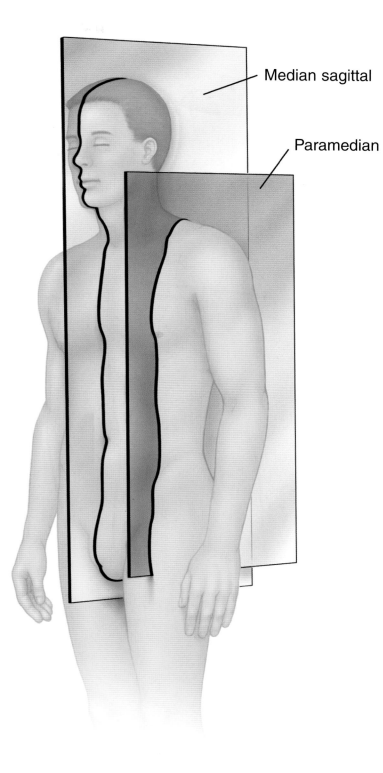

Figure 2. Median sagittal and paramedian planes.

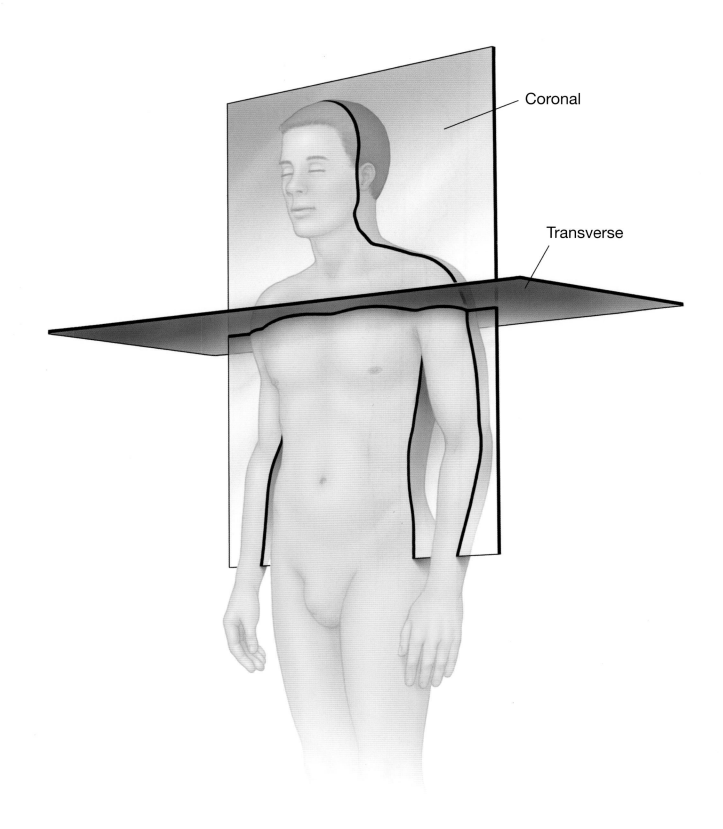

Figure 3. Coronal and transverse planes.

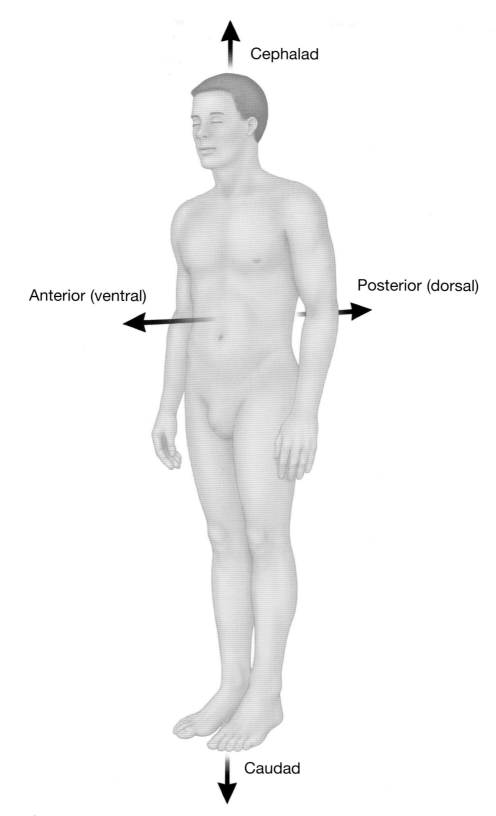

Figure 4. Basic surface orientations: cephalad, caudad, anterior, and posterior.

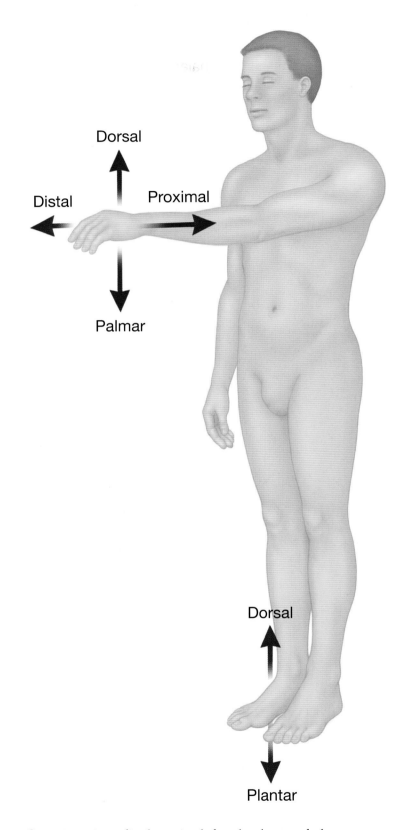

Figure 5. Basic surface orientations: distal, proximal, dorsal, palmar, and plantar.

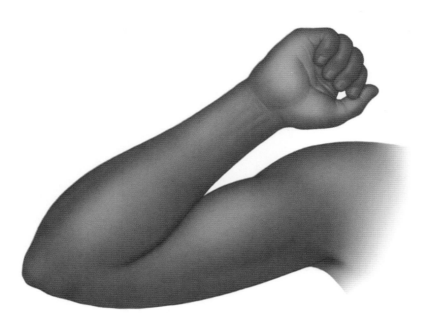

Flexion

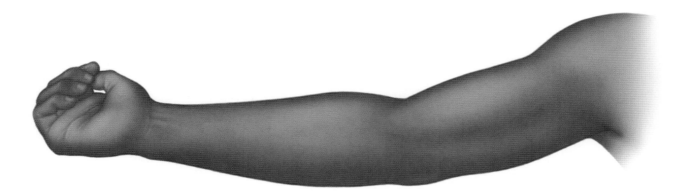

Extension

Figure 6. Upper extremity flexion and extension.

- *Extension*: movement in the sagittal plane in the posterior direction; generally describes the posterior movement of a joint
- *Abduction*: movement in the coronal plane away from the body
- *Adduction*: movement in the coronal plane toward the body

- *Rotation*: movement of the upper or lower extremity around its long axis in either a medial or a lateral direction
- *Supination*: lateral rotation of the upper extremity resulting in the palmar surface facing anteriorly
- *Pronation*: medial rotation of the upper extremity resulting in the palmar surface facing posteriorly

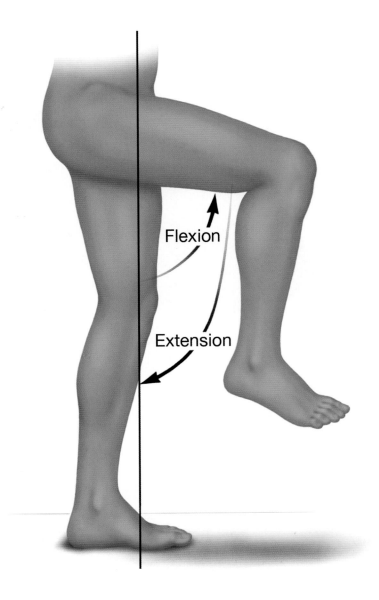

Figure 7. Lower extremity flexion and extension.

- *Eversion*: movement of the foot resulting in the plantar surface facing laterally
- *Inversion*: movement of the foot resulting in the plantar surface facing medially

Brachial Plexus Anatomy

The optimal use of regional anesthetic techniques for upper extremity surgical procedures requires a thorough knowledge of brachial plexus anatomy. Familiarity with the brachial plexus may also allow clinicians to use various regional techniques that may each provide distinct advantages to unique patient populations.

The most proximal portion of the brachial plexus is located within the posterior triangle of the neck. The anatomical borders of this triangle include the clavicle inferiorly, the trapezius muscle posteriorly, and the sternocleidomastoid muscle anteriorly. The platysma muscle, deep fascia, and skin complete the subcutaneous

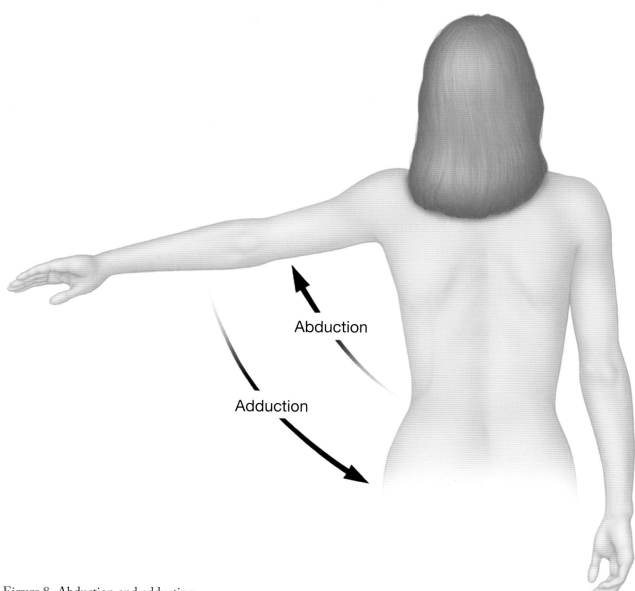

Figure 8. Abduction and adduction.

and surface anatomy of the triangle. The plexus is formed by the union of the anterior (ventral) primary rami of cervical nerves five through eight (C5-C8) and the greater part of the first thoracic nerve (T1). Variable contributions may also be made from the fourth cervical (C4) and second thoracic (T2) nerves. The ventral rami are the *roots* of the brachial plexus (Figure 12). They are nearly equal in size but are variable in their mode of junction. The rami of C5 and C6 begin to course laterally and unite near the lateral

border of the middle scalene muscle to form the *superior trunk* of the plexus. The ramus of C7 becomes the *middle trunk*, and the C8 and T1 contributions unite behind the anterior scalene muscle to form the *inferior trunk* (Figure 12). The interscalene groove is defined as the region between the anterior and middle scalene muscles at the level of the cricoid cartilage (C6). This anatomical location allows clinicians easy and reliable access to the roots and trunks of the brachial plexus for anesthetic blockade.

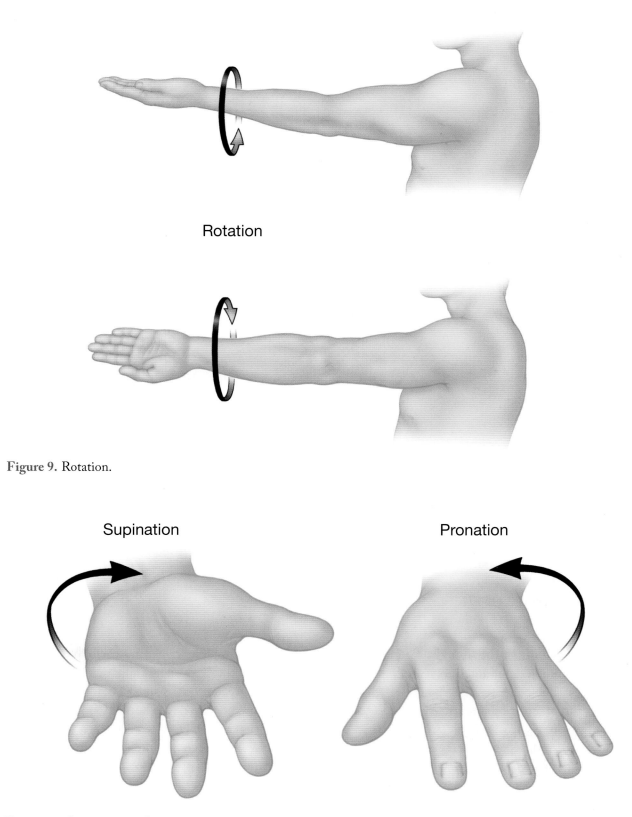

Figure 9. Rotation.

Figure 10. Supination and pronation.

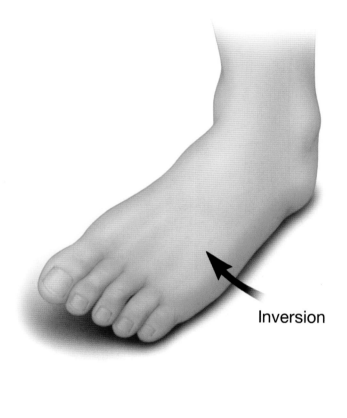

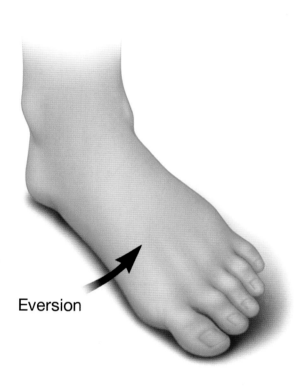

Figure 11. Inversion and eversion.

The three trunks, which lie within the lower portion of the posterior cervical triangle, continue to course laterally and inferiorly toward the first rib. At the lateral border of the first rib and just above or behind the middle third of the clavicle, the trunks undergo a primary anatomical division into *anterior* and *posterior* *divisions* (Figures 12 and 13). This division is important because the neural structures that will eventually supply the ventral (flexor) portion of the upper extremity are separated from those that will supply the dorsal (extensor) aspect. These divisions then enter the apex of the axilla and undergo yet another stage of reorganization into *cords*. The anterior divisions of the superior and middle trunks form the *lateral cord* of the plexus, the posterior divisions of all three trunks form the *posterior cord*, and the anterior division of the inferior trunk forms the *medial cord* (Figure 12). The cords are named according to their relationship to the second part of the axillary artery, which courses posterior to the pectoralis minor muscle (Figure 14).

At the lateral border of the pectoralis minor muscle, the three cords divide and give rise to the *terminal branches* of the plexus. Each cord possesses two major terminal branches and a variable number of minor intermediary branches (Figure 12). The cutaneous innervation of each

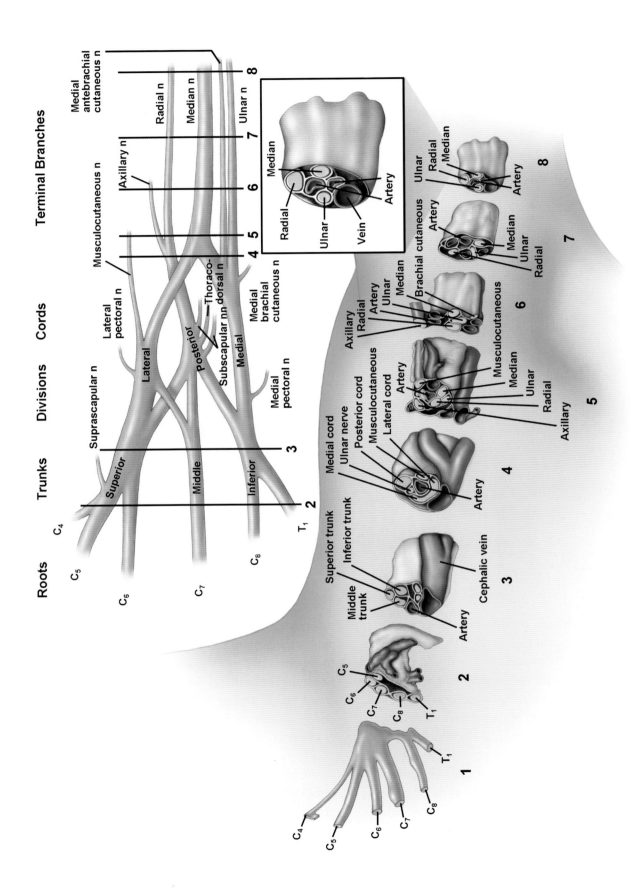

Figure 12. Brachial plexus anatomy.

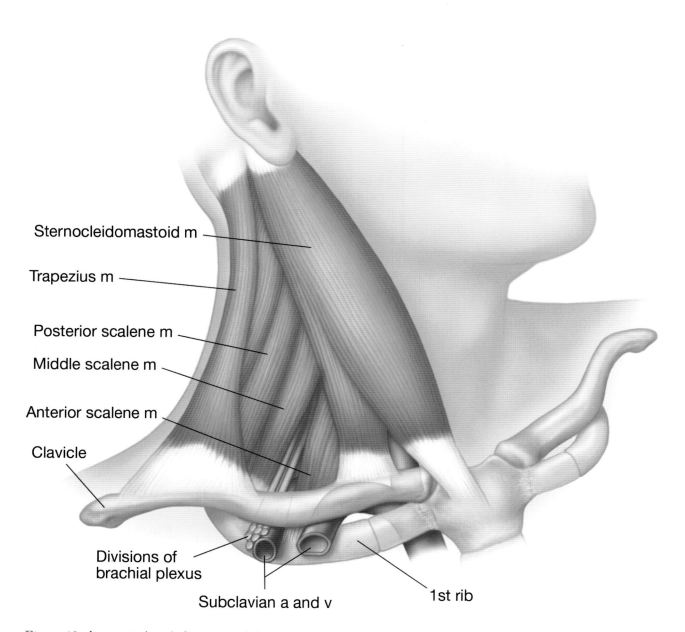

Sternocleidomastoid m

Trapezius m

Posterior scalene m

Middle scalene m

Anterior scalene m

Clavicle

Divisions of
brachial plexus

Subclavian a and v

1st rib

Figure 13. Anatomical neck dissection of the posterior cervical triangle.

major and minor branch is illustrated in Figure 15. The lateral cord has three branches:

- *Musculocutaneous nerve* (C4, C5, C6, and C7): major terminal branch that enters the coracobrachialis muscle, supplies the biceps musculature, and terminates as the lateral antebrachial cutaneous nerve of the forearm

- Lateral root of the *median nerve* (C5, C6, and C7): major terminal branch
- *Lateral pectoral nerve* (C5, C6, and C7): minor intermediary branch that pierces the clavipectoral fascia and supplies the pectoralis major muscle.

The posterior cord has five branches that generally supply the dorsal aspect of the upper extremity:

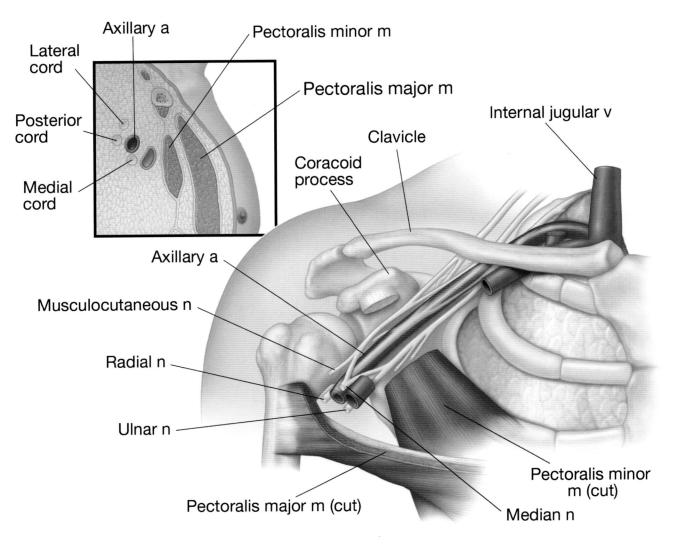

Figure 14. Infraclavicular neurovascular anatomy with cross-sectional view.

- *Axillary nerve* (C5 and C6): major terminal branch that innervates the deltoid and teres minor muscle groups and terminates by supplying the skin over the deltoid region of the shoulder and upper aspect of the arm
- *Radial nerve* (C5, C6, C7, C8, and T1): major terminal branch
- *Upper subscapular nerve* (C5 and C6): minor intermediary branch that supplies the subscapularis muscle
- *Thoracodorsal nerve* (C6, C7, and C8): minor intermediary branch that runs downward and laterally through the axillary fat to supply the latissimus dorsi muscle group

- *Lower subscapular nerve* (C5 and C6): minor intermediary branch that supplies the teres major muscle

Finally, the medial cord of the brachial plexus has five branches:

- *Ulnar nerve* (C7, C8, and T1): major terminal branch
- Medial root of the *median nerve* (C8 and T1): major terminal branch
- *Medial antebrachial cutaneous nerve* of the forearm (C8 and T1): major intermediary branch supplying the medial aspect of the forearm

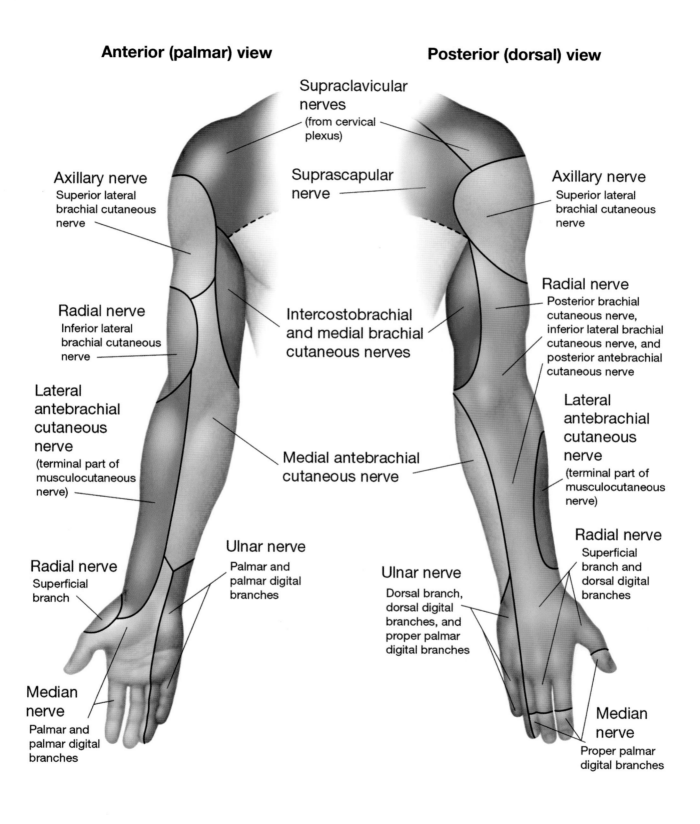

Figure 15. Upper extremity cutaneous innervation.

- *Medial cutaneous nerve* of the arm (C8 and T1): minor intermediary branch that supplies the medial aspect of the upper arm and a portion of the forearm. Within the axilla, it is joined by the *intercostobrachial nerve* (T2), which supplies the skin over the medial aspect of the arm and the floor of the axilla
- *Medial pectoral nerve* (C8 and T1): minor intermediary branch that passes through the pectoralis minor muscle into the pectoralis major, supplying both muscle groups

In addition to the brachial plexus itself, several vascular structures have profound clinical importance. Many of these vessels require avoidance, but others may be used as anatomical landmarks and intentionally punctured while performing regional techniques. The vertebral artery originates from the brachiocephalic and subclavian arteries on the right and left sides, respectively. It travels cephalad to enter a bony canal formed by the transverse processes at the level of C6 (Figure 16).

The phrenic nerve, which is derived from the C3 through C5 nerve roots, runs parallel to the vertebral artery at this location as it passes through the neck on the ventral surface of the anterior scalene muscle (Figure 16). As the cervical roots of the brachial plexus leave the transverse processes, they course immediately posterior to the vertebral artery. Thus, needle-tip location is of paramount importance when performing interscalene blockade to avoid potential intravascular injection. Additional vascular anatomical landmarks during interscalene blockade include the external jugular vein, which often overlies the interscalene groove at the level of C6. However, this should not be used as a reliable or consistent anatomical marker because of potential variability among individuals.

The subclavian artery enters the posterior cervical triangle of the neck and unites with the brachial plexus at the lateral border of the anterior scalene muscle. It courses behind the clavicle and comes into direct contact with the first rib posterior to the anterior scalene muscle and inferior to the inferior trunk of the plexus.

At this point, the divisions of the brachial plexus begin to develop and lie posterior and cephalad to the subclavian artery (Figure 16). In an emergency, or after inadvertent arterial puncture, the subclavian artery can be compressed against the first rib to control any bleeding that may occur.

At the lateral border of the first rib, the subclavian artery becomes the axillary artery, a critical anatomical landmark for axillary brachial plexus blockade. At the lateral border of the pectoralis minor muscle, the axillary artery is surrounded on three sides (lateral, posterior, and medial) by the corresponding named cords of the brachial plexus (Figure 14). As it enters the axilla, it assumes its characteristic location in relation to the terminal branches of the plexus: anterior to the radial nerve, posteromedial to the median nerve, and anterolateral to the ulnar nerve (Figure 12, inset). Once the axillary artery passes the inferior border of the teres major muscle, it becomes the brachial artery.

Normal Anatomical Variants

Anatomical variations within the plexus are extremely common and may be considered the rule rather than the exception. A common variant involves the contribution and distribution of the cervical nerve roots to the brachial plexus. As described above, the plexus is most often derived from the C5 through C8 and T1 nerve roots. However, variable contributions from the C4 and T2 nerve roots may also occur. In an anatomical study of 156 brachial plexuses, Kerr found that 62% had contributions from either C3 or C4. With this anatomy, contributions from T2 are generally absent and the branch from T1 is reduced. This is termed a *prefixed plexus*. Alternatively, a *postfixed plexus* is one in which the contribution from C5 is reduced or absent, whereas those of T1 and T2 become more dominant. McCann and Bindelglass reported that up to 60% of plexuses may be postfixed.

Bony abnormalities that greatly affect the plexus may also occur. Alterations in the bony anatomy within the lower part of the neck and thoracic inlet such as cervical

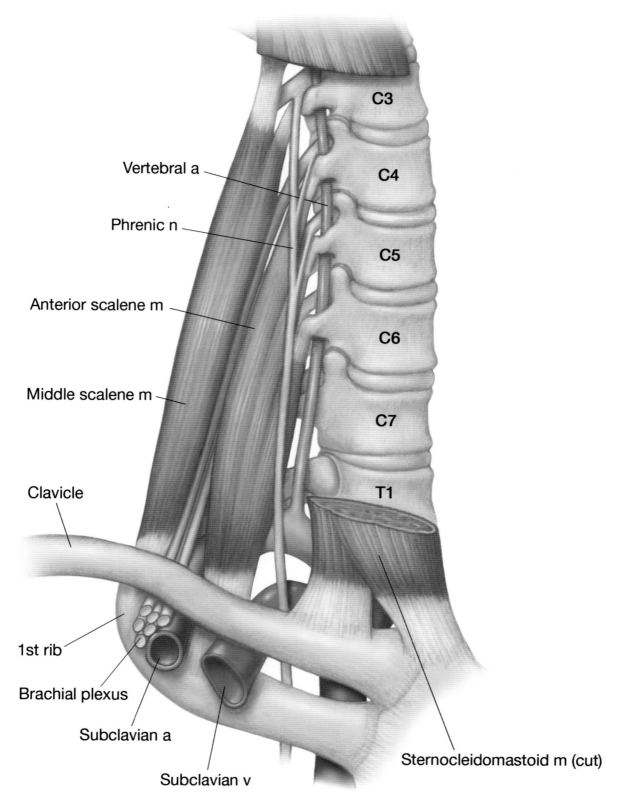

Figure 16. Neurovascular anatomy of the neck.

ribs and lesions of the first rib or clavicle may impinge on neural structures and cause neurologic symptoms. Cervical ribs occur in approximately 1% of the population, and only 10% become symptomatic. They are twice as common in females and occur unilaterally in 50% to 80% of cases. The ribs vary in length and may be connected to the first rib by a fibrous band. Reede showed that the brachial plexus may be affected by cervical ribs in two ways: 1) they may narrow the space between the posterior aspect of the first rib and anterior scalene muscle through which the neural structures and subclavian artery must pass or 2) they may be situated in such a manner that the neurovascular complex must pass over a bony ridge. In the latter case, the lower trunk of the plexus may rest firmly against the cervical rib, causing symptoms.

Additional causes of thoracic outlet syndrome may include the presence of a scalene minimus, or a variation in the relationship between the scalene muscles and neurovascular structures of the posterior triangle. The scalene minimus is an accessory muscle segment that is often derived from the anterior scalene muscle. It arises from the transverse process of C7 and inserts into the medial border of the first rib posterior to the subclavian artery and anterior to the inferior trunk of the plexus. Its size may range from a few fibers that strengthen the suprapleural membrane to a well-developed muscle body. In an anatomical dissection of 51 cadavers, Harry and colleagues found that the scalene minimus was present in 46%. Interestingly, the classically described anatomical relationship between the brachial plexus and scalene muscles was present in only 32% of cadavers bilaterally.

Axillary Sheath

The axillary sheath is a collection of connective tissue surrounding the neurovascular structures of the brachial plexus. It is a continuation of the prevertebral fascia separating the anterior and middle scalene muscles. Original descriptions of the sheath considered it to be a dense tubular structure extending from above the first rib to a point distal to the axilla where it fuses with the anterior surface of the medial intermuscular septum. It was believed that the axillary artery and vein and the median, ulnar,

and radial nerves were all lying loose within its center. The clinical implication was that conduction anesthesia of the upper extremity could be performed with a single injection at any site along the sheath, with local anesthetic *volume* being the primary determinant for successful blockade.

However, several investigators challenged the concept of a tubular axillary sheath. Thompson and Rorie and Partridge and colleagues proposed that the sheath is a multicompartmental structure, formed by thin layers of fibrous tissue surrounding the plexus and extending inward to create discrete fascial septae. As a result, individual fascial compartments are created for each nerve, which defined the anatomical limits for that neural structure (Figure 12, inset). They argued that these compartments may functionally limit the circumferential spread of injected solutions, thus requiring separate injections into each compartment for maximal blockade. However, proximal connections between compartments have been identified, which may account for the success of single-injection techniques. Therefore, although the compartmentalized description of the axillary sheath is generally well accepted, its clinical significance remains to be seen.

Nonbrachial Plexus Anatomy

The supraclavicular nerves of the cervical plexus are also of clinical importance for upper extremity and shoulder surgery. They are derived from the ventral rami of C3 and C4, which unite to form a common trunk that emerges from the midpoint of the sternocleidomastoid muscle at its posterior border (Figure 17). The supraclavicular nerve trunk descends posterior to the platysma and deep cervical fascia, where it divides into medial, intermediate, and lateral (posterior) branches. The three branches pierce the deep fascia just cephalad to the clavicle.

The *medial supraclavicular nerve* courses inferomedially across the external jugular vein and the clavicular and sternal heads of the sternocleidomastoid muscle to supply the skin as far as the midline and as low as the second rib. The *intermediate supraclavicular nerve*

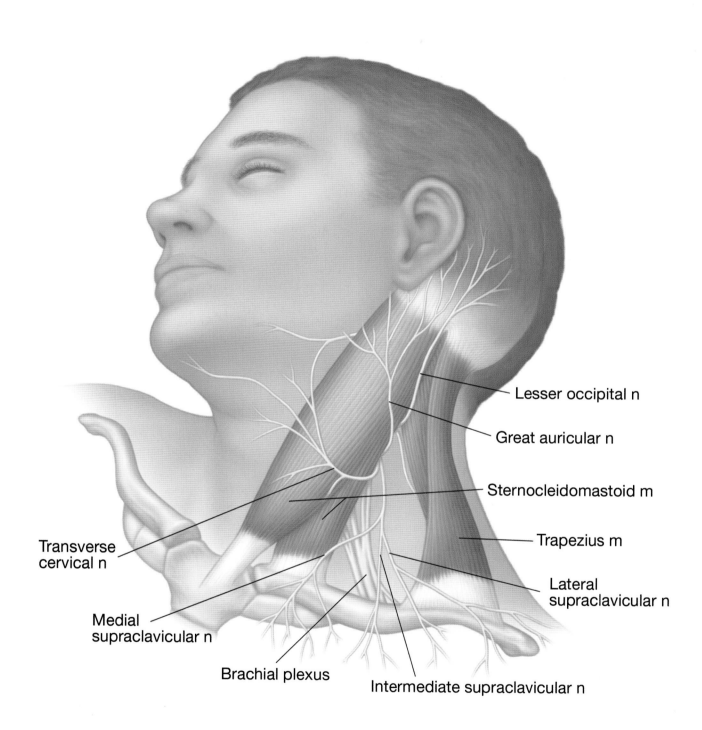

Figure 17. Superficial cervical plexus.

crosses the clavicle to supply the skin over the pectoralis major and deltoid muscles down to the level of the second rib, adjacent to the region supplied by the axillary and intercostobrachial nerves (Figure 15). Finally, the *lateral (posterior) supraclavicular nerve* descends superficially across the trapezius muscle and acromion to supply the skin of the upper and posterior aspects of the shoulder (Figure 15).

The *suprascapular nerve* may also innervate a portion of the upper extremity and shoulder. It is derived from the C5 and C6 nerve roots and originates from the superior trunk of the brachial plexus (Figure 12). It runs laterally deep to the trapezius and omohyoid muscles before entering the supraspinous fossa through the scapular notch. From here it passes laterally to the border of the scapular spine to reach the infraspinous fossa, where it branches to supply the supraspinatus (arm abduction) and infraspinatus (lateral rotation and partial abduction and adduction of the arm) musculature. The suprascapular nerve may also send sensory fibers to supply the shoulder and acromioclavicular joints and cutaneous innervation to the proximal third of the arm within the territory of the axillary nerve in approximately 10% of individuals (Figure 15).

Finally, the *intercostobrachial nerve* (i.e., ICB) is the remaining neural structure independent of the brachial plexus that has major clinical importance within the upper extremity. It is the lateral cutaneous branch of the second intercostal nerve, originating from the ventral rami of T2. It travels laterally, posterior to the pectoralis minor muscle, and enters the axilla anterior to the latissimus dorsi muscle. It continues through the axilla to the medial aspect of the arm, where it is joined by the medial cutaneous nerve. The two nerves pierce the deep fascia and supply the skin of the upper half of the posterior and medial aspects of the arm (Figure 15). The size and contribution from the intercostobrachial nerve are inversely proportional to the size and contribution from the medial cutaneous nerve. Of note, cutaneous innervation may be redundant within this region with a second intercostobrachial nerve that separates off from the lateral cutaneous branch of the ventral rami of T3.

This secondary intercostobrachial nerve also supplies the medial aspect of the upper arm and the floor of the axilla.

Lumbar Plexus Anatomy

The optimal use of regional anesthetic techniques for lower extremity surgical procedures requires a thorough knowledge of both lumbar and lumbosacral plexus anatomy. Familiarity with these two major nerve plexuses allows clinicians to use various regional techniques that provide distinct advantages to unique patient populations.

The lumbar plexus is derived from the anterior (ventral) primary rami of lumbar nerves one through four (L1-L4) with variable contributions from the 12th thoracic (T12) and 5th lumbar (L5) nerves (Figure 18). The ventral rami of these nerves converge to form the plexus anterior to the transverse processes of the lumbar vertebrae deep within the psoas major muscle or between the psoas major and quadratus lumborum muscles (Figure 19). The cephalad portion of the lumbar plexus (i.e., T12-L1) immediately divides into superior and inferior branches. The superior branch subsequently divides into the iliohypogastric and ilioinguinal nerves, and the inferior branch merges with a small branch from L2 to form the genitofemoral nerve (Figure 18).

The *iliohypogastric nerve* arises from the ventral rami of L1 and travels anterior to the quadratus lumborum muscle before penetrating the transversus abdominis muscle near the crest of the ilium. The nerve continues to course along the abdominal wall before terminating at the level of the pubic symphysis. The iliohypogastric nerve provides motor innervation to the abdominal musculature and ends in an anterior cutaneous branch to the skin of the suprapubic region and a lateral cutaneous branch to an area immediately adjacent to the iliac crest.

The *ilioinguinal nerve* arises from the ventral rami of L1 and travels anterior to the quadratus lumborum muscle and slightly inferior to the iliohypogastric nerve. Similar to the iliohypogastric nerve, the ilioinguinal nerve penetrates the transversus abdominis muscle near the crest of the ilium before piercing the posterior wall of the inguinal canal and

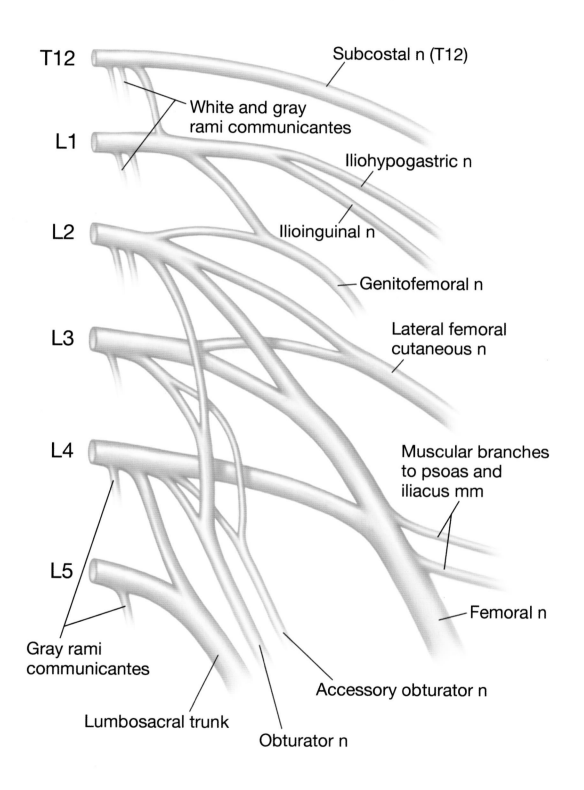

Figure 18. Lumbar plexus anatomy.

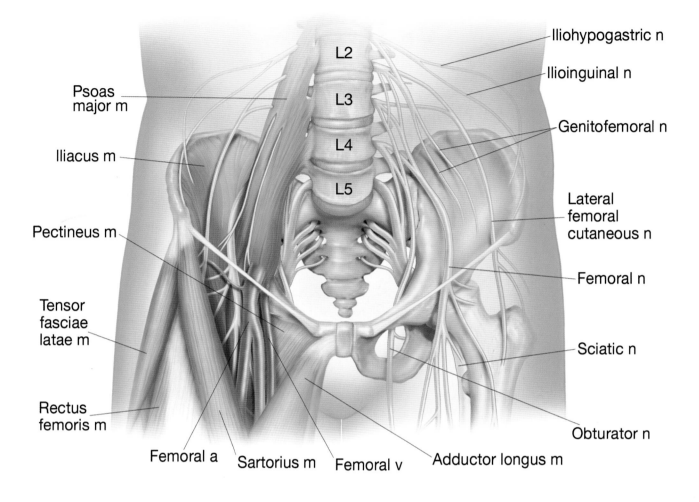

Figure 19. Anatomical location of the lumbar plexus in situ.

passing through the superficial inguinal ring. In males, the nerve terminates as cutaneous branches that supply the upper and medial aspect of the thigh, the root of the penis, and the anterior scrotum. In females, its cutaneous branches innervate the mons pubis and labia majora.

The *genitofemoral nerve* arises from the ventral rami of L1 and L2 and travels inferolaterally through the psoas major muscle where it divides into genital and femoral branches. The genital branch enters the inguinal canal through the deep inguinal ring before supplying the cremaster muscle and associated fascia.

It also provides cutaneous innervation to the skin and fascia of the scrotum, labia majora, and adjacent areas of the medial aspect of the thigh (Figure 20). The femoral branch continues under the inguinal ligament and pierces the anterior wall of the canal, where it innervates the skin over the femoral triangle lateral to that supplied by the genital branch and ilioinguinal nerve (Figure 20).

The caudad portion of the lumbar plexus (L2-L4) forms three major nerves of the lower extremity—the lateral femoral cutaneous, femoral, and obturator nerves

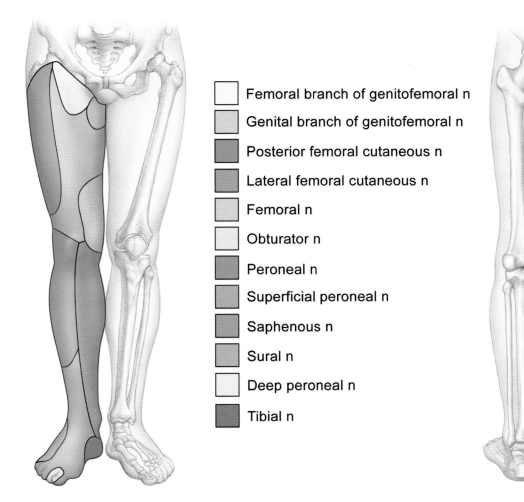

Femoral branch of genitofemoral n

Genital branch of genitofemoral n

Posterior femoral cutaneous n

Lateral femoral cutaneous n

Femoral n

Obturator n

Peroneal n

Superficial peroneal n

Saphenous n

Sural n

Deep peroneal n

Tibial n

Figure 20. Lower extremity cutaneous innervation.

(Figure 18). These major nerves exit the pelvis anteriorly and provide the primary innervation to the ventral aspect of the lower extremity.

The *lateral femoral cutaneous nerve* arises from the posterior divisions of the ventral rami of L2 and L3 (Figure 18). It courses along the posterior abdominal wall until it crosses the iliac crest into the pelvis, where it descends anterior to the iliacus muscle (Figure 19). The nerve passes under the lateral segment of the inguinal ligament—medial to the anterior superior iliac spine—before providing cutaneous innervation

to the proximal two-thirds of the lateral aspect of the thigh (Figures 20 and 21). The lateral femoral cutaneous nerve may also provide variable cutaneous innervation to the lateral aspect of the buttock distal to the greater trochanter.

The *obturator nerve* arises from the anterior division of the ventral rami of L2 to L4 (Figure 18). It descends toward the pelvis along the posteromedial border of the psoas major muscle, passes under the iliac vessels at the level of L5, and crosses inferior to the superior pubic ramus (Figure 19). The nerve accompanies the

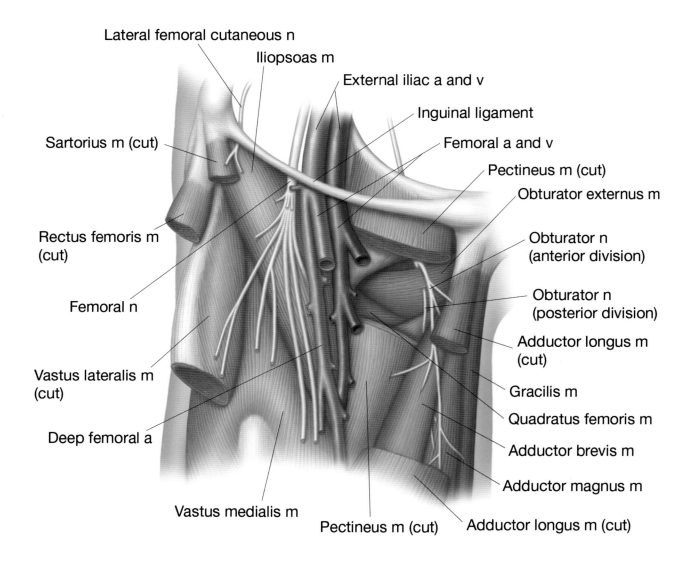

Figure 21. Neurovascular anatomy of the femoral region.

obturator artery and vein through the obturator canal and into the medial compartment of the thigh, where it branches into an anterior division and a posterior division. The *anterior division* of the obturator nerve courses deep to the pectineus and adductor longus muscles and anterior to the adductor brevis and obturator externus muscles before terminating within the gracilis muscle (Figure 21). The anterior division provides innervation to the superficial adductor muscles of the leg (i.e., adductor brevis, adductor longus, pectineus, and gracilis muscles), articular branches to the anteromedial hip capsule, and cutaneous branches to the skin overlying the posteromedial aspect of the thigh (Figure 20). However, cutaneous innervation has been shown to be extremely variable from one individual to another. The *posterior division* of the obturator nerve travels posterior to the adductor brevis muscle and anterior to the adductor magnus muscle (Figure 21). The posterior division provides innervation to the deep adductor muscles of the leg (i.e., obturator externus, adductor magnus, and adductor brevis muscles) and articular branches to the posterior knee joint. The posterior division of the obturator nerve has no cutaneous innervation.

The *femoral nerve* is the largest branch of the lumbar plexus and arises from the posterior division of the ventral rami of L2 to L4 (Figure 18). It descends through the pelvis along the lateral border of the psoas major muscle within the groove between the psoas and iliacus muscles. The nerve passes under the inguinal ligament—deep to the fascia iliaca—and enters the femoral triangle, where it lies lateral to the femoral artery and vein (Figure 21). Within the femoral triangle, the nerve divides into several major and minor muscular and cutaneous branches that innervate the anterior compartment of the leg. The two major branches of the femoral nerve are the anterior (superficial) and posterior (deep) divisions. The *anterior division* of the femoral nerve provides motor innervation to the sartorius and pectineus muscles and cutaneous innervation to the anterior and medial thigh (i.e., middle and medial cutaneous nerves) (Figure 20). The *posterior division* of the femoral nerve provides motor

innervation to the rectus femoris, vastus lateralis, vastus medialis, and vastus intermedius muscles and articular branches to the hip and knee joints. The saphenous nerve of the lower extremity is also derived from the posterior division. The *saphenous branch* of the femoral nerve follows the posterior surface of the sartorius muscle to its attachment on the tibia. At this location, the saphenous nerve divides into infrapatellar and distal cutaneous branches (Figure 22) that supply the medial aspect of the leg from the knee to the medial malleolus (Figures 20 and 23).

Lumbosacral Plexus Anatomy

The lumbosacral plexus is derived from the anterior (ventral) primary rami of the fourth lumbar nerve through the fourth sacral nerve (L4-S4) (Figure 24). It provides the primary sensory and motor innervation to the dorsal aspect of the upper leg and the majority of sensorimotor innervation below the knee. The posterior femoral cutaneous nerve and the sciatic nerve are two of the most relevant neural structures for lower extremity peripheral nerve blockade.

The *posterior femoral cutaneous nerve* is derived from the anterior and posterior divisions of the ventral rami of S1 to S3 (Figure 24). The nerve courses inferolaterally and exits the pelvis with the sciatic nerve through the greater sciatic foramen (Figure 25). It enters the gluteal region inferior to the piriformis muscle and descends posterior to the superior gemellus, inferior gemellus, obturator internus, and quadratus femoris muscles. The posterior femoral cutaneous nerve provides sensory innervation to the posterior thigh from the inferior gluteal region to the popliteal fossa (Figure 20). Perineal branches of the posterior femoral cutaneous nerve emerge at the level of the ischial tuberosity and course posterior to the biceps femoris and semitendinosus muscles (Figure 25).

The *sciatic nerve* is formed from the convergence of two major nerve trunks—the tibial and common peroneal nerves. The *tibial nerve* arises from the anterior divisions of the ventral rami of L4 to S3 (Figure 24).

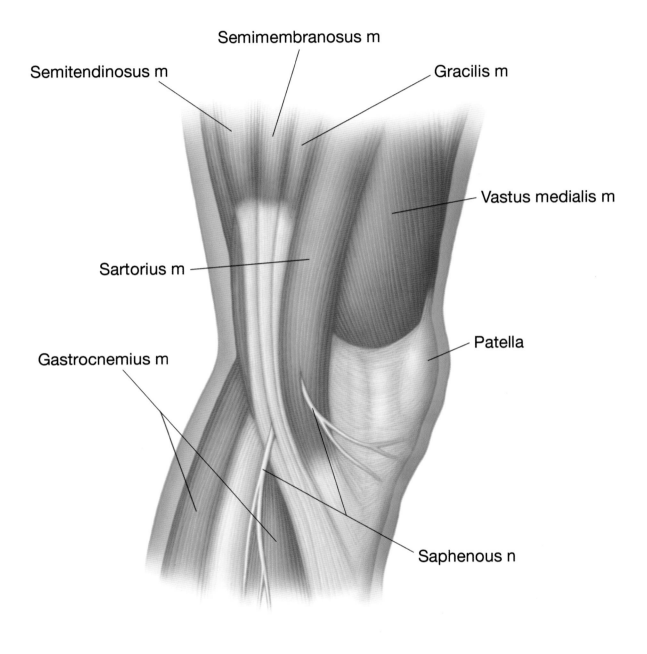

Figure 22. Saphenous neuroanatomy.

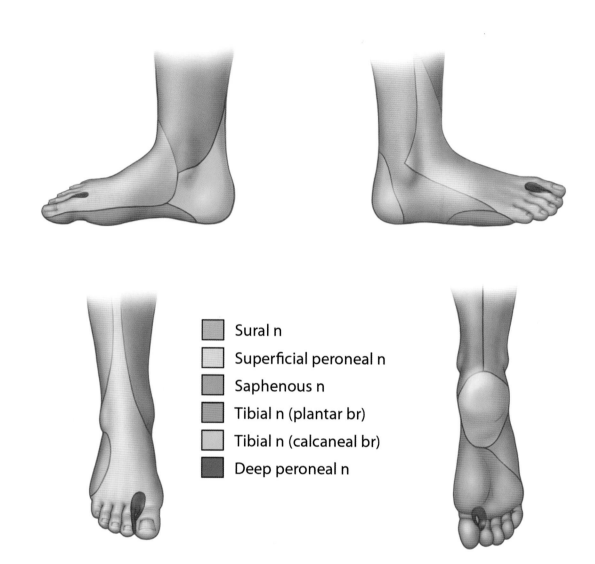

Figure 23. Cutaneous innervation of the foot and ankle.

Sural n

Superficial peroneal n

Saphenous n

Tibial n (plantar br)

Tibial n (calcaneal br)

Deep peroneal n

The *common peroneal nerve* is derived from the posterior divisions of the ventral rami of L4 to S2 (Figure 24). The sciatic nerve courses inferolaterally and exits the pelvis with the posterior femoral cutaneous nerve through the greater sciatic foramen (Figure 25). It enters the gluteal region inferior to the piriformis muscle and descends posterior to the superior gemellus, inferior gemellus, obturator internus, and quadratus femoris muscles lateral to the ischial tuberosity. The sciatic nerve enters the posterior thigh at the inferior border of the gluteus maximus muscle posterior to the adductor magnus muscle and anterior to the long head of the biceps femoris muscle. It descends to the popliteal fossa within the groove between the semimembranosus and semitendinosus muscles medially and the long head of the biceps femoris muscle laterally. En route to the popliteal fossa, the tibial component of the sciatic nerve provides motor innervation to the adductor magnus, biceps femoris (long head), semitendinosus, and semimembranosus muscles.

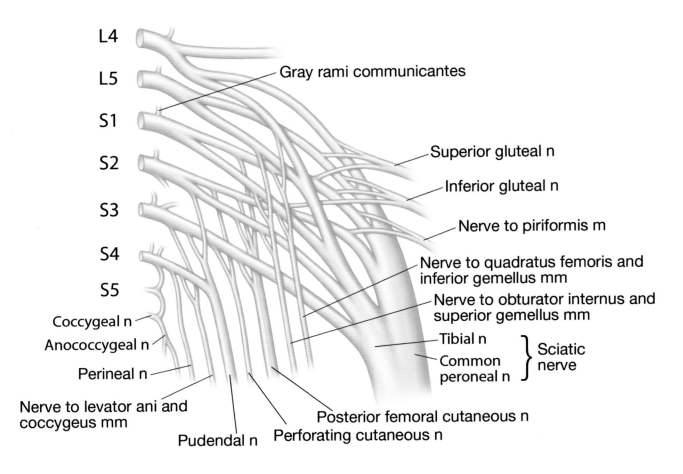

L4

L5

S1

S2

S3

S4

S5

Coccygeal n

Anococcygeal n

Perineal n

Nerve to levator ani and
coccygeus mm

Pudendal n

Gray rami communicantes

Superior gluteal n

Inferior gluteal n

Nerve to piriformis m

Nerve to quadratus femoris and
inferior gemellus mm

Nerve to obturator internus and
superior gemellus mm

Tibial n

Common
peroneal n

} Sciatic
nerve

Posterior femoral cutaneous n

Perforating cutaneous n

Figure 24. Lumbosacral plexus anatomy.

Within the popliteal fossa, the tibial and peroneal components of the sciatic nerve diverge into the tibial and common peroneal nerves. The popliteal artery and vein are located medial and deep to both the tibial and the common peroneal nerves (Figures 26 and 27). The *tibial nerve* exits the popliteal fossa and courses deep (i.e., anterior) to the soleus muscle, where it descends within the posterior compartment of the leg with the posterior tibial artery. The nerve and artery travel within the groove between the tibialis posterior and flexor digitorum longus muscles before passing posterior to the medial malleolus (Figure 28). At the level of the medial malleolus, the tibial nerve separates into the medial plantar, lateral plantar, and medial calcaneal nerves, which provide sensorimotor innervation to the plantar aspect of the foot (Figure 23). The *medial sural*

cutaneous nerve is a proximal branch of the tibial nerve that provides cutaneous innervation to the posterolateral aspect of the distal leg. It branches from the tibial nerve within the popliteal fossa and descends through the superficial compartment of the leg between the two heads of the gastrocnemius muscle. The medial sural cutaneous nerve becomes the *sural nerve* at the level of the mid-calf after receiving crossover innervation from the lateral sural cutaneous nerve (see below). The sural nerve descends the leg along the lateral border of the Achilles tendon and passes posterior to the lateral malleolus. At the level of the lateral malleolus, the sural nerve branches into the lateral calcaneal and lateral dorsal cutaneous nerves, which provide sensory innervation to the lateral aspect of the foot and ankle (Figure 23).

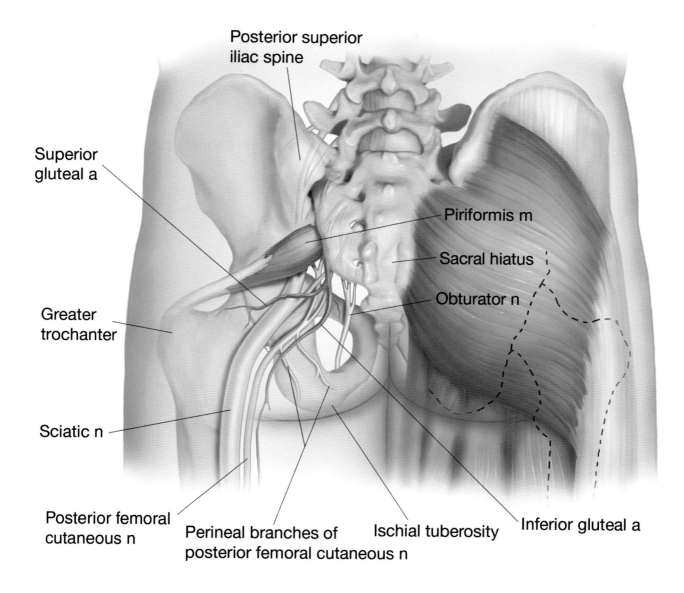

Figure 25. Sciatic neuroanatomy.

The *common peroneal nerve* courses inferolaterally along the border of the biceps femoris muscle and its tendon insertion onto the head of the fibula. At the inferior neck of the fibula, the common peroneal nerve divides into its deep and superficial components. The *deep peroneal nerve* travels within the anterior compartment of the leg with the anterior tibial artery between the tibialis anterior and extensor digitorum longus muscles. It crosses the ankle immediately lateral to the extensor hallucis longus tendon and medial to the extensor digitorum longus tendon (Figure 29). The deep peroneal nerve provides motor innervation to the tibialis anterior, extensor digitorum longus and brevis, and extensor hallucis longus and brevis muscles. It provides sensory innervation to the deep dorsal structures of the foot and the web space between the first and second toes (Figure 23). The *superficial peroneal nerve* travels within the lateral compartment of the leg between the peroneus longus and extensor digitorum

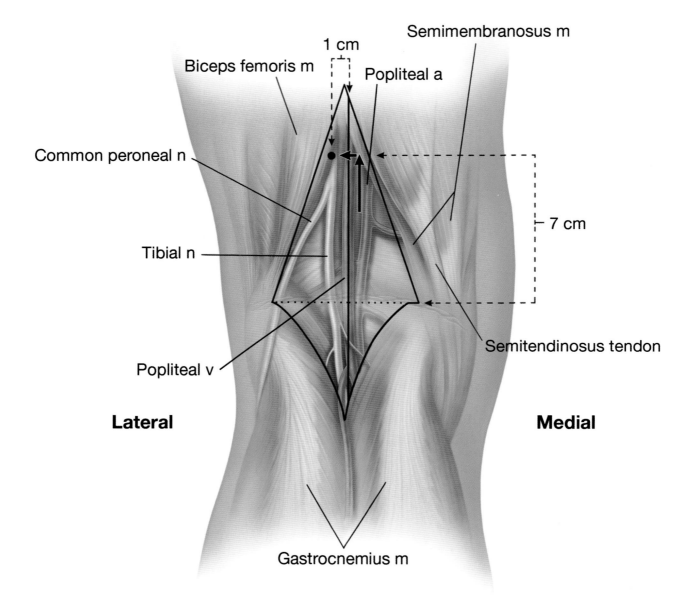

Figure 26. Neurovascular anatomy of the popliteal fossa.

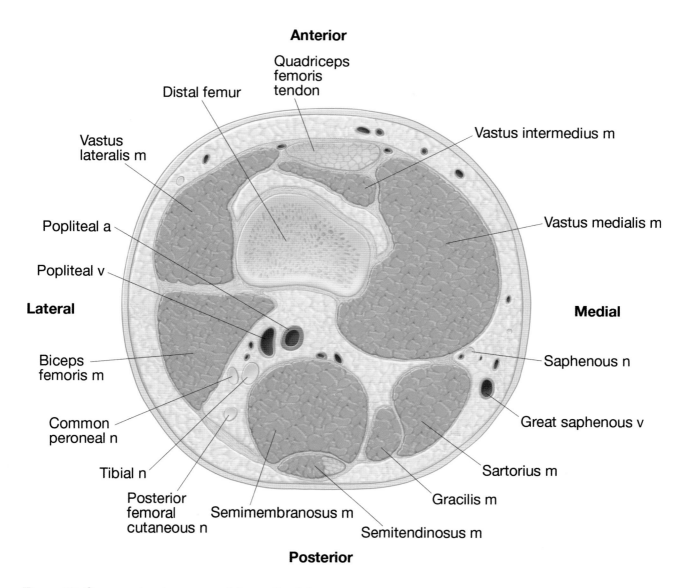

Figure 27. Cross-sectional anatomy of the popliteal fossa.

longus muscles and terminates in the foot anterior (i.e., superficial) and medial to the lateral malleolus (Figures 28 and 29). It provides motor innervation to the peroneus longus and brevis muscles and sensory innervation to the dorsal aspect of the foot (Figure 23). Finally, the *lateral sural cutaneous nerve* is a branch of the common peroneal nerve that originates in the popliteal fossa and travels within the lateral compartment of the leg. The lateral sural cutaneous nerve provides sensory innervation to the lateral knee and the anterolateral aspect of the proximal leg (Figure 20).

Peripheral Nerve Anatomy

The peripheral nervous system makes up less than 0.1% of all nerve tissue. The somatic peripheral nervous system, when defined anatomically by the presence of Schwann cells, includes the primary nerve roots, dorsal root ganglions, mixed spinal nerves, plexuses, nerve trunks, and the autonomic nervous system. Each peripheral nerve is composed of individual myelinated nerve fibers embedded within an endoneurial connective tissue layer and grouped into discrete bundles termed *fascicles*.

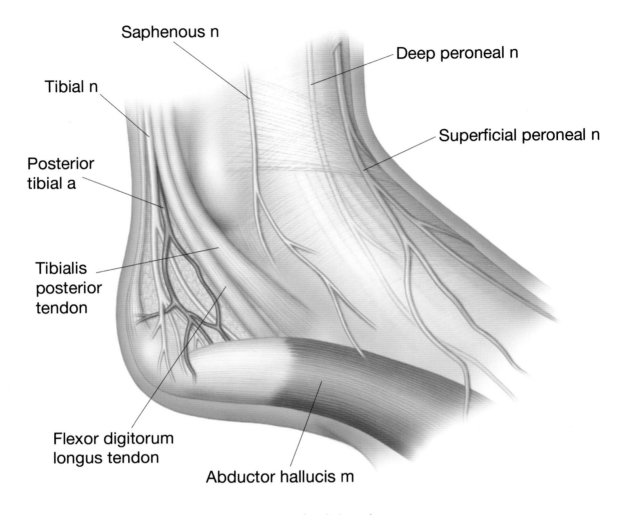

Figure 28. Neurovascular anatomy of the foot and ankle (medial view).

Each fascicle is surrounded by a perineurial membrane that regulates the microenvironment, or homeostatic milieu, of the myelinated nerve fibers. Nerve fascicles are surrounded by a connective tissue environment (i.e., perineural space) and encased by the outer epineurial membrane of the peripheral nerve (Figure 30).

The peripheral nervous system consists of both sensory and motor components. The cell bodies of sensory nerves are located within the dorsal root ganglion and those for motor nerves are located within the anterior horn of the spinal cord. Normal function of myelinated nerve fibers depends on the integrity of *both* the axon and its myelin sheath. Nerve action potentials "jump"

from one node of Ranvier to the next—propagating neural signal transmission. This rapid saltatory conduction depends on the insulating properties of the myelin sheath for proper and efficient functioning.

Sensory and Motor Innervation

The sensory and motor innervation of the upper and lower extremities may have profound clinical importance to practitioners using regional anesthetic techniques. A generalized understanding of the functional anatomy is necessary for several reasons: 1) to determine which cutaneous nerve distributions within a surgical field require conduction blockade, 2) to recognize which

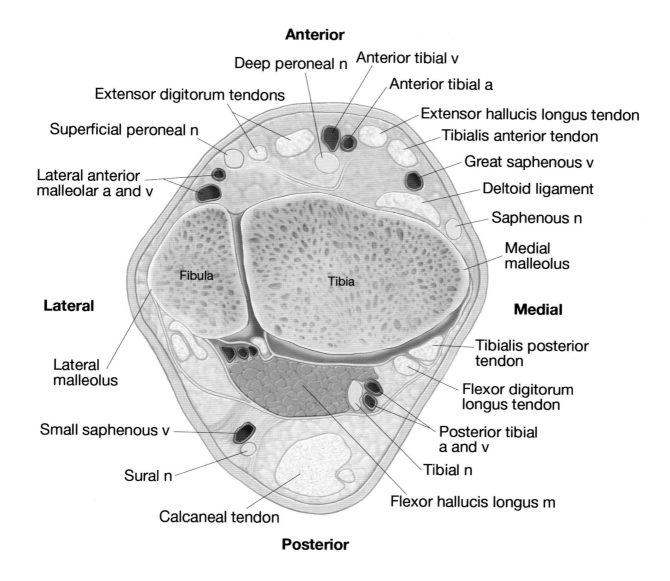

Anterior

Deep peroneal n   Anterior tibial v

Extensor digitorum tendons   Anterior tibial a

Superficial peroneal n   Extensor hallucis longus tendon

Tibialis anterior tendon

Lateral anterior malleolar a and v   Great saphenous v

Deltoid ligament

Saphenous n

Medial malleolus

Fibula   Tibia

Lateral   **Medial**

Lateral malleolus   Tibialis posterior tendon

Flexor digitorum longus tendon

Small saphenous v   Posterior tibial a and v

Sural n   Tibial n

Calcaneal tendon   Flexor hallucis longus m

Posterior

Figure 29. Cross-sectional anatomy of the ankle.

terminal nerve branches may require supplementation for a failed or partially failed block, 3) to assess the onset and efficacy of conduction blockade within specific nerve distributions, 4) to document the distribution of preoperative and postoperative neurologic deficits, and 5) to determine whether prolonged sensory or motor blockade after regional anesthesia may be attributed to delayed resolution of the block itself or whether a new neurologic deficit has occurred.

Dermatomes, Osteotomes, and Myotomes

A *dermatome* is an area of the skin supplied by nerve fibers originating from a single dorsal nerve root. This orientation is constant, regardless of the cutaneous nerves to which the spinal segmental fibers contribute. In general, dermatomes form cutaneous bands or strips of innervation that are named according to the spinal nerve that supplies them. Most illustrations suggest that dermatomal boundaries are sharply defined (Figures 31-33).

In reality, there is an abundance of overlap of innervation between adjacent dermatomes. Therefore, if there is a loss of afferent nerve function by one spinal nerve, overlap innervation from adjacent spinal nerves generally helps preserve partial sensation. However, when this occurs, there is an overall reduction in cutaneous sensation and sensitivity.

In contrast to dermatomes, segments of *cutaneous innervation* refer to regions of the body supplied by the fibers of a single peripheral nerve (Figures 15 and 20). Cutaneous innervation may innervate an area of skin that crosses multiple dermatomal levels. Most modern texts are in agreement about which areas of the skin are innervated by which peripheral nerves. However, slight variations remain as to the specific borders of many cutaneous nerve fields.

Osteotomes are the segments or portions of bones innervated by a single dorsal nerve root. The number of osteotome segments present within a given bone may depend on anatomical variants (Figures 32-34).

A *myotome* refers to a group of muscles that are primarily innervated by the motor fibers of a single nerve root. Although slight variation exists, myotomal patterns of distribution are relatively consistent from person to person (Figure 35).

Motor Function Assessment

The assessment of motor function is also necessary when attempting to localize lesions of the nervous system. The interruption of motor fibers may occur as a result of mechanical trauma, ischemia, infection, or metabolic disturbances and may lead to a lower motor neuron lesion that results in paresis or paralysis of the involved muscles. Atrophy of specific muscle groups and characteristic deformities generally follow this sequence of events. Motor assessment may also be used to determine the onset and success of neural blockade after regional techniques. For example, biceps and triceps motor weakness may be an indicator of musculocutaneous and radial nerve blockade, respectively. A summary of motor innervation to the upper and lower extremities is provided in Tables 1 and 2. Motor innervation of the foot and ankle is summarized in Table 3.

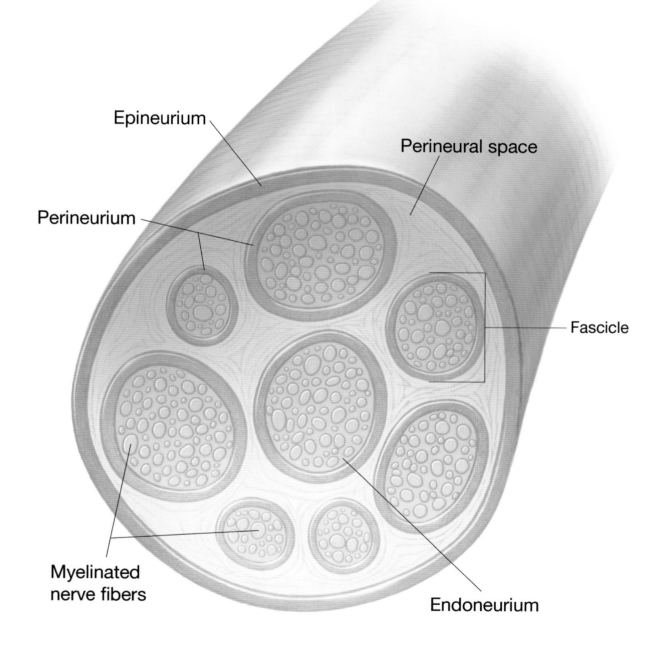

Figure 30. Peripheral nerve anatomy.

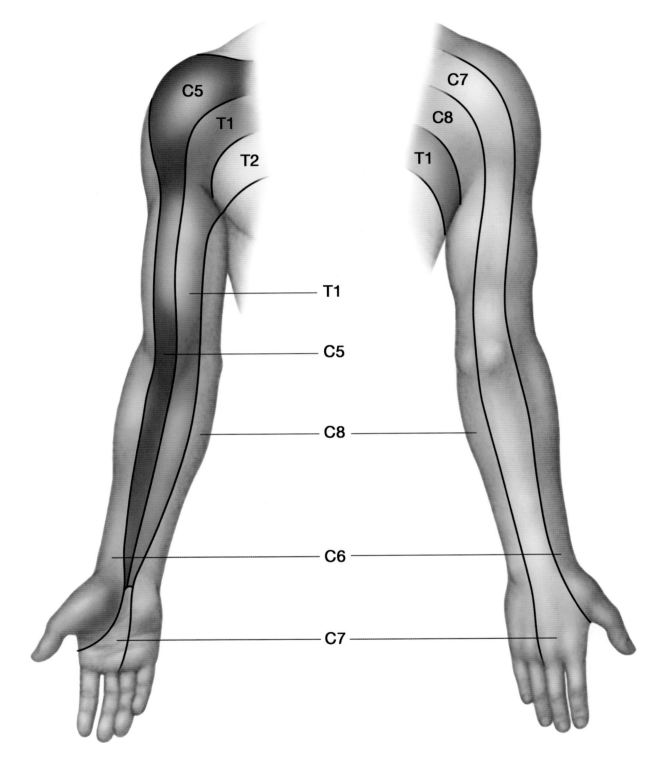

Anterior (palmar) view

Posterior (dorsal) view

Figure 31. Upper extremity spinal dermatomes.

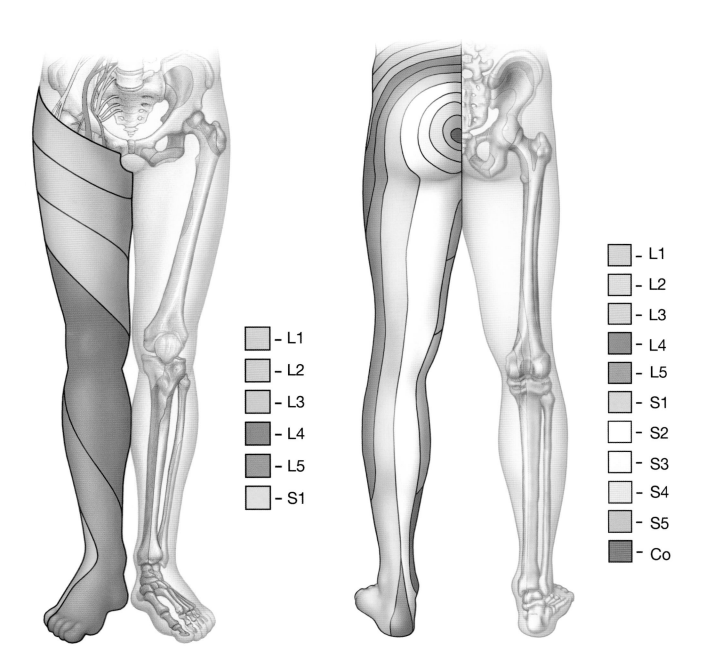

Figure 32. Spinal dermatomes and osteotomes of the lower extremity.

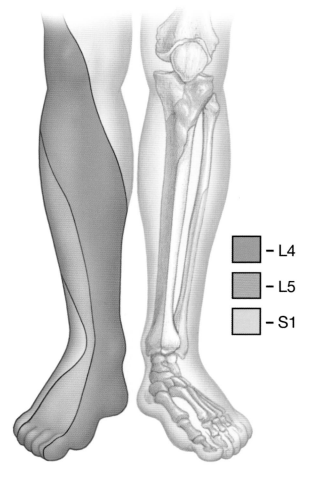

Figure 33. Spinal dermatomes and osteotomes of the foot and ankle.

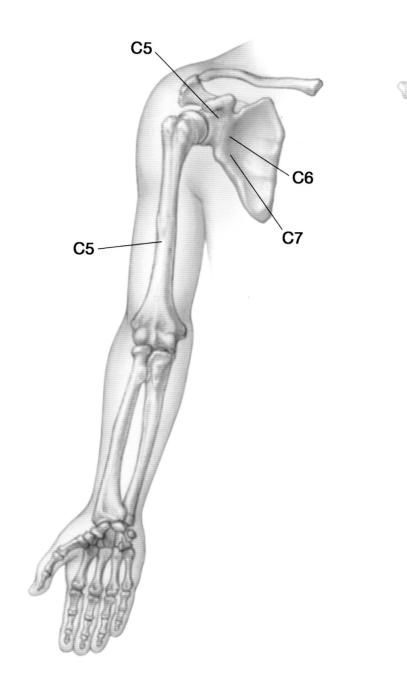
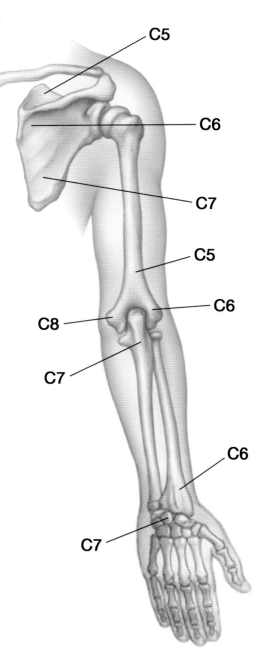

Figure 34. Upper extremity osteotomes.

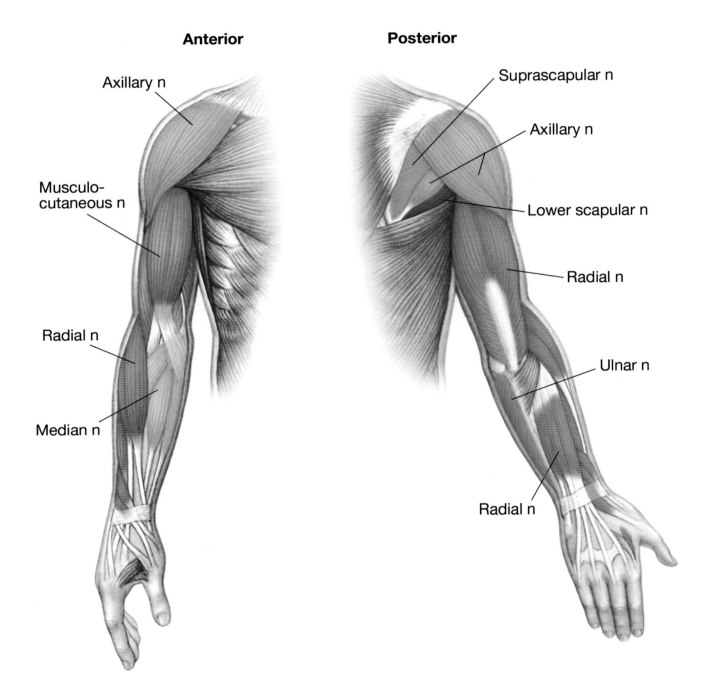

Figure 35. Upper extremity myotomes.

Table 1. Motor Innervation of the Upper Extremity

Nerve	Muscle group(s)	Function or action
Axillary (C5, C6)	Deltoid	Abducts arm, flexes and medially rotates arm (anterior fibers), extends and laterally rotates arm (posterior fibers)
	Teres minor	Rotates arm laterally, adduction
Suprascapular (C5, C6)	Supraspinatus	Abducts arm
	Infraspinatus	Rotates arm laterally, abduction (upper fibers), adduction (lower fibers)
Upper subscapular (C5, C6)	Subscapularis	Rotates arm medially; assists with flexion, extension, abduction, and adduction
Lower subscapular (C5, C6)	Teres major	Adducts, extends, and medially rotates arm
Musculocutaneous (C5, C6)	Coracobrachialis	Flexes and adducts the arm
	Biceps (long head)	Flexes arm and forearm
	Biceps (short head)	Supinates hand
	Brachialis	Flexes forearm
Radial (C5-C8)	Triceps (long head)	Extends and adducts arm
	Triceps (lateral head)	Extends forearm
	Triceps (medial head)	Extends forearm
	Brachioradialis	Flexes forearm
	Extensor carpi radialis	Extends and abducts hand
	Extensor digitorum	Extends fingers
	Extensor carpi ulnaris	Extends and adducts hand
	Supinator	Supinates forearm
	Abductor pollicis longus	Abducts and extends thumb
Median (C6-T1)	Pronator teres	Pronates and flexes forearm
	Flexor carpi radialis	Flexes and abducts hand at wrist
	Palmaris longus	Flexes hand at wrist
	Flexor digitorum superficialis	Flexes hand, first and second phalanges
	Flexor pollicis longus	Flexes hand and phalanges
	Pronator quadratus	Pronates forearm
Ulnar (C8, T1)	Flexor carpi ulnaris	Flexes and adducts hand at wrist
	Flexor digitorum profundus	Flexes all phalanges and hand at wrist
	Intrinsic hand muscles	Flex, extend, abduct, and adduct phalanges

Table 2.   Motor Innervation of the Lower Extremity

Nerve	Muscle group(s)	Function or action
Femoral (L2-L4)	Sartorius	Flexes and laterally rotates thigh, flexes and medially rotates leg
	Quadriceps	
	Rectus femoris	Flexes thigh, extends leg
	Vastus lateralis	Extends leg
	Vastus medialis	Extends leg
	Vastus intermedius	Extends leg
	Pectineus	Flexes thigh, adducts and laterally rotates thigh
Branch to iliopsoas (L2-L4)	Iliopsoas	Flexes and adducts thigh, laterally rotates thigh when extremity is not weight-bearing
Obturator (L2-L4)	Adductor longus	Adducts, flexes, and laterally rotates thigh
	Gracilis	Adducts thigh, flexes and medially rotates leg
	Adductor brevis	Adducts and flexes thigh
	Adductor magnus (oblique head)	Adducts and flexes thigh
	Obturator externus	Rotates thigh laterally
Superior gluteal (L5, S1)	Gluteus medius	Abducts thigh, rotates thigh medially (anterior fibers), rotates thigh laterally (posterior fibers)
	Gluteus minimus	Abducts and medially rotates thigh, flexes thigh (weakly)
	Tensor fasciae latae	Flexes, abducts, and medially rotates thigh
Inferior gluteal (L5-S2)	Gluteus maximus	Extends and laterally rotates thigh
Nerve to obturator internus (L5, S1)	Obturator internus	Abducts and laterally rotates thigh
	Superior gemellus	Abducts and laterally rotates thigh
Nerve to quadratus femoris (L5, S1)	Inferior gemellus	Abducts and laterally rotates thigh
	Quadratus femoris	Rotates thigh laterally
Nerve to piriformis (S1, S2)	Piriformis	Abducts and laterally rotates thigh
Sciatic		
Tibial (L4-S3)	Adductor magnus (vertical head)	Extends thigh
	Biceps femoris (long head)	Extends thigh, flexes and laterally rotates leg if knee is flexed
	Semitendinosus	Extends thigh, flexes and medially rotates leg
	Semimembranosus	Extends thigh, flexes and medially rotates leg
	Gastrocnemius	Flexes leg
	Plantaris	Flexes leg
	Popliteus	Flexes and medially rotates leg
Common peroneal (L4-S2)	Biceps femoris (short head)	Flexes leg

Table 3.   Motor Innervation of the Foot and Ankle

Nerve	Muscle group(s)	Function or action
Common peroneal		
Superficial peroneal (L5-S2)	Peroneus longus	Plantar flexes and everts foot
	Peroneus brevis	Plantar flexes and everts foot
Deep peroneal (L4-S1)	Tibialis anterior	Dorsiflexes and inverts foot
	Extensor hallucis longus	Extends great toe and everts foot
	Extensor digitorum longus	Extends toes, dorsiflexes and everts foot
	Extensor digitorum brevis	Extends medial four toes
Tibial (L4-S3)	Gastrocnemius	Plantar flexes and inverts foot
	Soleus	Plantar flexes and inverts foot
	Plantaris	Plantar flexes foot
	Tibialis posterior	Plantar flexes, adducts, and inverts foot
	Flexor hallucis longus	Flexes distal phalanx, inverts foot
	Flexor digitorum longus	Flexes toes, plantar flexes and inverts foot
Lateral plantar (S2, S3)	Quadratus plantae	Flexes toes
	Adductor hallucis (oblique and transverse head)	Adducts and flexes proximal phalanx and great toe
	Abductor digiti minimi	Flexes and abducts proximal phalanx and small toe
Medial plantar (S1-S3)	Abductor hallucis	Flexes and abducts great toe
	Flexor hallucis brevis	Flexes proximal phalanx and great toe
	Flexor digitorum brevis	Flexes toes

Suggested Reading

Brown DL. Atlas of regional anesthesia. 2nd ed. Philadelphia: Saunders; c1999. Chapter 2, Upper extremity block anatomy; p. 13-22. Chapter 9, Lower extremity anatomy; p. 75-84.

De Jong RH. Axillary block of the brachial plexus. Anesthesiology. 1961 Mar-Apr;22:215-25.

Harry WG, Bennett JD, Guha SC. Scalene muscles and the brachial plexus: anatomical variations and their clinical significance. Clin Anat. 1997;10(4):250-2.

Kerr AT. The brachial plexus of nerves in man: the variations in its formation and branches. Am J Anat. 1918;23:285-395.

McCann PD, Bindelglass DF. The brachial plexus: clinical anatomy. Orthop Rev. 1991 May;20(5):413-9.

Pansky B. Review of gross anatomy. 6th ed. New York: McGraw-Hill; c1996. Unit 3, Upper extremity; p. 231-324. Unit 6, Lower extremity; p. 497-584.

Partridge BL, Katz J, Benirschke K. Functional anatomy of the brachial plexus sheath: implications for anesthesia. Anesthesiology. 1987 Jun;66(6):743-7.

Reede DL. MR imaging of the brachial plexus. Magn Reson Imaging Clin N Am. 1997 Nov;5(4):897-906.

Thompson GE, Rorie DK. Functional anatomy of the brachial plexus sheaths. Anesthesiology. 1983 Aug;59(2):117-22.

Williams PL, Warwick R, Dyson M, Bannister LH. Gray's anatomy. 37th edition. New York: Churchill Livingstone; c1989. p. 768-76.

SECTION
III

Ultrasound-Guided
Regional Anesthesia

The use of ultrasound in regional anesthesia is increasing because of technologic improvements in image quality and growing recognition of its clinical utility. Ultrasonography is ideally suited to regional anesthetic techniques for upper extremity surgery because the brachial plexus is sufficiently superficial to allow excellent imaging. Moreover, the proximity of neural structures to pleura and vascular structures is such that direct visualization offers a distinct advantage. In contrast, ultrasound-guided lower extremity regional techniques may be more challenging because of the deeper anatomical location of many neurovascular structures (e.g., sciatic nerve). When successfully performed, ultrasound-guided regional anesthesia techniques allow neural localization and real-time observation of both needle placement and distribution of local anesthetic around neural targets.

Most anesthesiologists have had little formal training in ultrasonography or its applications in regional anesthesia. In simple terms, the learning curve involves relative mastery of three distinct skill sets:

1. Familiarity with the fundamentals of ultrasound and equipment used during ultrasonography
2. Understanding sonoanatomy and recognizing the appearance of neural structures during ultrasonography
3. Acquisition of technical proficiency in performing neural blockade

Together, these skills allow anesthesiologists to use and adjust ultrasound equipment, identify relevant anatomy, and safely inject local anesthetic around neural structures (Figure 1).

The next three chapters provide a foundation for understanding the relevant aspects of each requisite skill set. Regardless of the amount of information gathered from published sources, safe and successful execution of ultrasound-guided regional techniques is directly proportional to the amount of time spent training and practicing the various skills. There is no substitute for studying ultrasound images, scanning human anatomy, and developing hand-eye coordination on phantom gel or alternative models. Comfort with these preclinical skills will lead to a more successful experience for both patient and provider.

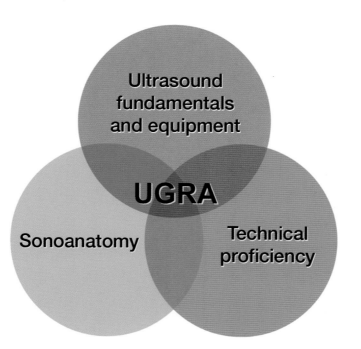

Figure 1. Skill sets needed for ultrasound-guided regional anesthesia (UGRA).

CHAPTER

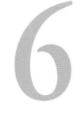

Ultrasound Fundamentals and Equipment

Adam K. Jacob, M.D.

Historical Perspective

Ultrasonography is one of the most commonly used diagnostic and therapeutic imaging methods in medicine. The use of ultrasound in medicine evolved from SONAR (SOund NAvigation and Ranging) technology, first described in the late 19th century. Karl Dussik, a neurologist and psychiatrist at the University of Vienna, pioneered the use of ultrasound in medicine while attempting to locate brain tumors and cerebral ventricles by measuring the transmission of ultrasound beams through the skull. He and his brother, physicist Friedrich Dussik, published their first experiments on "hyperphonography" in 1947.

The first application of ultrasonography in regional anesthesia was reported by la Grange and colleagues in 1978. They described the use of Doppler ultrasound to localize the third division of the subclavian artery during supraclavicular blockade. In 1989, Ting and Sivagnanaratnam used ultrasound to evaluate the spread of local anesthetic within the neurovascular sheath during axillary brachial plexus block. Similarly, in 1994, Kapral and colleagues used real-time ultrasonography to guide cannula placement and show the spread of local anesthetic during supraclavicular block. Since that time, several investigations have examined the utility of ultrasound-guided peripheral nerve blockade. Clinical applications, ease of use, block-onset times, clinical efficacy, and block duration have been examined for most regional anesthetic techniques.

Ultrasound Fundamentals

The Sound Wave
Sound is the result of mechanical energy transmitted by pressure waves through matter. In modern ultrasound systems, pressure waves are created by applying rapidly alternating electric fields to piezoelectric materials (i.e., lead zirconate titanate). In response to the electric fields, the piezoelectric material contracts or expands. Thus, rapidly alternating electric fields cause crystal vibrations and the emission of pressure waves. The pressure waves produce density zones of compression and decompression (rarefaction) as molecules oscillate about their normal,

unperturbed locations. Because the oscillation of molecules is repetitive, the term *cycle* is used to describe any sequence of changes in molecular motion that recurs at regular intervals. The *frequency* of a wave is the number of oscillations, or cycles, in 1 second and is measured in units called *hertz* (Hz). Normal human hearing occurs in the frequency range of 20 to 20,000 Hz. The term *ultrasound* refers to sound waves with frequencies above the range of human hearing (i.e., more than 15-20 kHz). *Wavelength* is a measure of distance between successive equivalent density zones, and *amplitude* measures the pressure magnitude, or height, of a wave at maximum compression or rarefaction (Figure 1).

Sound Wave Propagation and Tissue Interaction
Once an ultrasound wave is produced, the beam is transmitted through the tissue by a series of elastic oscillatory deformations. The initial pressure increase causes movement of particles adjacent to the source, which in turn produces motion in neighboring particles, and so on. As the energy propagates through the body, it encounters various tissue types and interfaces. A fraction of the beam's energy is reflected back to the transducer as it encounters each interface. The transducer converts this reflected sound energy back into electric energy and

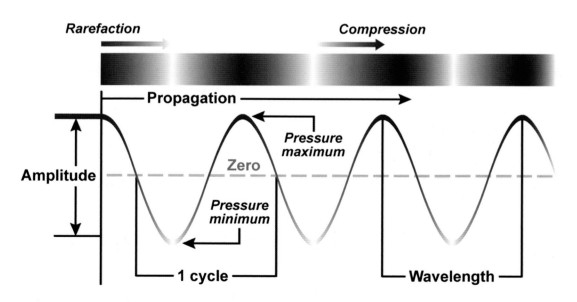

Figure 1. Characteristics of sound waves: frequency, wavelength, and amplitude.

yields a digital image after progression through a series of signal filters and amplifiers.

All tissues have their own unique physical properties that govern the transmission and attenuation of ultrasound. This is known as *acoustic impedance* (Z). Specifically, acoustic impedance refers to the resistance of a medium to the propagation of sound waves. Each tissue (e.g., muscle, fat, bone) has its own unique acoustic impedance (Table 1).

Acoustic impedance can greatly influence the quality of an ultrasound image. For example, when an ultrasound beam passes through one tissue medium (e.g., fat) and then encounters another tissue medium (e.g., muscle), the difference in impedance affects the amount of energy reflected back to the transducer and thus the image. To obtain a reasonable ultrasound image with good resolution, at least 1% of a beam must be reflected by the interface of two tissues, allowing a substantial portion of the energy to be transmitted to deeper tissues (Figure 2).

The fraction of reflected sound energy is also dependent on the wave's *angle of incidence*. The angle of incidence is the angle at which the ultrasound beam strikes its intended target. Maximal energy is reflected back to the transducer at an incident angle of 90°. If the angle of incidence is more or less than 90°, then only a fraction of the incident energy is reflected back to the transducer (Figure 3). Adjusting the probe to approximate a 90° angle of incidence to a target increases the overall image quality.

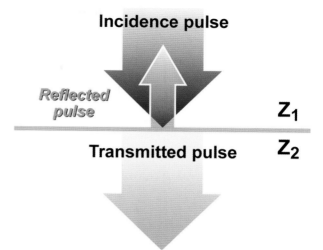

Figure 2. Sound wave reflection and transmission.

Ultrasound energy decays, or attenuates, as it propagates into tissue. The amount of attenuation depends on the attenuation coefficient (α) of the tissue, depth of ultrasound penetration (r), and ultrasound frequency (f).

$$\text{Attenuation (dB)} = \alpha \left(\frac{dB}{MHz \cdot cm} \right) \times r(cm) \times f(MHz)$$

The attenuation coefficient represents the amount of energy absorbed by a tissue medium. Similar to acoustic impedance, different tissues have various amounts of attenuation (Table 2). The attenuation equation also illustrates the relationship between depth of penetration and ultrasound frequency. This relationship is an important and fundamental concept of ultrasonography.

Penetration Versus Resolution

A common dilemma in ultrasound imaging is the inverse relationship between depth of tissue penetration and image quality (i.e., resolution). In general, a high-frequency ultrasound wave provides a large amount of detailed information (i.e., high resolution) at shallow depths. However, these high-frequency waves cannot penetrate to deeper tissue layers because of attenuation and loss of signal reflection back to the transducer. Conversely, low-frequency waves provide less information (i.e., poor resolution) but can penetrate to deeper tissue levels with minimal attenuation. The result is a

Table 1. Tissue Acoustic Impedance	
Medium	**Impedance, Z**
Air	0.0004
Fat	1.38
Water	1.50
Blood	1.60
Muscle	1.70
Bone	6.50

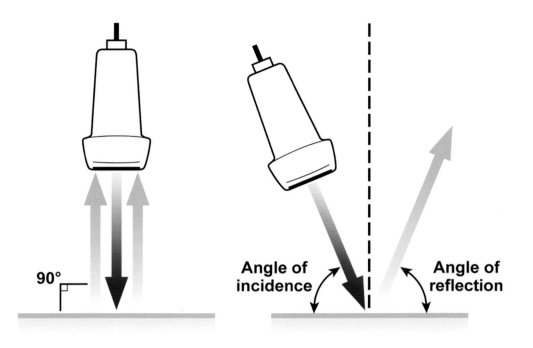

Figure 3. Angle of incidence and angle of reflection of sound waves.

simple but critically important concept of ultrasound imaging: high-frequency probes are used to produce high-quality images at shallow tissue depths (<4 cm), whereas low-frequency probes (with decreased resolution) are required for deeper imaging.

Artifacts

Even though ultrasound can provide useful information about structural anatomy, various artifacts potentially

Table 2.   Tissue Attenuation Coefficient

Medium	Attenuation coefficient
Water	0.0002
Blood	0.18
Muscle	0.2-0.6
Soft tissue	0.3-0.8
Fat	0.5-1.8
Tendon	0.9-1.1
Bone	13-26

compromise image quality. The anesthesiologist performing regional anesthesia should be aware of several common artifacts that can lead to misinterpretation of images. Most imaging artifacts arise from equipment malfunction, operator error, or unavoidable interactions of basic principles. *Reverberation*, or multiple reflection artifact, is common during regional anesthetic blockade. Reverberation occurs when a portion of the sound pulse returning to the transducer is reflected back into the patient (Figure 4). That retransmitted pulse strikes the same interface and is reflected back to the transducer a second time, producing a type of echo. Clinically, reverberation occurs when reflected energy from the needle shaft is reflected off the transducer face and retransmitted into the patient. The artifact appears as multiple needle shafts in parallel (Figure 5).

Another artifact commonly identified during ultrasound-guided regional blockade is *shadowing* (i.e., attenuation or dropout). This typically appears as a hypoechoic or anechoic zone extending deep from a strongly attenuating *or* reflecting interface (Figure 6). During ultrasound-guided nerve blocks, shadowing commonly occurs while

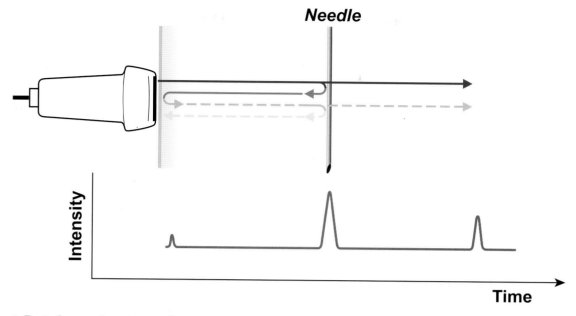

Figure 4. Basis for reverberation artifact.

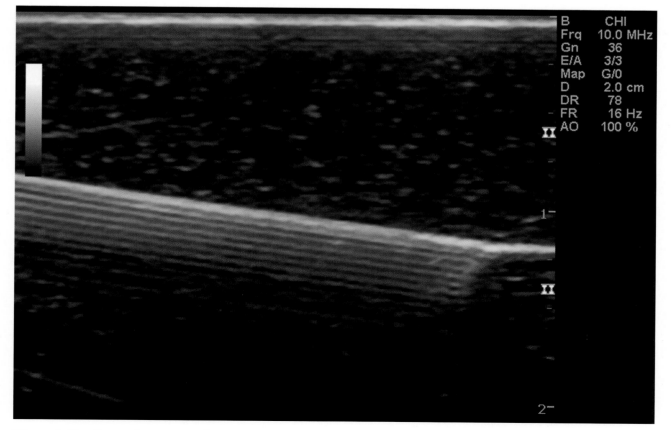

Figure 5. Needle reverberation artifact.

viewing structures deep to the needle or vessel walls, during poor transducer-to-skin contact, or when air bubbles are inadvertently injected into the field of view and the structures deep to the air become obscured or lost in shadow (Figures 7 and 8).

Acoustic enhancement is the opposite artifact of shadowing. During acoustic enhancement, a hyperechoic region appears beneath tissue with relatively low signal attenuation (Figure 9). This type of artifact commonly appears deep to arteries and veins (Figure 10).

Compound Imaging
Conventional ultrasonography uses multiple piezoelectric crystals arranged in either linear or curved arrays. Each element transmits an ultrasound beam perpendicular to the face of the transducer. With the aid of computer processing, the elements transmit beams in rapid succession and produce an ultrasound plane that shows the tissue

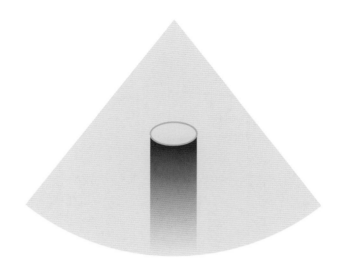

Figure 6. Basis for acoustic shadowing artifact.

beneath the transducer (Figure 11). Although this technology provides relatively good structural detail, the image is subject to artifacts.

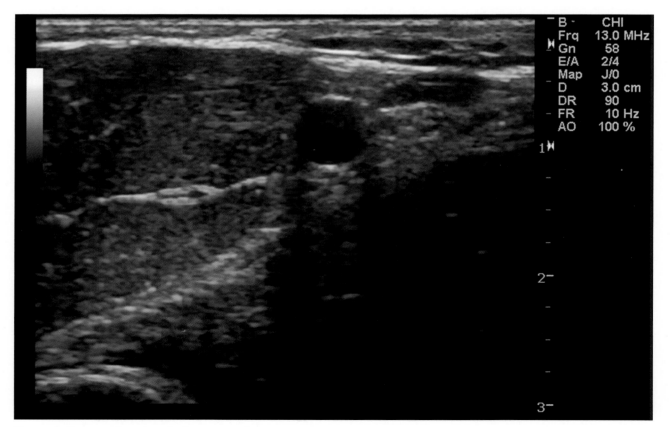

Figure 7. Perivascular edge shadowing artifact.

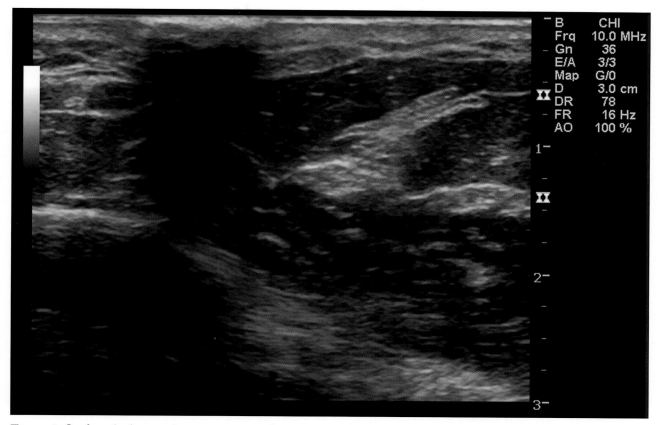

Figure 8. Surface shadowing due to contact artifact.

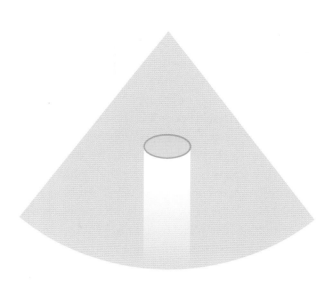

Figure 9. Basis for acoustic enhancement artifact.

In contrast, *compound imaging* is available on most modern ultrasound machines. It is a sonographic technique that uses electronic beam steering to rapidly acquire several overlapping, coplanar images of a structure from different viewing angles. These single-angle scans are averaged to form a new multiangle compound image. With averaging of these independent frames from different viewing angles, inconstant artifacts in each frame area are suppressed and constant signals from real structures are reinforced (Figure 12).

Thus, compound imaging produces better image quality than conventional ultrasonography primarily because of reductions in various acoustic artifacts. Images are less dependent on the incident angle and better depict tissue boundaries. In general, compound ultrasonography produces more realistic images of different tissues (Figure 13).

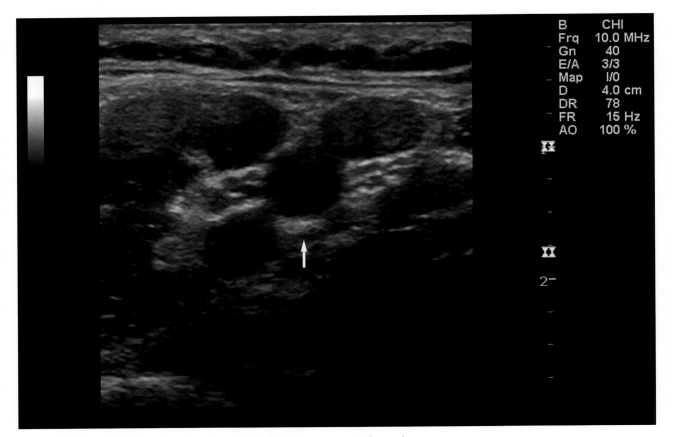

Figure 10. Acoustic enhancement artifact posterior to the artery (arrow).

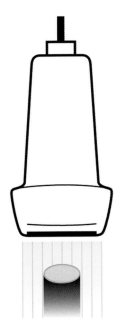

Figure 11. Conventional (linear) ultrasonography.

Ultrasound Equipment and Supplies

Probe Selection

Various probe sizes, shapes, and frequencies are available with modern ultrasound platforms. Different probes possess unique features to allow optimal imaging and ergonomics depending on the application. Three aspects of probe design should be considered when selecting the optimal probe for an imaging application: *frequency*, *array*, and *footprint*. As described above, probe frequency determines both image quality and depth of penetration. Most structures of interest in the upper extremity (e.g., brachial plexus) are easily imaged with a probe capable of transmitting frequencies from 7 to 14 MHz or higher. In contrast, lower extremity imaging may require the use of lower-frequency probes. Transducer arrays are linear, curvilinear, or phased. Linear-array probes are the most common probes used for upper extremity (i.e., superficial)

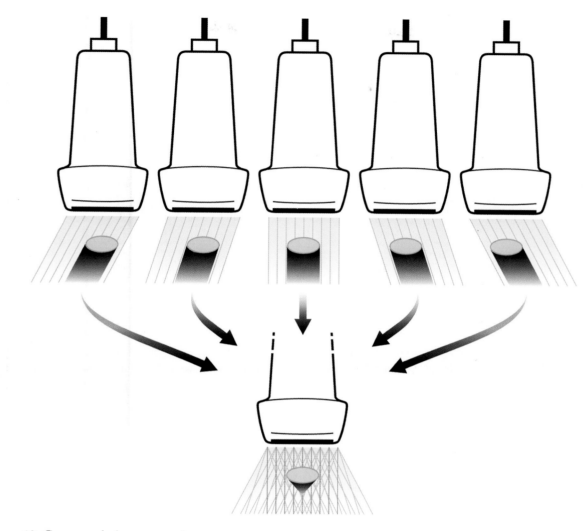

Figure 12. Compound ultrasonography.

regional anesthetic techniques (Figure 14). Curved-array probes (Figure 15) are more useful for deeper imaging (i.e., lumbar plexus and sciatic blockade).

The ultrasound footprint represents the surface area of the probe that contacts the skin. The larger the footprint, the larger the surface area that is covered and imaged. It may seem intuitive to choose a probe with the largest footprint for every imaging application. However, surface anatomy may dictate the upper limits of footprint size. For example, the size of the supraclavicular fossa can be limited by the relative size and position of the clavicle and may not allow a probe with

a large footprint. Ultrasound machines adapted specifically to regional anesthesia often have multiple transducers with variable-size footprints. The optimal footprint is best decided on the basis of the application, the patient, and the proceduralist.

Optimizing the Image

Once the proper probe has been selected and the scanning started, several features on the ultrasound machine can be adjusted to optimize the image. Specifically, the frequency, depth, gain, and focus position can be modified to suit the application and highlight the structure(s) of interest.

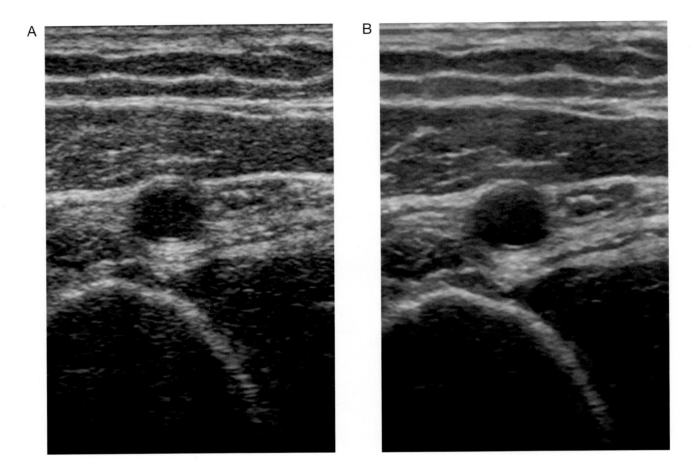

Figure 13. Brachial plexus imaging with conventional ultrasonography (A) and with compound ultrasonography (B).

Frequency

Ultrasound probes are designed to operate over a broad range of frequencies. The frequency is typically adjustable on the console of most ultrasound machines. The frequency usually can be changed by either rotating a dial or using a toggle button to switch between frequencies. Regardless, it is important to remember that high-frequency ultrasound is effective for producing high-quality images (i.e., high resolution) at shallow depths. Most machines and transducers emit a spectrum of frequencies, the highest density of frequencies being the variable that is adjusted.

Depth

The image depth reflects the distance of tissue penetration and is noted as centimeter markings on the left or right side of the viewing screen. As with frequency, depth is typically adjusted either by rotating a dial or by depressing a toggle button. There is no best depth for a given application. In general, the structure of interest should be located in the center of the image (top to bottom). Most structures of interest in the upper extremity (e.g., brachial plexus) can be clearly imaged at a depth of 2 to 3 cm.

Gain

Gain is the increase in signal power by an amplifier. It functions to amplify an ultrasound signal by mathematically adjusting the ratio of signal output to input. In general terms, it changes the overall brightness (or darkness) of the image. Most ultrasound systems have a gain dial to fine-tune the overall brightness of the

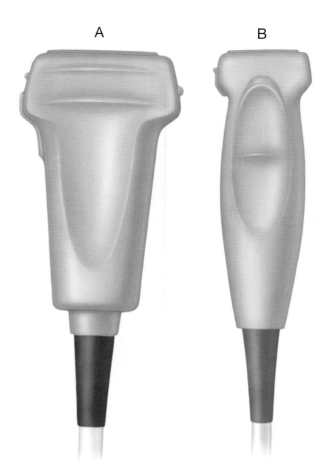

Figure 14. Linear-array ultrasound probes. A, 38-mm footprint. B, 25-mm footprint.

a value within 3 dB of the maximum along the transducer axis. Practically speaking, this represents the zone where image resolution is greatest. Most ultrasound machines allow the focal zone to be adjusted to a desired depth. Ideally, the focal zone should be located at a depth that includes the structure(s) of interest.

Conducting Gel

Ultrasound frequencies used for medical applications are poorly transmitted by air. Therefore, a conduction medium similar in acoustic properties to those of anatomical tissue needs to be used. This is commonly a thick fluid or gel-like material. The ultrasound coupling gel displaces air and fills contours between the ultrasound transducer and the body surface into which the sound is being directed. Although coupling gel can be sterilized, it offers no antimicrobial barrier between the patient and the transducer. Therefore, a

image and specific dials or slider bars to adjust gain as a function of image depth. As with depth, there is no best gain. During ultrasound-guided techniques, image gain should be adjusted to whatever seems best to the proceduralist.

Focusing and Focal Zone

Ultrasound beams are comprised of three zones or fields: the near field, the focal zone, and the far field (Figure 16). The beam emerges from the transducer as multiple ultrasound waves together. These waves combine via constructive interference to form a central region of greatest uniform intensity. The point of greatest beam uniformity and intensity occurs in the focal zone. The focal zone is technically defined as the region where the intensity has

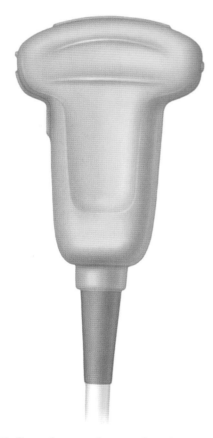

Figure 15. Curved-array ultrasound probe.

Sound intensity profile

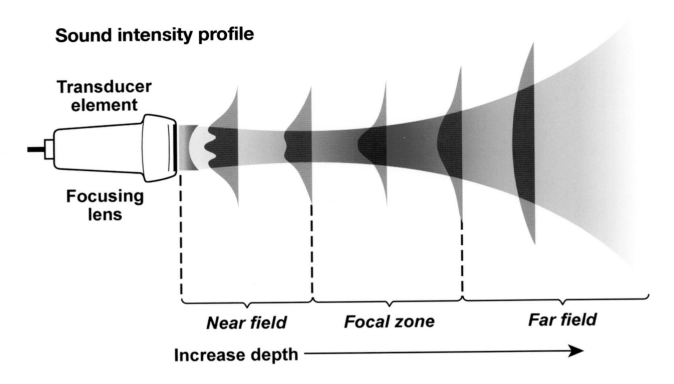

Figure 16. Ultrasound zones: near field, focal zone, and far field.

latex rubber or synthetic elastomer probe cover should be applied over the transducer to prevent transmission of microorganisms.

Ultrasound-Probe Stand
Many regional anesthetic techniques require an assistant to perform tasks such as aspiration with a syringe, injection of local anesthetic, or adjustment of the current of a peripheral nerve stimulator. Although the addition of real-time ultrasonography to regional anesthesia has its advantages, one potential drawback is the additional equipment necessary during the technique. This often requires additional personnel. One potential solution to this dilemma is the use of an ultrasound-probe stand. The probe stand can be useful because it allows a proceduralist to position the probe for imaging while keeping both hands free to manipulate the needle, syringe, or catheter required for the technique (Figure 17).

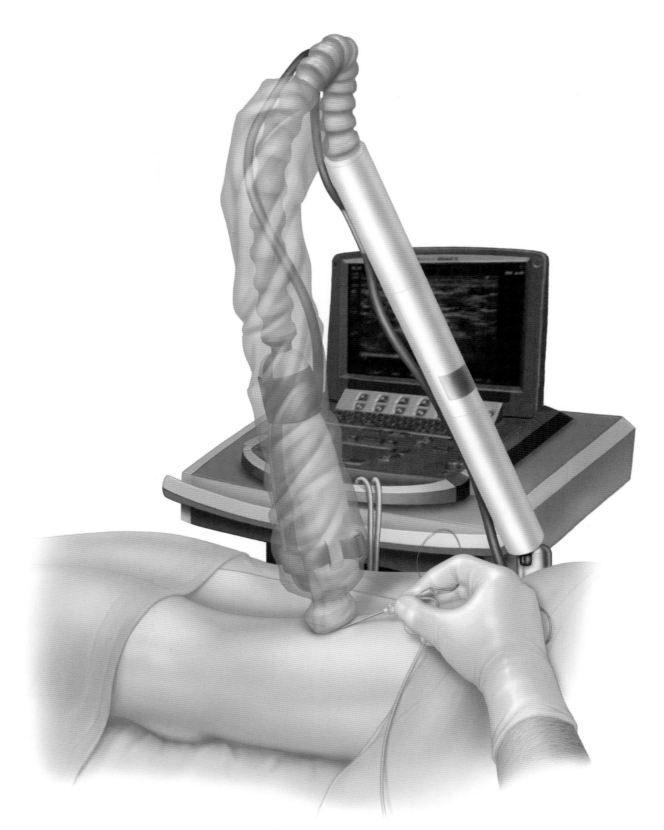

Figure 17. Ultrasound-probe stand.

Suggested Reading

Dabu A, Chan VWS. A practical guide to ultrasound imaging for peripheral nerve blocks. c2004. p. 7-21.

Dussik KT. On the possibility of using ultrasound waves as a diagnostic aid. Neurol Psychiat. 1942;174:153-68.

Hedrick WR, Hykes DL, Starchman DE. Ultrasound physics and instrumentation. 4th edition. St. Louis: Elsevier Mosby; c2005. Chapter 1, Basic ultrasound physics, p. 1-22.

Kapral S, Krafft P, Eibenberger K, Fitzgerald R, Gosch M, Weinstabl C. Ultrasound-guided supraclavicular approach for regional anesthesia of the brachial plexus. Anesth Analg. 1994 Mar;78(3):507-13.

la Grange P, Foster PA, Pretorius LK. Application of the Doppler ultrasound bloodflow detector in supraclavicular brachial plexus block. Br J Anaesth. 1978 Sep;50(9): 965-7.

Sites BD, Brull R, Chan VW, Spence BC, Gallagher J, Beach ML, et al. Artifacts and pitfall errors associated with ultrasound-guided regional anesthesia. Part I: understanding the basic principles of ultrasound physics and machine operations. Reg Anesth Pain Med. 2007 Sep-Oct;32(5):412-8.

Sites BD, Brull R, Chan VW, Spence BC, Gallagher J, Beach ML, et al. Artifacts and pitfall errors associated with ultrasound-guided regional anesthesia. Part II: a pictorial approach to understanding and avoidance. Reg Anesth Pain Med. 2007 Sep-Oct;32(5):419-33.

Ting PL, Sivagnanaratnam V. Ultrasonographic study of the spread of local anaesthetic during axillary brachial plexus block. Br J Anaesth. 1989 Sep;63(3):326-9.

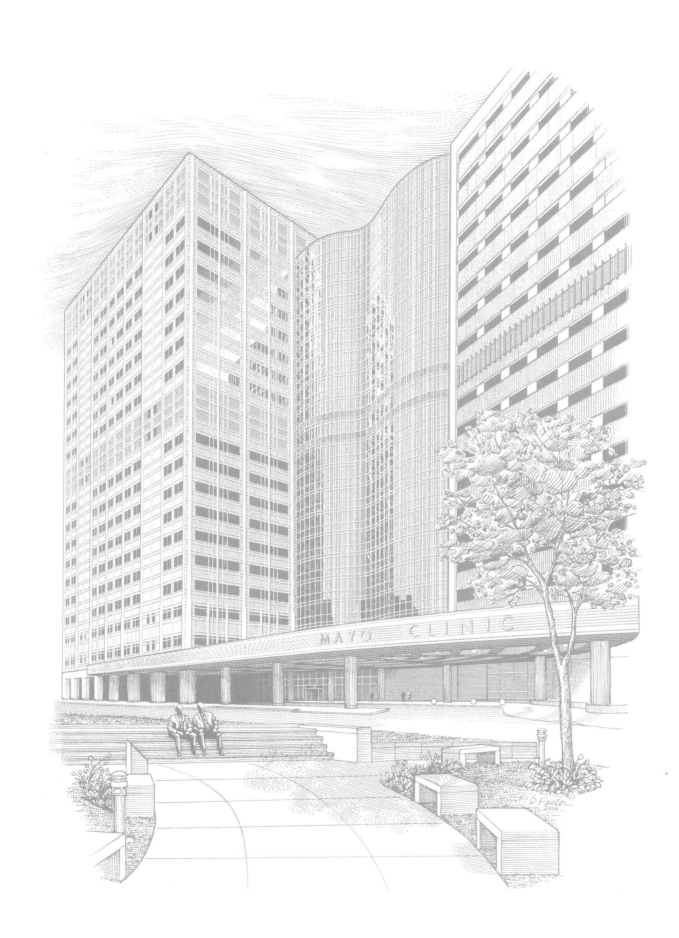

CHAPTER

7

Sonoanatomy of the Upper and Lower Extremity

Hugh M. Smith, M.D., Ph.D.

Ultrasound-guided regional anesthesia is the practice of applied anatomy. A detailed knowledge of neuroanatomy and the relationships of nerves to other structures is critical to successfully perform ultrasound-based procedures. In addition to anatomical knowledge, a comprehensive understanding of ultrasound equipment, probe selection, image optimization, and scanning technique is also essential to the proceduralist.

Visible anatomical structures such as bone, tendon, fascia, muscle, nerve, and vessels all have a characteristic ultrasound appearance. The physics of sound-wave attenuation and reflection, in conjunction with innate differences in tissue densities, allows sonographic distinction and identification of anatomical structures. These structures may be described using a glossary of specific ultrasound terms:

- *Echogenicity*: capacity of a structure within the path of an ultrasound beam to reflect back sound waves
- *Hyperechoic*: relatively brighter than the surrounding tissues

- *Hypoechoic*: relatively darker than the surrounding tissues
- *Heterogeneous*: variation or difference in echogenicity
- *Homogeneous*: sameness or lack of difference in echogenicity
- *Artifact*: false image, aberration or distortion of the true anatomy
- *Interface*: boundary between two substances that transmit sound at different velocities

Bone, tendon, fascia, and fibrous connective tissue surrounding nerves tend to appear brighter, or hyperechoic (Figure 1). Muscles possess an intermediate density and are commonly outlined by fascial layers. In contrast to these anatomical structures, vessels appear dark, or hypoechoic. Arteries can be distinguished from veins by their non-compressible, round, and pulsatile appearance. Veins tend to be more oval and collapsible with moderate probe pressure. Nerve tissue in proximal locations (e.g., interscalene and supraclavicular) appears hypoechoic, whereas more distal neural structures appear honeycombed and hyperechoic (e.g., axillary, femoral, popliteal) (Figure 1).

Image Optimization

Various elements, including probe selection, machine adjustments, and scanning technique influence image quality, neural localization, and overall success of a block. Probe selection is critically important and should be based on the depth and location of the planned procedure. In general, high-frequency linear transducers are sufficient for the vast majority of upper extremity nerve blocks. Linear transducers with smaller footprints can be useful in tight spaces such as the supraclavicular fossa. Familiarity with basic image adjustments, as well as features unique to the ultrasound equipment in use, is equally important. For example, depth, gain, and frequency are essential adjustments for obtaining basic images. However, the ability to manipulate and

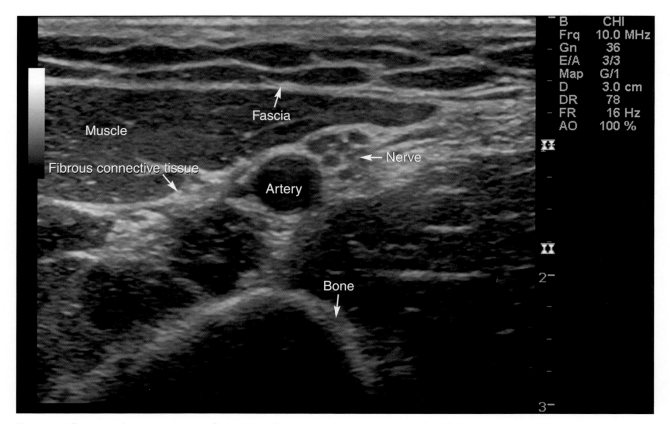

Figure 1. Sonographic appearance of anatomical structures.

appropriately adjust dynamic range, compound imaging, harmonics, and gray-scale features can provide additional resolution and improvement in image quality on some ultrasound machines. Dedicating time to master scanning and image optimization is an investment rewarded with consistently better picture quality.

Sonographic Scanning Techniques

The importance of ultrasound scanning, or the ability to manipulate the ultrasound probe to obtain and optimize images of neurovascular structures, cannot be overemphasized. Scanning involves elements of gel application, probe contact, pressure variation, hand position, and probe movements to acquire high-quality images. The position of the ultrasound monitor and ergonomics are also important considerations.

Monitor Position

Proper positioning of the ultrasound monitor should be the first consideration when preparing to perform an ultrasound-guided regional procedure. For most techniques, the proceduralist should be positioned on the side of the patient to be blocked. The ultrasound monitor is then placed directly opposite the proceduralist, on the contralateral side of the patient (Figure 2). This orientation provides the best viewing of the ultrasound screen while allowing a comfortable hand position for probe and needle control.

Ergonomics

Sitting on an adjustable chair or stool is the most stable ergonomic position. The transducer should be held in a relaxed hand, low on the probe, and close to the scanning lens. If possible, the scanning hand and forearm of the proceduralist should rest in a comfortable position on the patient or bed for stability. This position eliminates muscle fatigue and enhances the ability to perform the fine motor movements necessary for imaging and needle visualization.

Pressure

Many inexperienced ultrasonographers fail to use sufficient probe pressure during scanning and image acquisition. Fear of causing discomfort to the patient is a common concern but is rarely justified during routine scanning techniques. Image quality improves greatly when firm pressure and full probe contact are maintained. However, varying the intensity of probe pressure is important for distinguishing collapsible venous structures from arteries and neural targets.

Probe Orientation

Nearly all ultrasound transducers and monitors possess markings that indicate probe-monitor orientation. By convention, most probes use a vertical line or other marker to correlate with an emblem or dot on the left side of the ultrasound screen. It is generally recommended to orient the vertical line cephalad when scanning in a sagittal plane and to the right of the patient when scanning in a coronal plane. This orientation provides mirror images when opposite sides of the body are scanned and ensures that the image on the ultrasound screen is anatomically correct (Figure 3). However, some ultrasonographers prefer to orient the probe so that the image appearing on the monitor is the same—regardless of which side of the body is scanned. This orientation requires that the vertical line, or probe marker, is always positioned in a lateral anatomical position. The advantage of this approach is that pattern recognition and teaching are simpler if the anatomical relationships are consistent. For example, orienting the probe with the vertical marker directed laterally for both right and left axillary views always shows the musculocutaneous nerve on the left side of the axillary artery (Figure 4).

Scanning Movements

Movements of the probe can be divided into five motions: *sliding, angling, rotating, tilting,* and *pressure* (Figure 5). *Sliding* refers to proximal or distal probe movements while maintaining constant transducer angle, tilt, and rotation. This movement is useful for tracing the path of a nerve and aids identification. *Angling* refers to tipping the probe away from perpendicular. Nerves and other structures may not always travel parallel to the skin. Therefore, optimal imaging may require probe angling to acquire a precise perpendicular cross-section of the neural target. Optimal imaging occurs when the angle of incidence and target are 90° to one another. *Rotating* the probe refers to spinning the probe around its long axis.

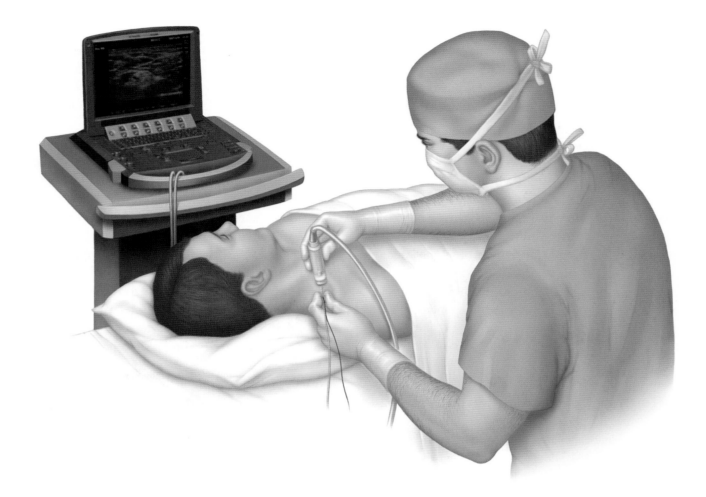

Figure 2. Orientation of the ultrasound monitor, patient, and proceduralist.

This movement is helpful for optimizing images seen in cross-section and for aligning the ultrasound beam with the full length of the needle. *Tilting* refers to applying pressure to the edge of the probe farthest away from the needle in order to improve the angle of incidence and visualization of the needle. *Tilting* and *angling* are distinct movements. *Tilting* is tipping the probe from end to end. *Angling* is tipping the probe from side to side. *Pressure* is the amount of downward displacement applied to the probe.

Anisotropy

An important ultrasound phenomenon with clinical utility involves probe *angling* and the principle of anisotropy.

Anisotropy essentially means directional dependence. In ultrasonography, anisotropy pertains to anatomical structures that are visible only when the ultrasound beam is directed within limited angles of incidence. For example, the median nerve and flexor tendon are both visible within the upper left field of Figure 6 B when the ultrasound probe is at a 90° angle of incidence. However, when the probe is angled to approximately 70°, the median nerve remains visible but the tendon in the upper left field of the image is not (Figure 7 B). This anisotropy, or directional dependence, is useful for distinguishing structures that may otherwise have similar sonographic appearance.

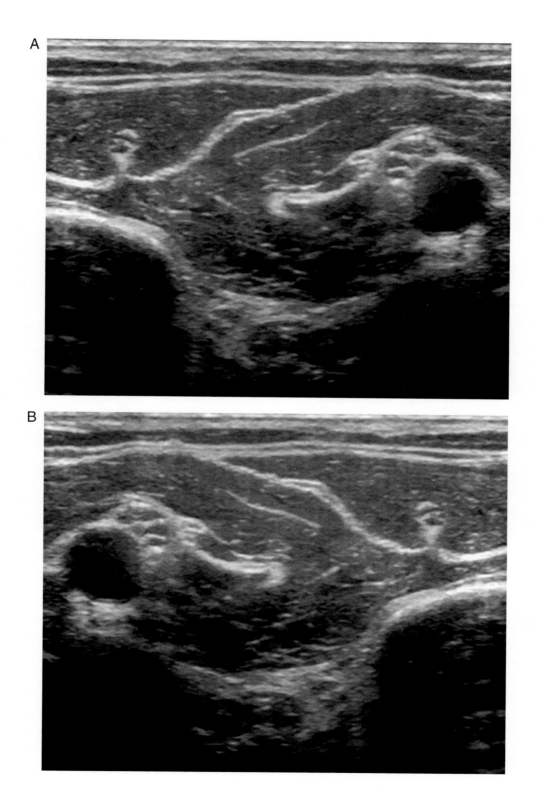

Figure 3. Mirror ultrasound images obtained with standard (right-directed vertical probe marker) probe orientation.
A, Right-sided axillary view. B, Left-sided axillary view.

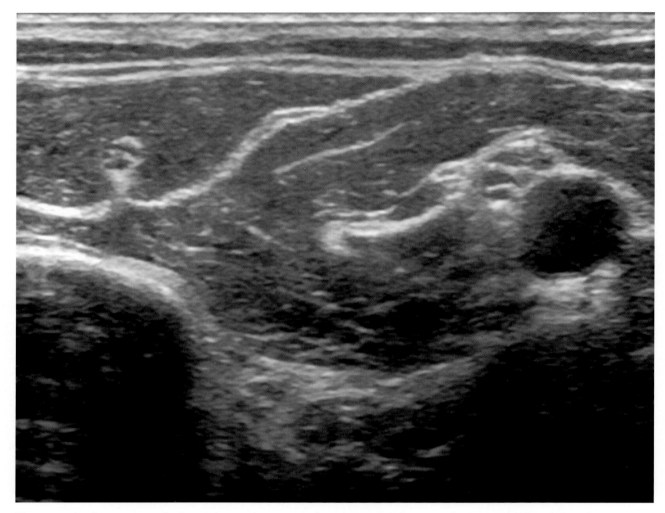

Figure 4. Axillary view with the probe marker oriented in the lateral direction (right- and left-sided axillary views will be the same).

Ultrasound Atlas of the Upper Extremity

Brachial Plexus Imaging

Once learned, the unique neural patterns of the brachial plexus can be easily recognized in most patients. With the exception of the interscalene view, all images of the proximal brachial plexus are associated with a neurovascular bundle—including a large, prominent artery that functions as a reliable anatomical landmark. Once vascular identification occurs, knowing the position(s) of neural structures relative to the vessel enables nerve target localization. Identifying the artery as a central landmark also allows clinicians to use the analogy of a clock face for describing nerve positions (i.e., as numbers on the face of a clock). This is an effective method for communicating nerve locations to assistants, learners, or observers. If image quality is poor, wide-angle scanning may allow surrounding structures to be identified (e.g., muscles and bones). Identifying adjacent structures that are familiar to the ultrasonographer may assist with initial orientation and allow the proceduralist to then "focus in" on neural targets. Experienced ultrasonographers are able to not only readily identify structures that are clearly visible but also manipulate the probe and machine settings (e.g., depth, gain, dynamic range, compound imaging, harmonics,

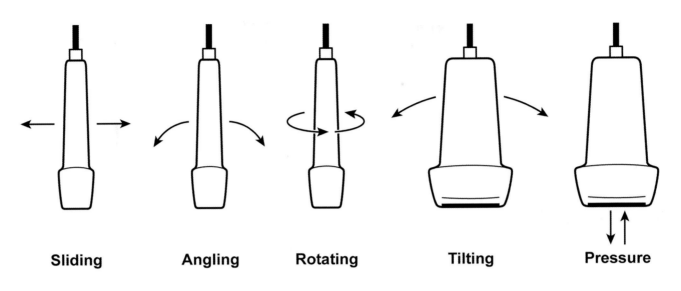

Sliding   **Angling**   **Rotating**   **Tilting**   **Pressure**

Figure 5. Ultrasound probe movements.

gray scale) to make visible anatomical structures that cannot be clearly seen, but are known to be present.

Supraclavicular View

Images of the supraclavicular neurovascular complex are obtained by placing the transducer parallel to the clavicle within the supraclavicular fossa (Figure 8). The patient should be supine with the head rotated away from the side to be blocked. A small towel roll or folded blanket is placed between the patient's scapulae, parallel to the long axis of the spine, to allow the shoulder to drop down and open up the supraclavicular fossa. The transducer should have a slight caudal angulation, directing the ultrasound beam underneath the clavicle toward the first rib.

Anatomical structures that are visible include the first rib and lung inferiorly, the subclavian artery and vein immediately superior to the first rib, and the distal trunks or proximal divisions of the brachial plexus immediately lateral to the artery (Figure 9). The middle and anterior scalene muscles may be visible anterior (superficial) to the plexus and artery. In most patients, the brachial plexus is located between 1 and 3 cm from the skin surface. The depth on the ultrasound machine should be adjusted so that the first rib is completely in view.

At the supraclavicular level, the brachial plexus has the sonographic appearance of dark circular structures clustered together, reflecting the homogeneous axon bundles of nervous tissue (Figure 9). An investing fascia enclosing the plexus is often visible, particularly after the injection of local anesthetic solution.

Infraclavicular View

As the brachial plexus emerges from beneath the clavicle, it travels posterior to the pectoralis muscles as an intact neurovascular bundle. For the infraclavicular view, the patient is positioned supine with the head in a neutral position, and the probe is oriented in a sagittal plane just inferior to the clavicle (Figure 10).

The axillary artery and vein are visible immediately deep to the pectoralis minor fascia. The medial, posterior, and lateral cords of the brachial plexus are oriented around the axillary artery—approximating the 3-, 6-, and 9-o'clock face positions (Figure 11). The neurovascular structures are typically between 2 and 4 cm deep, but the depth varies depending on the thickness of the pectoralis musculature. The plexus is not as visible within the infraclavicular region as it is on the interscalene and supraclavicular views. The *divisions* have rejoined to form the

A

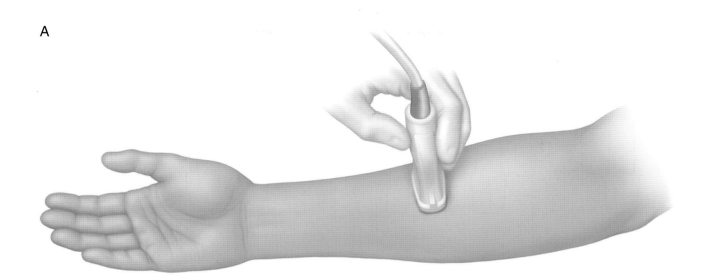

B

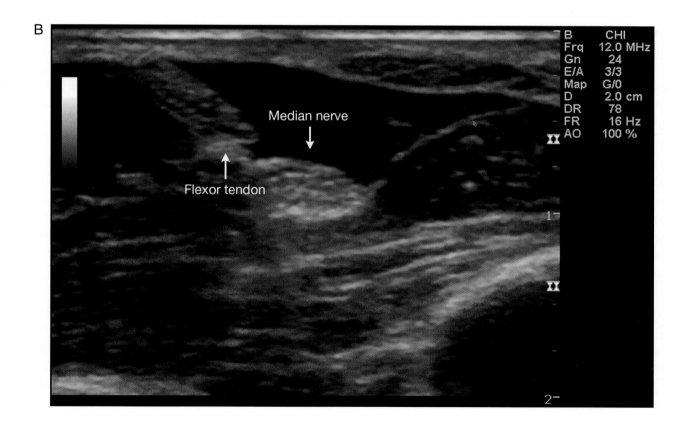

Figure 6. Ultrasound probe angle of incidence at 90°. A, Probe orientation. B, Ultrasound image of median nerve and flexor tendon.

A

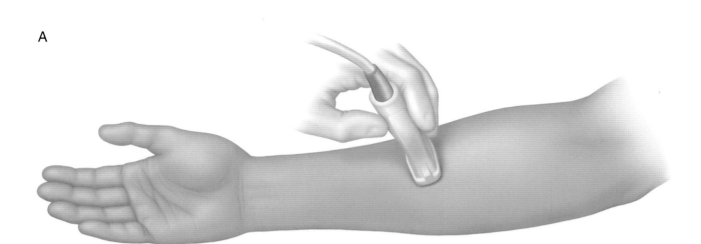

B

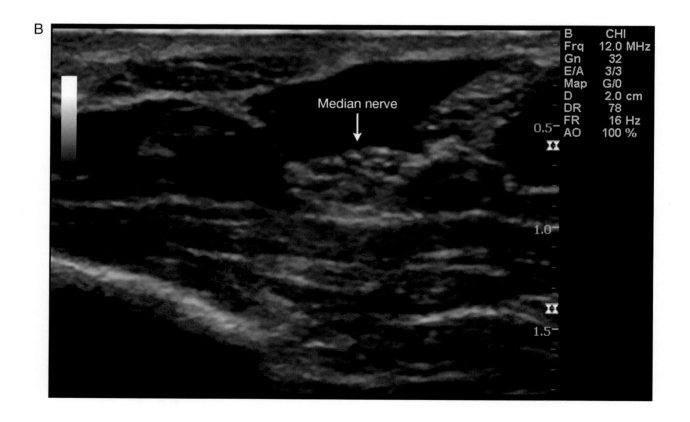

Figure 7. Ultrasound probe angle of incidence at 70°. A, Probe orientation. B, Ultrasound image of median nerve.

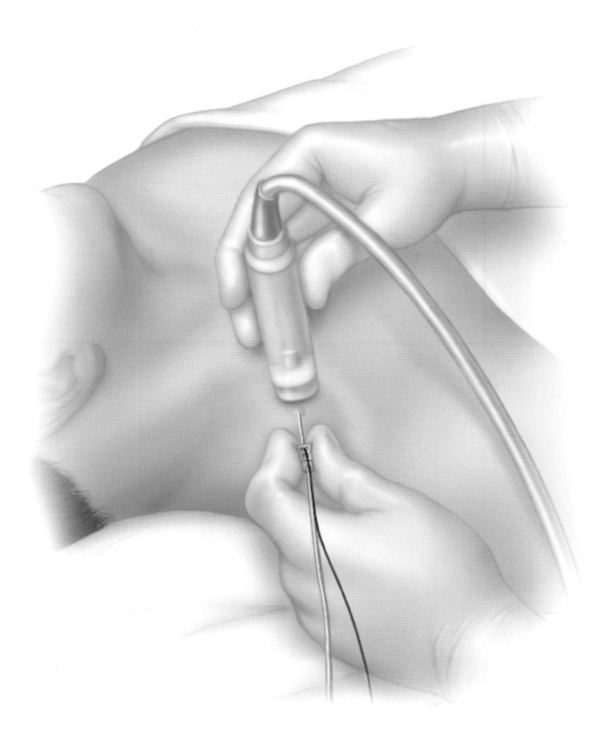

Figure 8. Supraclavicular ultrasound probe position.

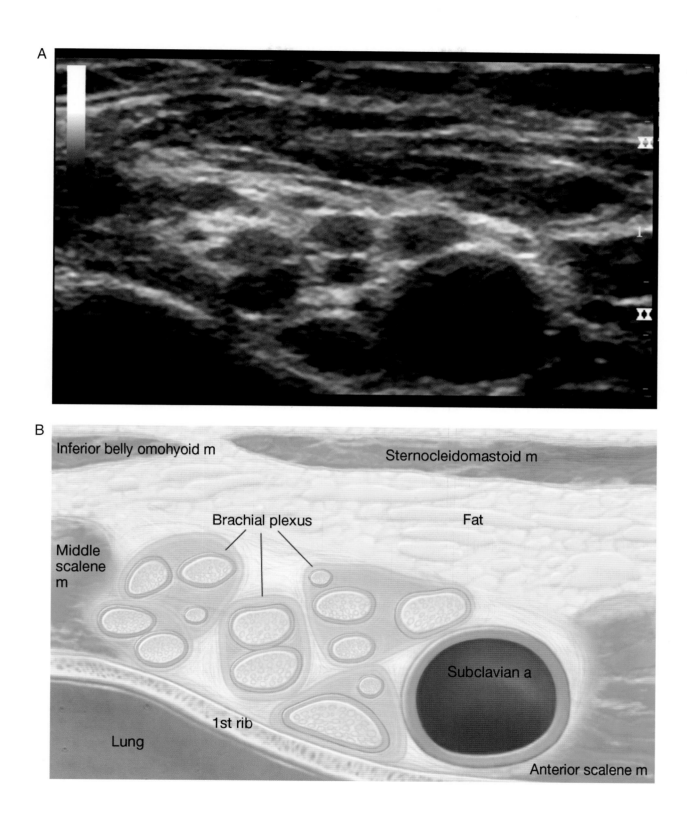

Figure 9. Supraclavicular view of the brachial plexus. A, Ultrasound image. B, Corresponding anatomical illustration.

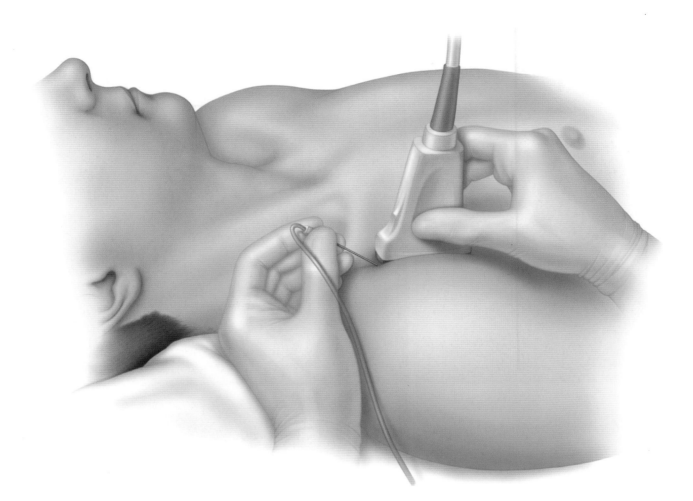

Figure 10. Infraclavicular ultrasound probe position.

cords of the brachial plexus, which no longer appear as hollow, hypoechoic structures. Rather, fibrous connective tissue, in combination with incomplete cross-sectional imaging, gives the cords a more solid, hyperechoic appearance (Figure 11).

Axillary View

Similar to the supraclavicular and infraclavicular views, the nerves of the brachial plexus in the axillary view are observed in relation to a central artery. With the patient's arm abducted and flexed at the elbow, the probe is positioned near the axillary crease in cross-section to the limb (Figure 12). Scanning movements in the proximal and distal directions may facilitate nerve identification. With the probe orientation marker directed cephalad, the image should be adjusted so that the artery is centrally located on the screen and the musculocutaneous and median nerves are located to the left of the artery. The ulnar nerve is usually seen above (anterior) and to the right (medial) of the artery, near the axillary vein. The radial nerve is frequently found deep to the ulnar nerve, between the 3- and 6-o'clock positions relative to the axillary artery (Figure 13). However, considerable anatomical variation exists among all neural structures within the axilla (Figures 14 and 15).

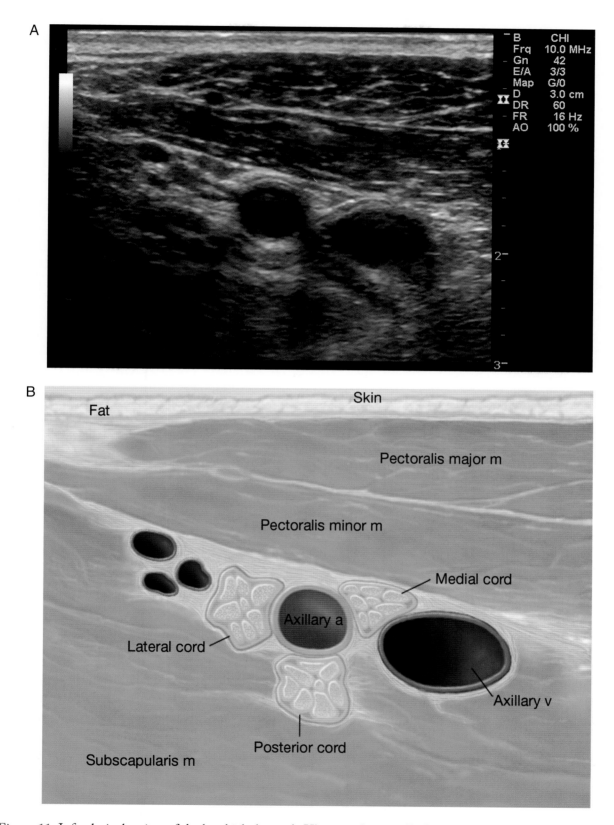

Figure 11. Infraclavicular view of the brachial plexus. A, Ultrasound image. B, Corresponding anatomical illustration.

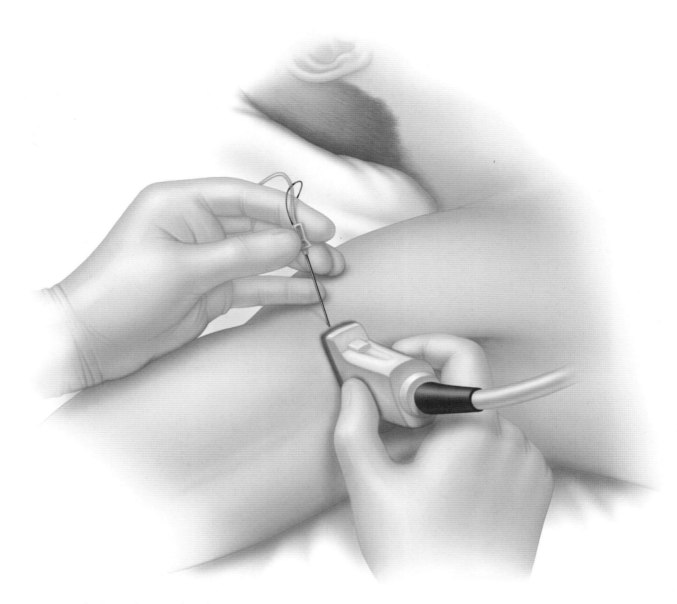

Figure 12. Axillary ultrasound probe position.

Nerve stimulation may be used in conjunction with ultrasound guidance to reliably identify neural structures. Characteristic motor responses may be elicited under direct visualization using low (<0.5 mA) stimulating currents. Similar to the infraclavicular region, neural structures within the axilla appear significantly different than those in more proximal locations. The cross-sectional appearance of nerves in the axilla is classically described as honeycombed—with dark (hypoechoic)

neural fascicles positioned within the inner core and bright (hyperechoic) connective tissue around the periphery of the nerve (Figures 14 and 15). This honeycomb appearance is preserved throughout the distal arm and forearm.

Interscalene View
For scanning the interscalene region, the patient should be positioned supine with the head rotated away from

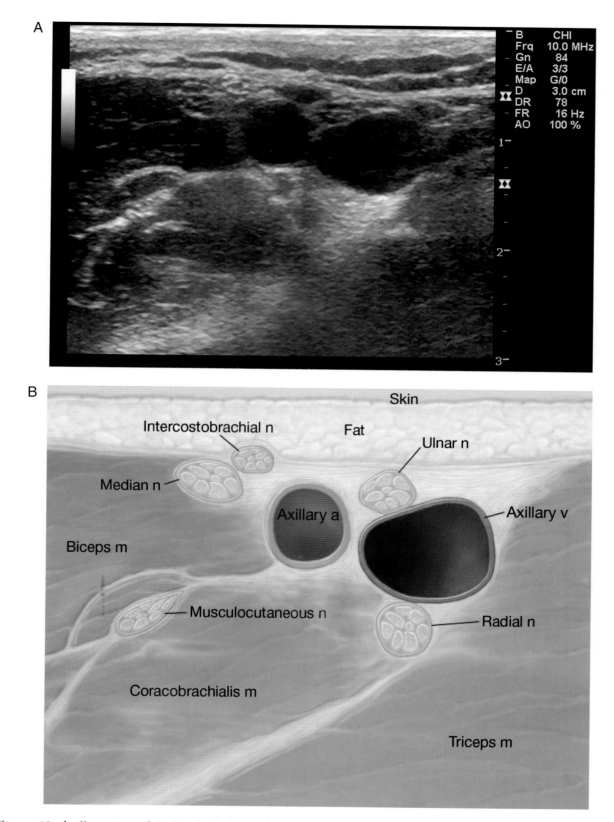

Figure 13. Axillary view of the brachial plexus. A, Ultrasound image. B, Corresponding anatomical illustration.

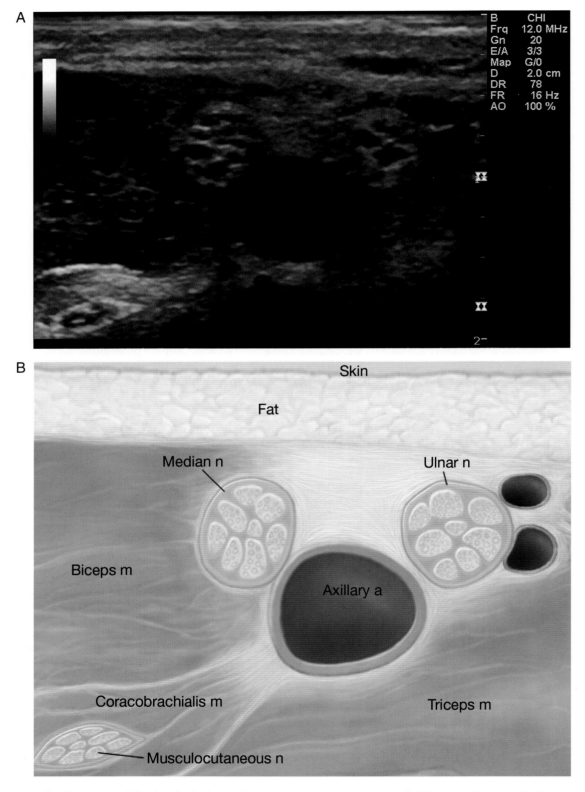

Figure 14. Axillary view of the brachial plexus, showing anatomical variation. A, Ultrasound image. B, Corresponding anatomical illustration.

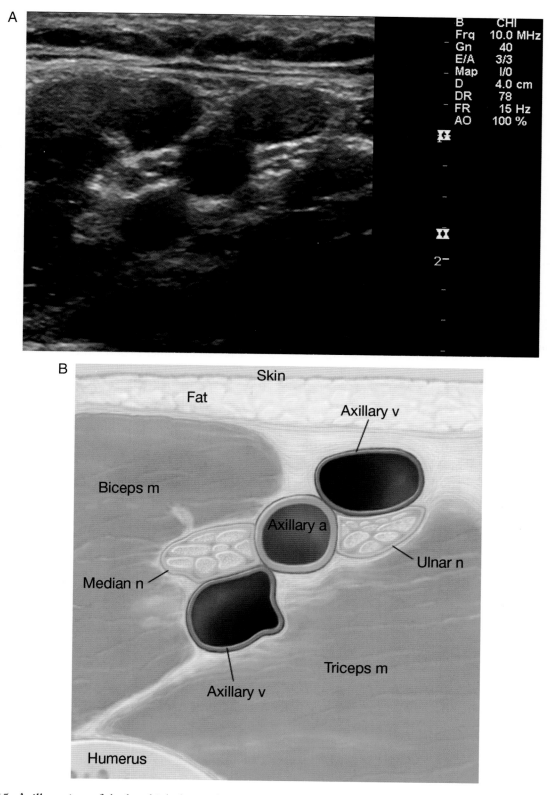

Figure 15. Axillary view of the brachial plexus, showing anatomical variation. A, Ultrasound image. B, Corresponding anatomical illustration.

the side to be blocked. Despite the superficial location of the brachial plexus within this region, interscalene imaging can be difficult, particularly compared with more distal regions of the brachial plexus. Inexperienced ultrasonographers often attempt to image the trunks of the brachial plexus by placing the probe on the lateral aspect of the neck, directly over the interscalene groove—as they would for a landmark-based technique. However, because the trunks travel in a medial to lateral direction and from a deep to superficial location, the beam of the ultrasound probe needs to be rotated slightly laterally and tilted caudad to optimally image the plexus in complete cross-section (Figure 16).

The interscalene view is most easily obtained by beginning within the supraclavicular fossa. The brachial plexus is identified within this region and then traced cephalad until the scalene muscles are seen clearly framing the plexus. Sonographically, the trunks appear as dark (hypoechoic) circular structures oriented vertically and often angling toward the midline (Figure 17). Although classic anatomy textbooks depict the brachial plexus as superior, middle, and inferior trunks within this region, the plexus may appear more subdivided when viewed with ultrasound imaging (Figure 18).

In most adult patients, the average depth to the superior trunk of the brachial plexus is between 0.5 and 2 cm. In approximately 50% of patients, the readily identifiable tapered edge of the sternocleidomastoid muscle lies directly above the superior trunk of the plexus.

Peripheral Nerve Imaging
The sonographic appearance of the radial nerve in a supracondylar location is typically elliptical, or even linear (Figure 19). The radial nerve is seen anterior to the humerus and should be traced proximally and distally to confirm its identity. The median and ulnar nerves are easily located by scanning over their associated neurovascular bundles. The median nerve travels with the brachial artery and vein as it courses through the midhumeral region. The bicipital aponeurosis at the elbow can partially obscure the view of the

median nerve at this location. Therefore, the nerve is best scanned at the supracondylar, or even midhumeral, level (Figure 20).

Most peripheral nerves can be viewed in either a cross-sectional or longitudinal plane. For example, the median nerve can be imaged in transverse (Figure 6 B) or longitudinal (Figure 21) section as it courses posterior to the flexor digitorum superficialis muscle within the forearm.

The ulnar nerve can be viewed either above the elbow or within the mid forearm. Cross-sectional scanning from an anterior to medial location just above the elbow passes over the ulnar nerve (Figure 22). With distal tracing, the ulnar nerve is seen getting closer to the humerus and eventually entering the ulnar canal.

The terminal branches of the brachial plexus are easily scanned within the forearm. In fact, the median nerve between the carpal tunnel and the mid forearm is an excellent nerve for novice ultrasonographers to trace and learn the classic appearance of neural structures. Furthermore, this anatomical region may be used as an ultrasound "constant." For example, for evaluating different ultrasound machines, it is useful to scan the same neural structures within the same anatomical region to facilitate a fair and easy comparison of equipment.

Ultrasound Atlas of the Lower Extremity

Lumbar and Lumbosacral Plexus Imaging
Ultrasound imaging of the lower extremity primarily involves the femoral and sciatic nerves and their associated terminal branches. Although ultrasound views of the more proximal lumbar plexus and ultrasound-guided psoas compartment blockade have also been described, the depth of the lumbar plexus and associated poor imaging have prevented the widespread use of ultrasound with this block technique. In contrast, ultrasound-guided femoral, sciatic, and popliteal blockade are being performed with increasing frequency.

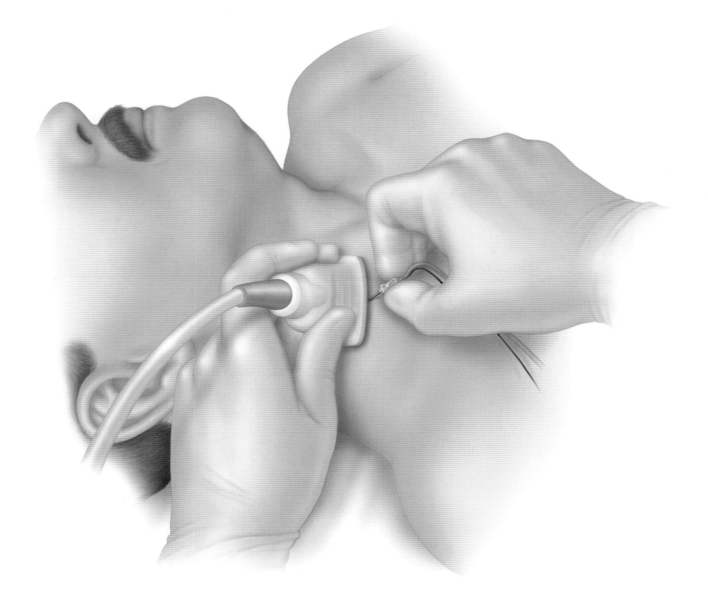

Figure 16. Interscalene ultrasound probe position.

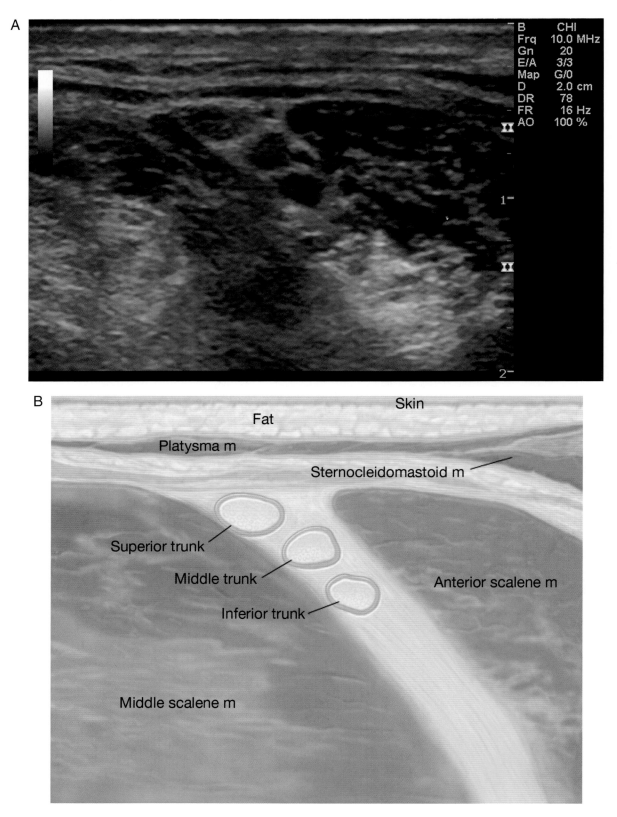

Figure 17. Interscalene view of the brachial plexus. A, Ultrasound image. B, Corresponding anatomical illustration.

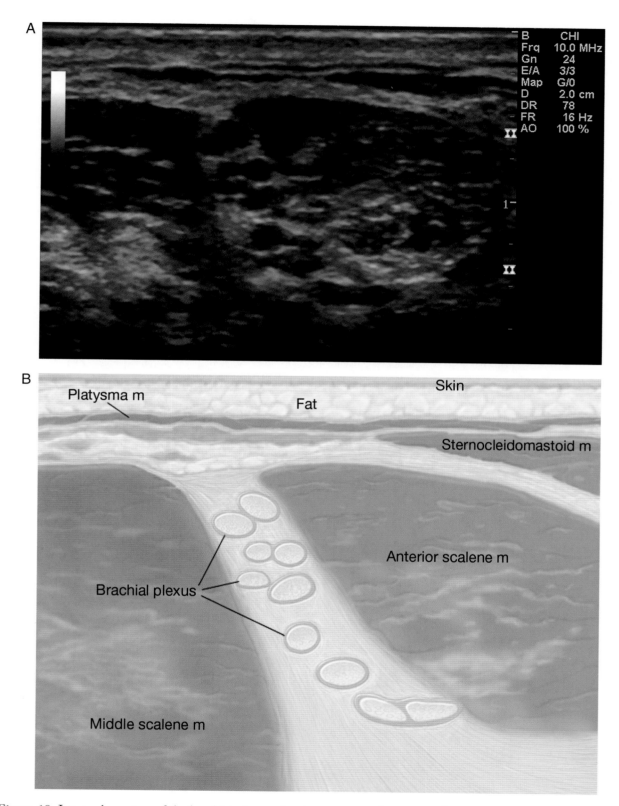

Figure 18. Interscalene view of the brachial plexus, showing anatomical variation. A, Ultrasound image. B, Corresponding anatomical illustration.

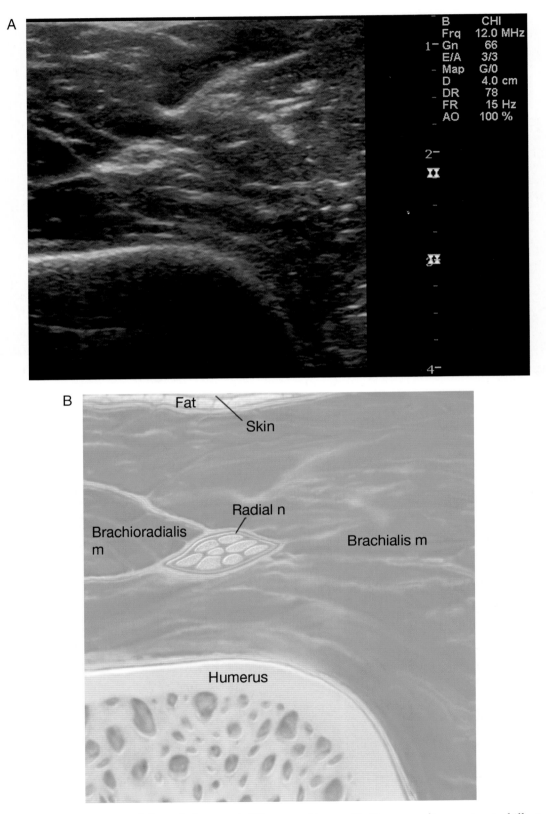

Figure 19. Supracondylar view of the radial nerve. A, Ultrasound image. B, Corresponding anatomical illustration.

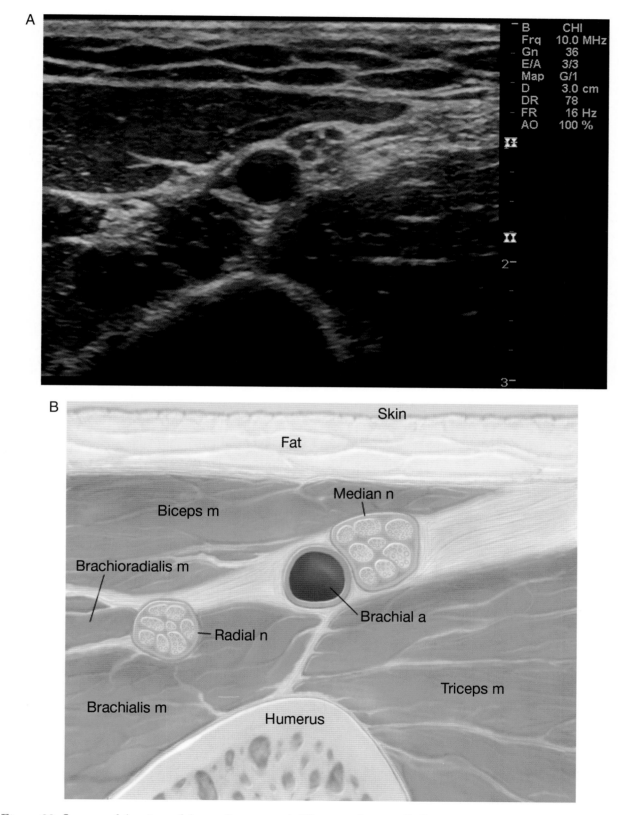

Figure 20. Supracondylar view of the median nerve. A, Ultrasound image. B, Corresponding anatomical illustration.

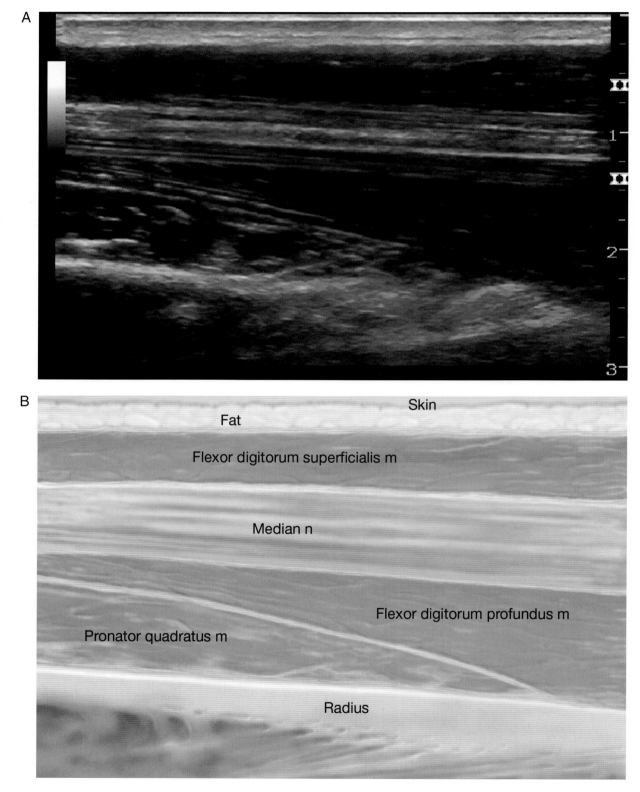

Figure 21. Longitudinal view of the median nerve within the forearm. A, Ultrasound image. B, Corresponding anatomical illustration.

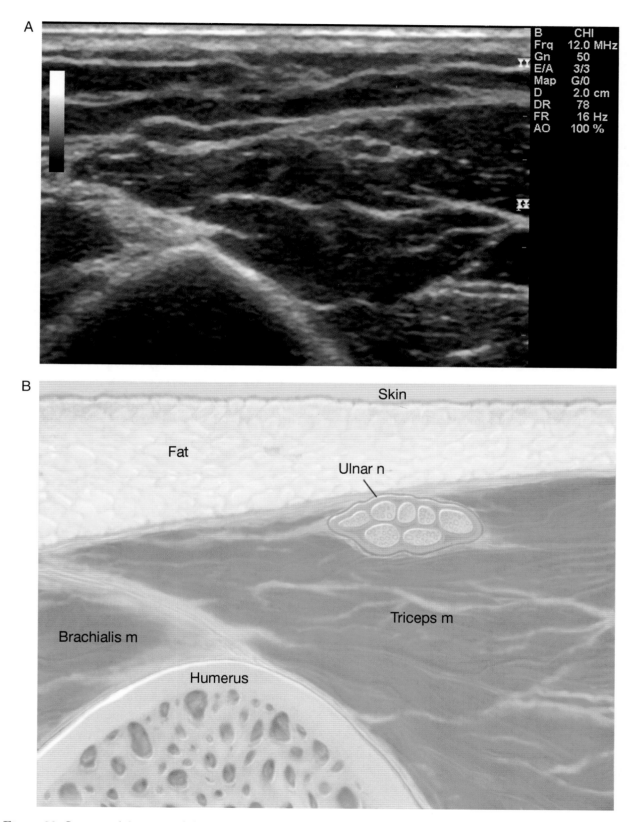

Figure 22. Supracondylar view of the ulnar nerve. A, Ultrasound image. B, Corresponding anatomical illustration.

The sonographic appearance of neural structures within the lower extremity often differs from that of many upper extremity views. For example, neural structures within the proximal aspect of the upper extremity (e.g., interscalene and supraclavicular) generally appear hypoechoic, whereas neural structures within the distal aspects of the upper extremity and the lower extremity appear honeycombed and uniformly hyperechoic. Similar to the upper extremity, vascular and bony landmarks are also important anatomical considerations when performing lower extremity ultrasound-guided regional techniques.

Femoral View
Ultrasound images of the femoral nerve are obtained with the patient in a supine position and the lower extremity in a neutral or slightly abducted orientation. The ultrasound probe is placed perpendicular to the long axis of the limb at the level of the inguinal skin crease (Figure 23). The femoral nerve, femoral artery, and femoral vein have a consistent anatomical relationship and are arranged from lateral to medial. This orientation allows the highly visible vascular structures (i.e., femoral artery and vein) to be used as guiding landmarks when attempting to identify the femoral nerve. The femoral artery can be easily identified as a large round, noncompressible, pulsatile, hypoechoic structure lateral to the femoral vein. Doppler ultrasound functions can also be used to confirm the vascular identity of both the artery and the vein. The femoral nerve is a hyperechoic structure located lateral to the artery and immediately deep to the fascia iliaca. The sonographic appearance of the nerve may vary depending on the location of the ultrasound probe. For example, at the level of the inguinal ligament, the nerve generally appears as a triangular or wedge-shaped hyperechoic structure with central honeycombing (Figure 24). However, at the level of the inguinal skin crease, the femoral nerve may appear more circular as the anterior and posterior divisions begin to form (Figure 25).

In most adult patients, the average depth of the femoral nerve is between 2 and 4 cm from the skin surface.

However, the depth at which the nerve is identified may be highly dependent upon the patient's body habitus.

Sciatic View (Subgluteal)
Several approaches to the sciatic nerve (e.g., posterior, parasacral, subgluteal, anterior) using traditional nerve stimulation techniques have been described. However, ultrasound-guided sciatic nerve blockade is generally performed within the subgluteal region because of optimal sonographic imaging. Ultrasound images of the sciatic nerve are obtained with the patient in the lateral position with the nondependent hip and knee slightly flexed (Figure 26). The ultrasound probe is placed perpendicular to the long axis of the limb on the posterior surface of the proximal aspect of the thigh immediately distal to the gluteal muscles (Figure 27). In most patients, a low-frequency curvilinear probe is necessary to obtain optimal images of the sciatic nerve. However, in patients with a small body habitus, a high-frequency linear probe may also produce adequate images.

The sciatic nerve emerges from the pelvis between the piriformis and superior gemellus muscles and courses anterior (i.e., deep) to the gluteus maximus muscle and posterior (i.e., superficial) to the quadratus femoris muscle. The ischial tuberosity and greater trochanter of the femur are two easily identifiable bony landmarks that create an anatomical frame of reference during sciatic imaging. The sciatic nerve is located lateral to the ischial tuberosity and medial to the greater trochanter. The intertrochanteric crest or lesser trochanter of the femur may also be seen laterally and slightly more distal. During ultrasound imaging, the ischial tuberosity and greater trochanter appear as bright hyperechoic structures with the sciatic nerve positioned between the two bony landmarks. The nerve itself may appear flattened, or linear, as it is compressed between the layers of the quadratus femoris and gluteus maximus muscles (Figure 28). In most adult patients, the sciatic nerve is located 4 to 6 cm from the skin surface. However, the depth at which the nerve is identified is highly dependent on the patient's body habitus. In some patients, the posterior femoral cutaneous nerve may also be seen adjacent to the sciatic nerve.

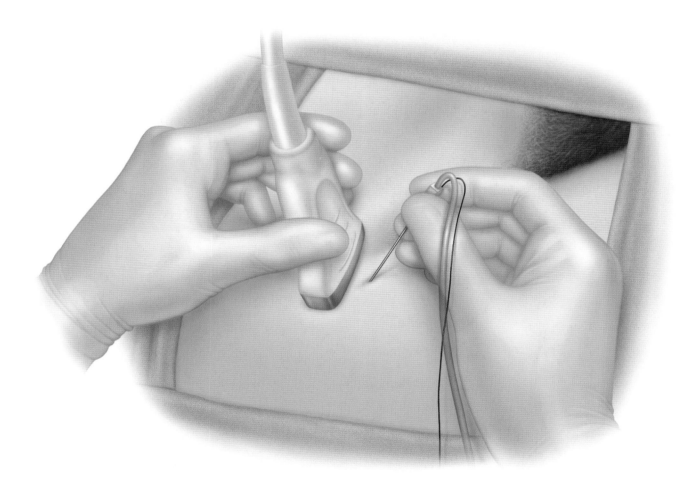

Figure 23. Femoral ultrasound probe position.

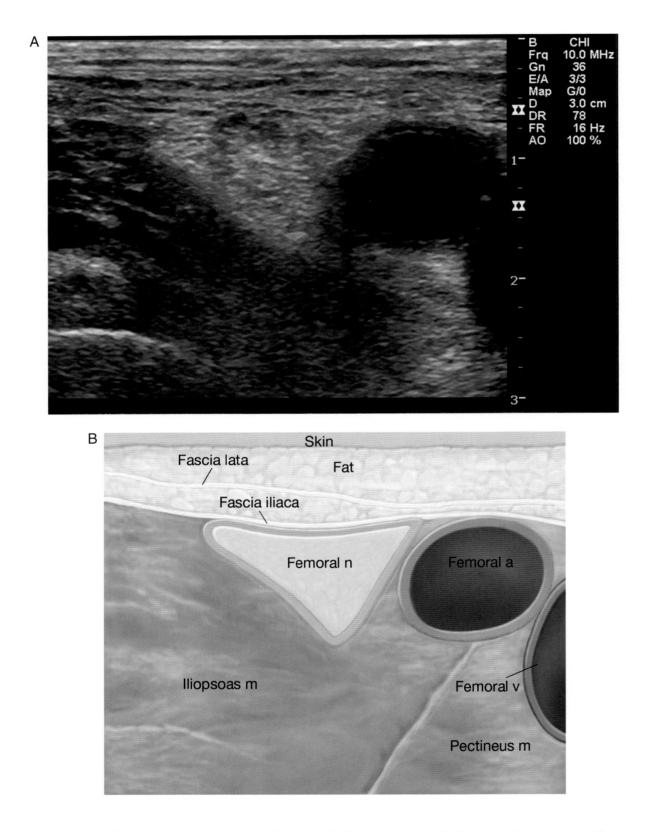

Figure 24. Femoral nerve anatomy at the inguinal ligament. A, Ultrasound image. B, Corresponding anatomical illustration.

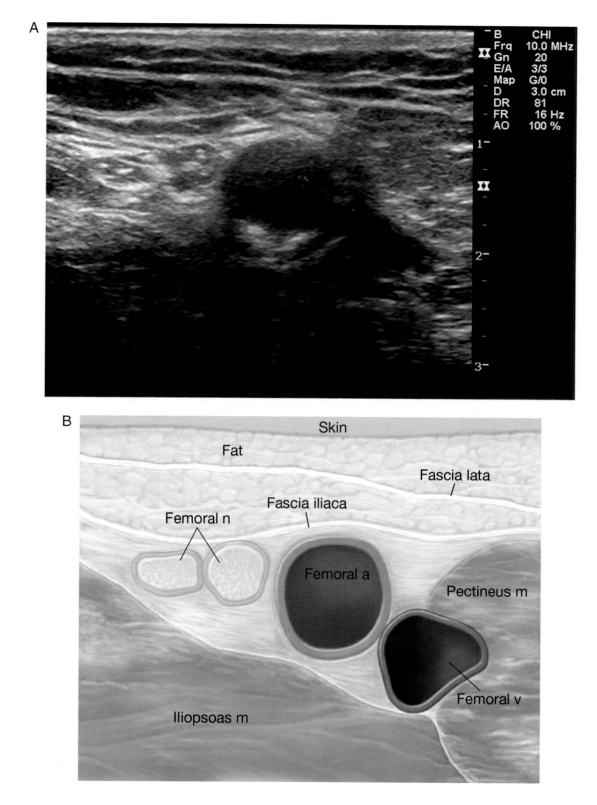

Figure 25. Femoral nerve anatomy at the inguinal skin crease. A, Ultrasound image. B, Corresponding anatomical illustration.

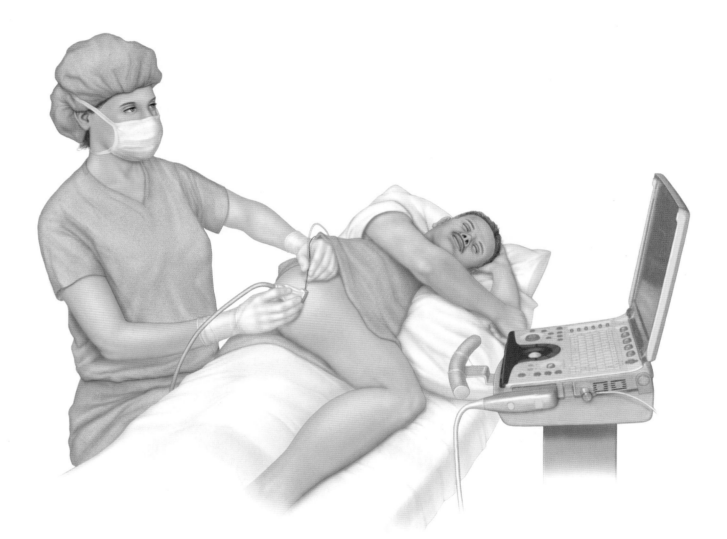

Figure 26. Patient-provider orientation during ultrasound-guided sciatic nerve blockade.

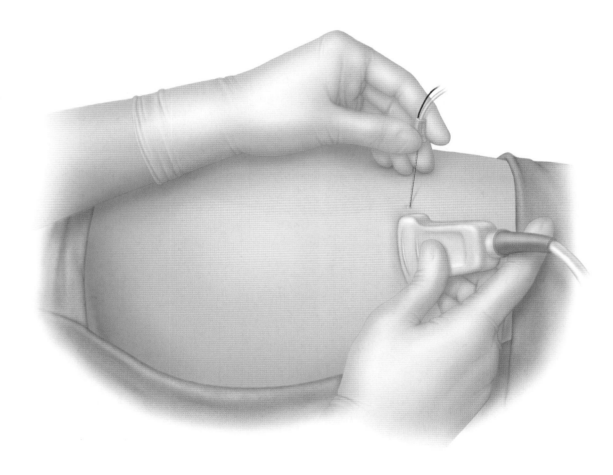

Figure 27. Sciatic ultrasound probe position.

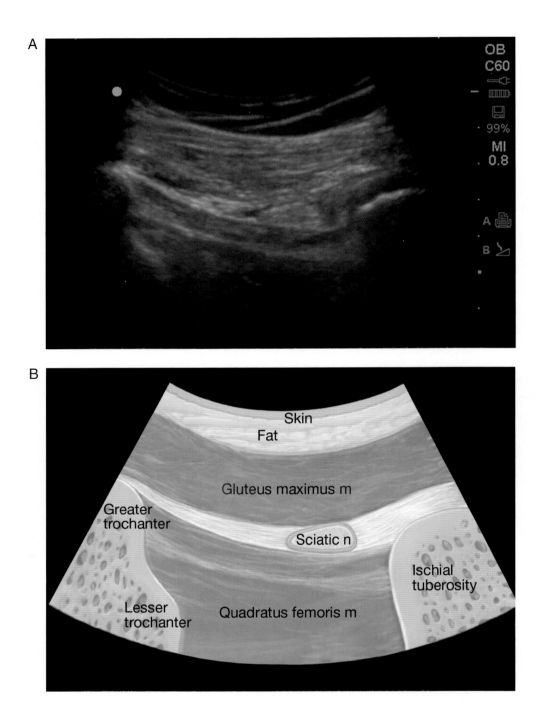

Figure 28. Subgluteal view of the sciatic nerve. A, Ultrasound image. B, Corresponding anatomical illustration.

Popliteal View (Tibial and Common Peroneal)

The sciatic nerve descends the leg within the groove between the semimembranosus and semitendinosus muscles medially and the long head of the biceps femoris muscle laterally. As the nerve approaches the popliteal fossa, it begins to separate into its tibial and common peroneal components. Within the popliteal fossa, the tibial and common peroneal nerves are located lateral and superficial (i.e., posterior) to both the popliteal artery and vein—two easily identifiable vascular landmarks.

Ultrasound images of the sciatic nerve within the popliteal fossa may be obtained with the patient in either the supine or the prone position. When the supine position is used, the extremity must be sufficiently elevated to allow adequate space under the leg for probe placement within the popliteal fossa. A more common approach is to have the patient prone with the leg in a neutral position. The ultrasound probe is placed perpendicular to the long axis of the limb on the posterior surface of the knee at the popliteal crease. This probe position allows providers to use either a posterior out-of-plane needle approach (Figure 29) or a lateral in-plane approach (Figure 30). At the level of the popliteal crease, both the popliteal artery and the femur should be readily identifiable. The sciatic nerve is a round hyperechoic structure with central honeycombing that is located superficial and slightly lateral to the popliteal artery (Figure 31). Scanning in a distal direction shows the hyperechoic sciatic nerve separating into its tibial and common peroneal components (Figure 32). The tibial nerve is typically 2 to 4 cm from the skin surface and located medial and deep to the common peroneal nerve. In addition, the tibial nerve tends to be larger in diameter than the common peroneal nerve.

As the sciatic nerve descends the leg, it travels from a deep to superficial location within the extremity. Therefore, an ideal cross-sectional view of the sciatic nerve is difficult to obtain if the ultrasound probe is positioned perpendicular to the surface of the skin. To improve the angle of incidence—and therefore the image—the transducer should be angled cephalad 50° to 70° with the skin (i.e., directing the ultrasound beam caudad) to ensure a perpendicular intersection between the ultrasound beam and the neural target.

Saphenous View

The saphenous nerve of the lower extremity is derived from the posterior division of the femoral nerve. It is the only nerve from the lumbar plexus to provide cutaneous innervation below the knee. As the saphenous nerve descends the leg, it follows the posterior surface of the sartorius muscle to its tendinous insertion on the tibia. At the medial border of the patella, the nerve divides into infrapatellar and distal cutaneous branches that provide sensory innervation to the medial aspect of the leg from the knee to the medial malleolus.

Ultrasound visualization of the saphenous nerve may be performed either above or below the knee. To visualize the saphenous nerve below the knee, the ultrasound probe is placed perpendicular to the long axis of the limb on the medial aspect of the proximal leg. At this location, the saphenous vein should be easily identified and used as an anatomical landmark. Excessive downward pressure on the probe collapses the vein and prevents it from being readily visible. The anatomical relationship between the saphenous nerve and the saphenous vein is highly predictable. The small, round hyperechoic nerve is consistently located posterior (i.e., deep) and medial to the vein (Figure 33). Because the saphenous nerve is both small and superficial, a high-frequency linear probe is recommended for optimal imaging.

To visualize the saphenous nerve above the knee, the ultrasound probe is placed perpendicular to the limb on the medial aspect of the distal thigh. The nerve is identified as a round hyperechoic structure within the fascia medial to the vastus medialis muscle (Figure 34). It is beneficial to be familiar with both anatomical locations of the saphenous nerve because the sonographic image quality may differ significantly from patient to patient and from location to location (i.e., above versus below the knee).

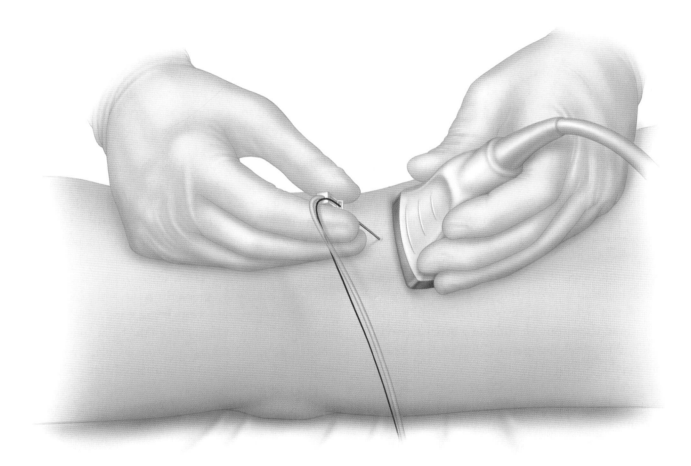

Figure 29. Popliteal ultrasound probe position, showing a posterior needle approach.

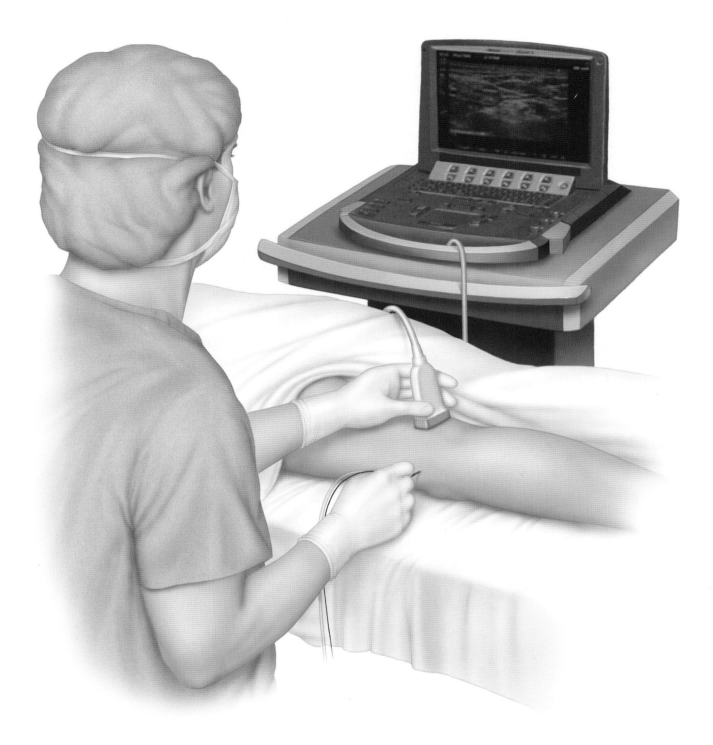

Figure 30. Popliteal ultrasound probe position, showing a lateral needle approach.

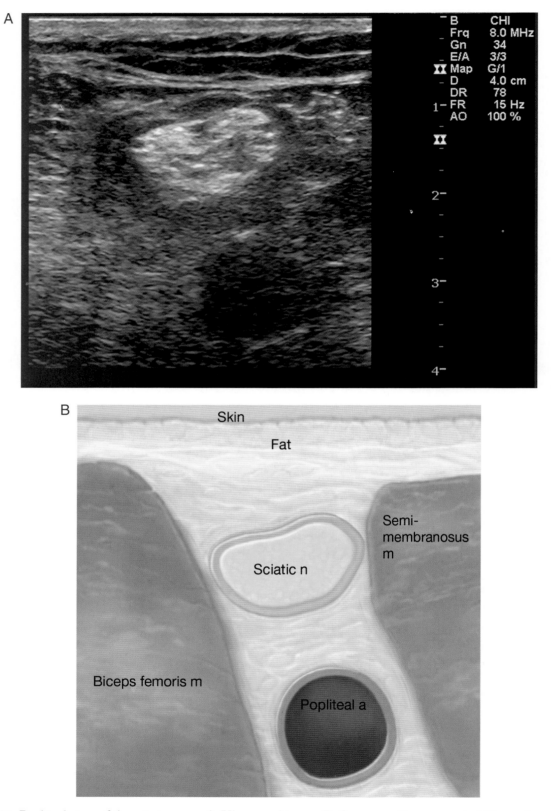

Figure 31. Popliteal view of the sciatic nerve. A, Ultrasound image. B, Corresponding anatomical illustration.

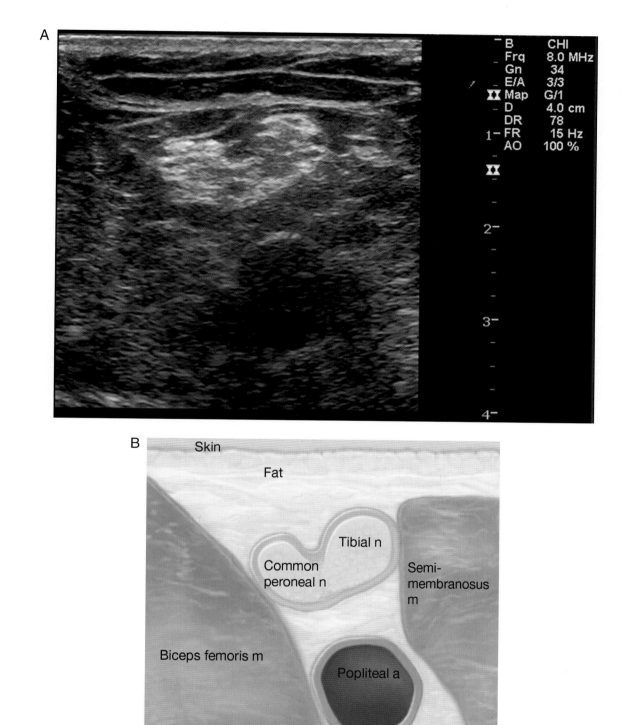

Figure 32. Popliteal view of the tibial and common peroneal nerves. A, Ultrasound image. B, Corresponding anatomical illustration.

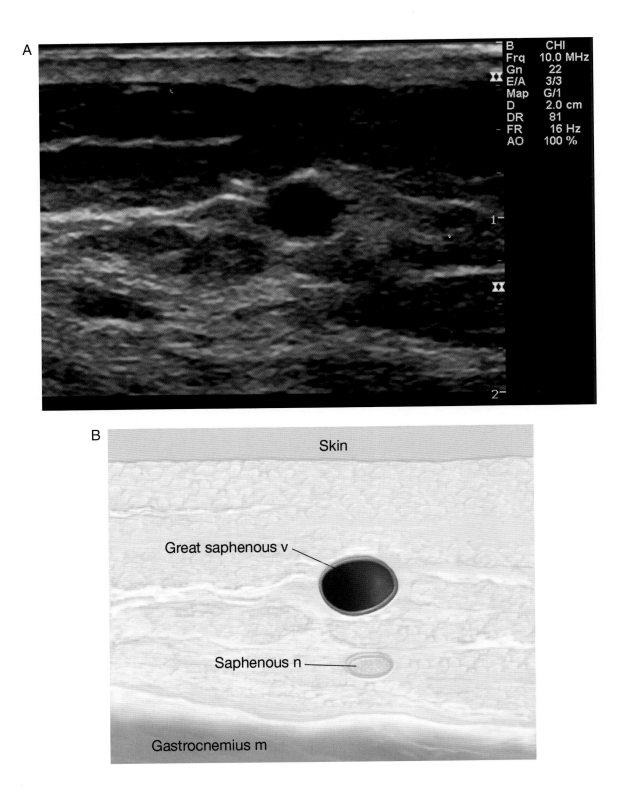

Figure 33. Paravenous view of the saphenous nerve. A, Ultrasound image. B, Corresponding anatomical illustration.

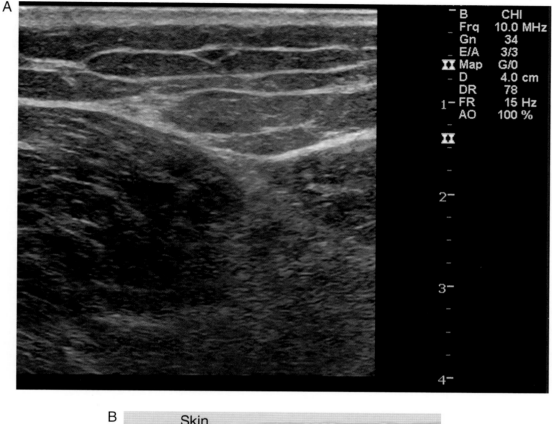

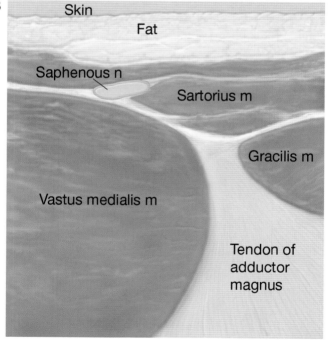

Figure 34. Transsartorial view of the saphenous nerve. A, Ultrasound image. B, Corresponding anatomical illustration.

Suggested Reading

Chan VW, Perlas A, Rawson R, Odukoya O. Ultrasound-guided supraclavicular brachial plexus block. Anesth Analg. 2003 Nov;97(5):1514-7.

De Andrés J, Sala-Blanch X. Ultrasound in the practice of brachial plexus anesthesia. Reg Anesth Pain Med. 2002 Jan-Feb;27(1):77-89.

Demondion X, Herbinet P, Boutry N, Fontaine C, Francke JP, Cotten A. Sonographic mapping of the normal brachial plexus. AJNR Am J Neuroradiol. 2003 Aug;24(7):1303-9.

Greher M, Kapral S. Is regional anesthesia simply an exercise in applied sonoanatomy? Aiming at higher frequencies of ultrasonographic imaging. Anesthesiology. 2003 Aug;99(2):250-1.

Kapral S, Krafft P, Eibenberger K, Fitzgerald R, Gosch M, Weinstabl C. Ultrasound-guided supraclavicular approach for regional anesthesia of the brachial plexus. Anesth Analg. 1994 Mar;78(3):507-13.

Krombach J, Gray AT. Sonography for saphenous nerve block near the adductor canal. Reg Anesth Pain Med. 2007 Jul-Aug;32(4):369-70. Erratum in: Reg Anesth Pain Med. 2007 Nov-Dec;32(6):536.

Perlas A, Chan VW, Simons M. Brachial plexus examination and localization using ultrasound and electrical stimulation: a volunteer study. Anesthesiology. 2003 Aug;99(2):429-35.

Sandhu NS, Capan LM. Ultrasound-guided infraclavicular brachial plexus block. Br J Anaesth. 2002 Aug;89(2):254-9.

Sinha A, Chan VW. Ultrasound imaging for popliteal sciatic nerve block. Reg Anesth Pain Med. 2004 Mar-Apr;29(2):130-4.

Yang WT, Chui PT, Metreweli C. Anatomy of the normal brachial plexus revealed by sonography and the role of sonographic guidance in anesthesia of the brachial plexus. AJR Am J Roentgenol. 1998 Dec;171(6):1631-6.

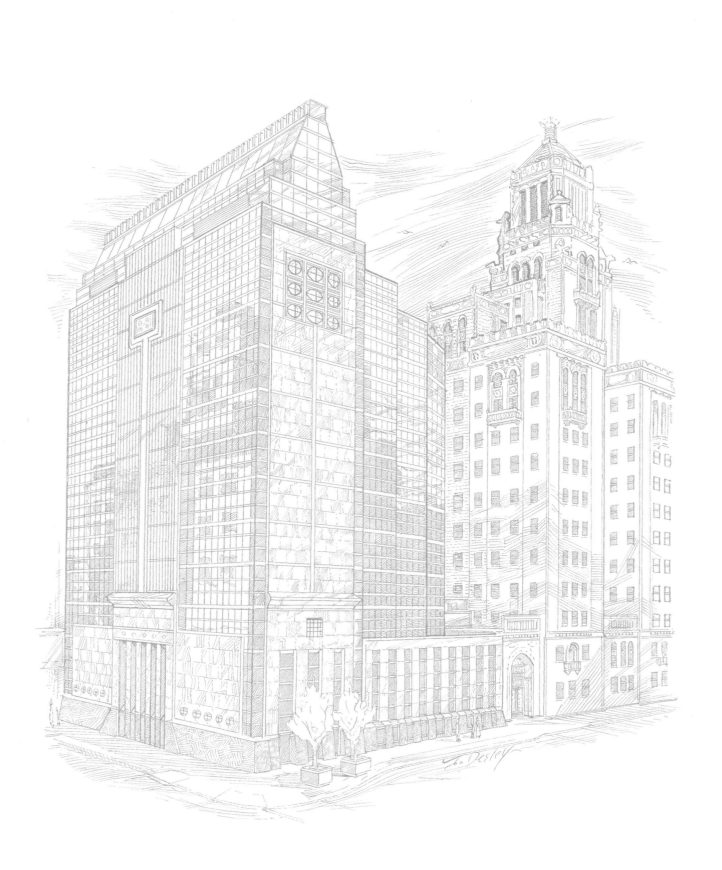

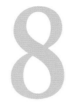
Clinical Applications of Ultrasound-Guided Regional Anesthesia

Hugh M. Smith, M.D., Ph.D.

Nearly every segment of neuroanatomy—from the trunks of the brachial plexus to the terminal branches of the lower extremity—can be visualized and blocked using high-resolution ultrasonography. This capability no longer requires providers to be dependent on traditional, landmark-based methods of neural localization. Although ultrasound-guided regional techniques may be performed at nearly any level, efficient blockade using a minimum number of needle punctures is best performed at proximal locations where nerves are bundled closely together. These proximal sites may also be associated with major vasculature, pleura, and other anatomical structures that clinicians hope to avoid while performing peripheral blockade. Therefore, the ability to visualize the needle in real time and accurately deposit local anesthetic around perineural structures may theoretically improve the safety and success of upper and lower extremity regional techniques.

The previous two chapters outlined the fundamental principles of ultrasound technology and the sonoanatomy of the upper and lower extremity. This chapter completes the learning triad by exploring the technical proficiency and clinical applications of ultrasound-guided regional anesthetic techniques (Figure 1). Developing the manual dexterity and coordination to advance a needle during real-time visualization may be facilitated by understanding several technical aspects of ultrasound guidance.

Ultrasound-Guided Regional Anesthesia

The performance of ultrasound-guided regional anesthetic techniques can be divided into six essential steps:

1. *Preparation*: Position the patient and prepare the ultrasound equipment and regional block tray
2. *Visualization*: Identify and optimize images of relevant anatomy
3. *Approximation*: Determine the optimal needle approach and puncture site. Bring the needle into proximity with the nerve
4. *Interrogation*: Interrogate neural targets with nerve stimulation to confirm their identity (optional)
5. *Deposition*: Deposit local anesthetic circumferentially around the neural target, repositioning the needle as needed to produce satisfactory spread
6. *Evaluation*: Assess the degree of sensorimotor blockade to determine success or the need for block supplementation

Mastery of ultrasound-guided regional procedures requires a familiarity with and progression through each of the six essential steps.

Step 1: Preparation

Preparation includes patient positioning, monitor placement, application of a sterile cover over the transducer, and preparation of the regional equipment (block tray, required needles and catheters, local anesthetics, sterile dressing). Patients are placed in a position that allows optimal anatomical scanning, proceduralist ergonomics, and patient comfort. The ultrasound machine is commonly placed next to the patient opposite the side to be blocked. A stool or small chair for the proceduralist provides stable positioning during the block. The skin should be widely prepped and draped with sterile towels or paper drapes. Fenestrated drapes may restrict the movement of the ultrasound probe and are not easily adjusted or repositioned. Before the sterile cover (adhesive cover or sterile sheath) is placed over the probe, sterile gel should be applied to the skin, and all needles (skin infiltration and block needles), catheters, and local anesthetics placed within easy reach.

Proper aseptic technique requires placing a sterile cover over the lens of the ultrasound probe. How this is accomplished depends on the ultrasound equipment and whether a flat or convex lens is used on the scanning surface of the probe. For example, probes with lenses that are flush with the scanning surface can be effectively covered with a clear adhesive cover (e.g., Opsite or Tegaderm dressing) (Figure 2 A). Under these conditions, no gel is required between the probe and the cover. However, the cover should be stretched tightly and secured to the probe without creating air pockets, bubbles, or wrinkles. In contrast, probes that use an elevated lens must be placed within a sterile sheath or sleeve with ultrasound scanning

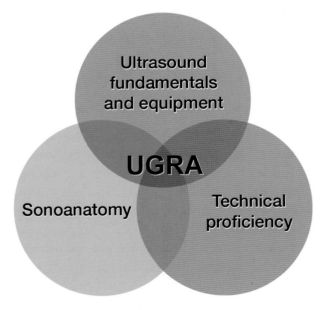

Figure 1. Skill sets needed for ultrasound-guided regional anesthesia (UGRA).

gel (Figure 2 B). The use of an adhesive cover on a probe with an elevated lens invariably leads to the formation of air bubbles and contact artifact. In general, any wrinkle, air bubble, or gel insufficiency can lead to contact artifacts that will substantially diminish the image quality.

Step 2: Visualization

Scanning to identify relevant anatomy should commence once preparation is complete. Scanning movements include sliding, angling, rotating, tilting, and changes in downward probe pressure (Figure 3). The correct scanning movements and probe orientation are those that produce the best image of the relevant neuroanatomy and the path between the skin and neural target. Because the majority of neural targets in the brachial plexus are associated with vascular structures (e.g., supraclavicular, infraclavicular, axillary), an artery is typically the easiest landmark to identify. Vascular structures are usually best seen in cross-section, with probe pressure distinguishing between arterial and venous anatomy. Mild to moderate probe pressure easily collapses venous structures while maintaining the integrity of arterial vasculature. However, considerable pressure can collapse arteries and help distinguish them from nerves.

It is important to identify precisely where the neural targets are optimally seen and then mark the location on the skin or stabilize the probe at that site. Once the optimal image is obtained, it may be difficult or even impossible to maintain the image with either patient or provider movement. After the needle enters the tissue, small, subtle hand movements (predominantly proximal and distal sliding) are often all that are necessary to keep the needle and neural target(s) in view.

Step 3: Approximation

Needle approximation includes determining how best to bring a needle into proximity to a nerve. Two basic approaches are commonly used during ultrasound-guided regional anesthesia—the *in-plane* (IP) and *out-of-plane* (OOP) approaches. The selected approach will determine whether the needle is seen along its entire length (in-plane) or in cross-section (out-of-plane). If the needle is inserted and advanced parallel to the

ultrasound probe, the needle is considered to be in-plane with the ultrasound beam (Figure 4). In contrast, the out-of-plane approach involves inserting the needle perpendicular to the ultrasound probe, effectively imaging a small cross-sectional segment of the needle as it passes through the ultrasound beam (Figure 5).

Each approach produces a different image of the needle and has distinct advantages and disadvantages. In-plane needle imaging allows complete visualization of the needle and the associated safety advantage of being able to see the needle throughout the procedure. However, it is technically difficult to maintain complete beam-needle alignment. In addition, the in-plane approach may result in greater patient discomfort because the needle typically traverses through a longer course of tissue planes than with out-of-plane approaches. Out-of-plane needle techniques are most useful for superficial targets or cannulating vessels. Compared with in-plane needle imaging, out-of-plane approaches do not produce good needle visualization because the ultrasound beam cuts cross-sectionally through the needle, leaving only a small bright hyperechoic sphere reflecting its location (Figure 5 B). Although this is easily seen in a homogeneous artificial gel model, the varying densities of human tissue create more visual challenges. Furthermore, the hyperechoic sphere confirms only that the ultrasound beam has "sliced" through the needle somewhere along its shaft—providing no information about the precise location of the tip. During the out-of-plane approach, position of the needle tip can be estimated by the downward appearance of tissue displacement during needle advancement. Proceduralists must become adept at scanning down the shaft of the needle to determine precisely where the needle ends. When the cross-sectional image of the needle disappears, the ultrasound beam has just traveled past the distal tip of the needle.

During needle approximation, advancement of the needle should occur only when the shaft of the needle (in-plane approach) or distal needle tip (out-of-plane approach) is visualized in its entirety. Ideally, this should occur along the entire trajectory to the neural target. Equally important is precisely how the needle approaches the nerve.

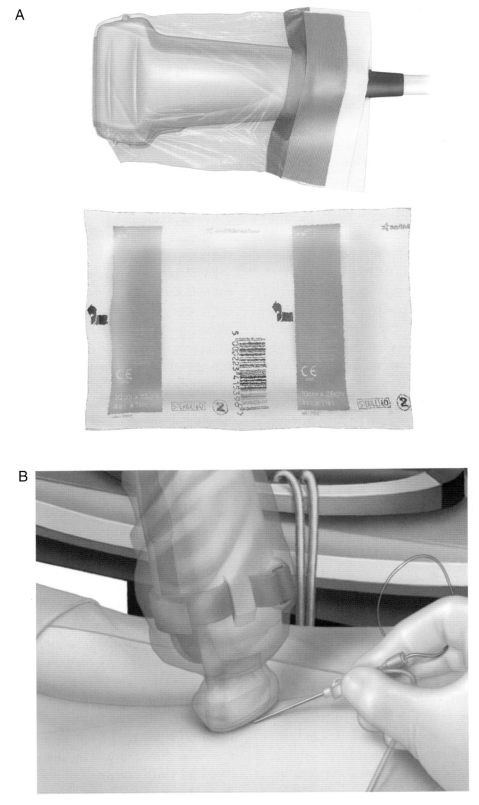

Figure 2. Sterile ultrasound probe covers. A, Adhesive cover. B, Sleeve cover.

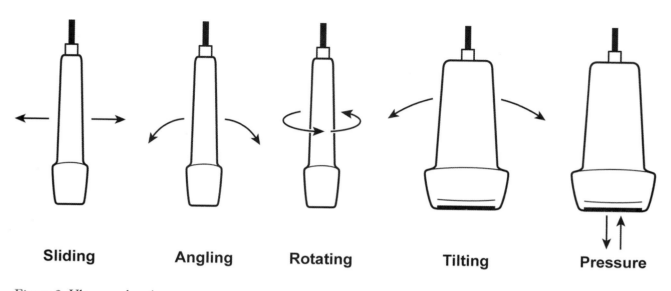

Sliding   Angling   Rotating   Tilting   Pressure

Figure 3. Ultrasound probe movements.

Given that complete needle visualization is unlikely to occur at all times, providers should avoid directing the needle toward the center of the neural target. For example, if the needle is advanced toward the middle of the nerve while the tip is in poor view, inadvertent neural injury may occur from needle trauma or intraneural injection. Rather, the needle should be directed toward the top or bottom of the nerve if it is approaching from a lateral or medial direction or to the right or left of the nerve if it is approaching from a vertical direction. The use of *hydrodissection*, or the separation of tissue planes through the injection of local anesthetic or other fluid through the needle, and routinely withdrawing the needle away from the nerve just before injection helps prevent direct needle-to-nerve contact.

Step 4: Interrogation

Nerve stimulation to interrogate anatomical structures has clinical utility in several situations: 1) when it is unclear whether the anatomical structure in question is a nerve or other anatomical tissue, 2) when distinguishing nerves by motor response has important clinical consequences (e.g., surgery within a specific cutaneous distribution), or 3) when neural tissue is not seen because of poor image quality. In the last case, nerve stimulation may discover the location of a neural target while ultrasound

is used to guide the needle to common anatomical locations. The injection of local anesthetic commonly makes previously undetectable nerves visible because the fluid collection functions as an acoustic window that separates the nerve from surrounding tissues of similar density and appearance.

The interrogation of nerves may also have educational value. Confirming nerve location by stimulation and identification of corresponding motor responses may help learners understand the anatomical position and sonographic appearance of neural structures. In addition, nerve interrogation may help providers develop confidence in their ultrasonography skills, particularly when first learning ultrasound-guided techniques. However, as a provider's skill level increases, nerve stimulation may become less useful, or even detrimental, under select clinical conditions. For example, nerve stimulation requires additional procedural time and direct needle contact with the nerve, which may theoretically increase the risk of nerve injury by direct needle contact. Interrogation is rarely necessary during ultrasound-guided blockade of the proximal brachial plexus (e.g., interscalene and supraclavicular blockade) because neural targets are generally large and easily visible within these regions. Nerve stimulation provides little benefit for these proximal procedures.

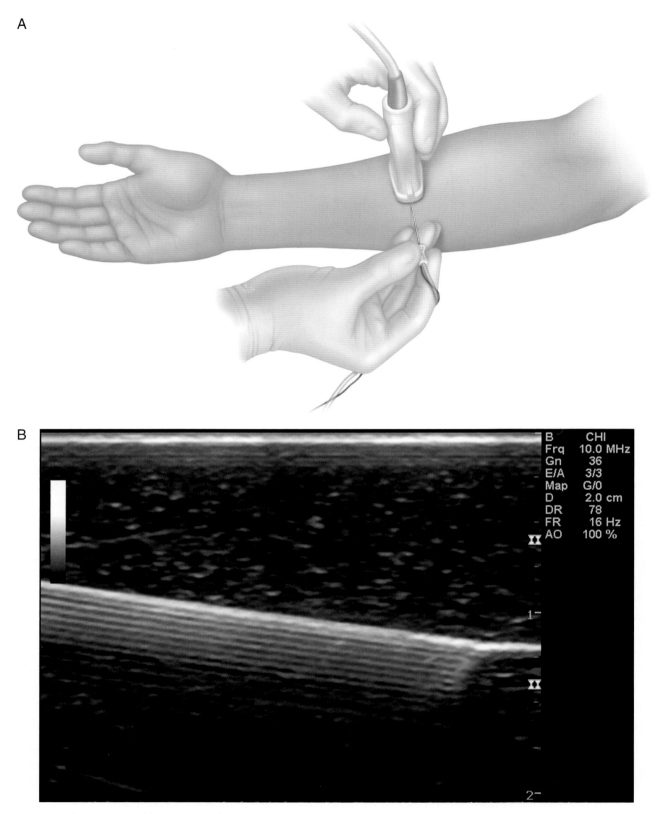

Figure 4. In-plane needle approach. A, Needle-probe orientation. B, Ultrasound image.

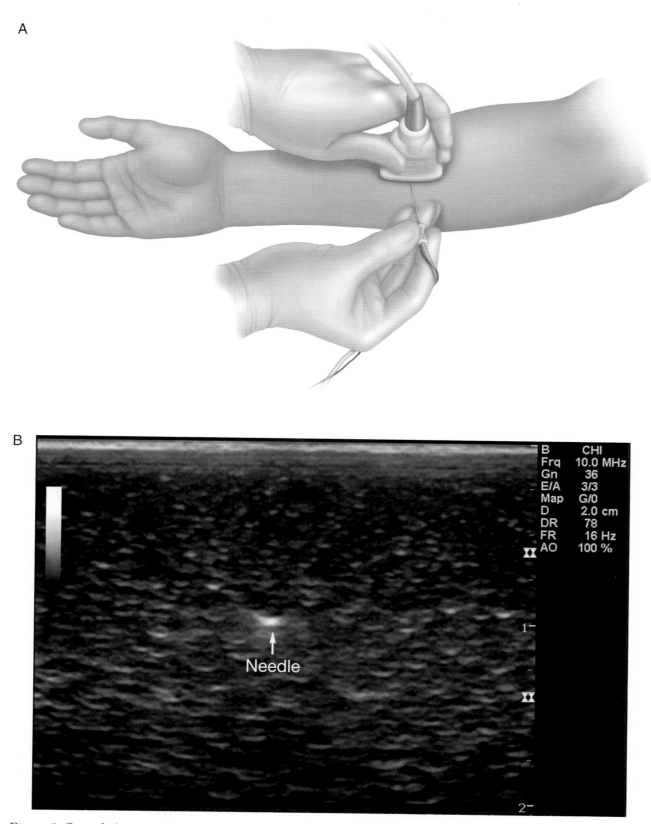

Figure 5. Out-of-plane needle approach. A, Needle-probe orientation. B, Ultrasound image.

Proceduralists who routinely use nerve stimulation in conjunction with ultrasound soon discover that failure to elicit a motor response can occur frequently. In fact, failed neural stimulation may occur between 13% and 23% of the time. This phenomenon has yet to be fully explained. However, its occurrence suggests that further investigation is warranted regarding the precise mechanism(s) and limitations of traditional peripheral nerve stimulation techniques.

Step 5: Deposition
Ultimately, the objective of any ultrasound-guided regional technique is to place the needle in a position that allows deposition of local anesthetic around a nerve. The result of a successful ultrasound-guided block is the circumferential spread of local anesthetic around the nerve (Figure 6). This has euphemistically been referred to as a "donut" sign. The practice of directing the needle anterior or posterior to the nerve to avoid inadvertent needle-to-nerve contact may reduce the risk of unrecognized intraneural injection (Figure 6).

Frequently, initial attempts to deposit local anesthetic around a nerve identify a fascial boundary that prevents complete circumferential spread. Under these conditions, the needle should be repositioned within the plane of the neural target to ensure that local anesthetic adequately surrounds the nerve. When entirely surrounded by local anesthetic, the nerve appears to float within the dark hypoechoic fluid collection (Figure 6 B). The local anesthetic volume required to produce complete circumferential spread is surprisingly low under many circumstances. For example, a few milliliters of local anesthetic is all that is needed to completely surround the terminal branches of the brachial plexus. Proponents of ultrasonography suggest that volume reduction is a potential safety advantage of ultrasound-guided techniques. However, current data are insufficient to definitively support these claims of increased safety.

Step 6: Evaluation
The evaluation of all regional blocks is an essential component of learning ultrasound-guided regional techniques. Repeated failures or deficiencies within a specific nerve distribution may indicate that the provider needs to review ultrasound sonoanatomy, optimize needle approximation, ensure proper neural interrogation, or confirm the spread of local anesthetic. Furthermore, the early identification of a failed or incomplete block allows the provider adequate time to consider all rescue options. For example, ultrasound-guided block supplementation, local infiltration by the surgeon, or conversion to general anesthesia may all be considered.

Practitioners of regional anesthesia will inevitably be faced with the occasional failed or incomplete peripheral nerve block. Anatomical variation, provider inexperience, and technical limitations may all contribute to inadequate or incomplete anesthesia. Rescue blockade, or block supplementation, can salvage an incomplete block and prevent patients from requiring a general anesthetic. However, block supplementation of a partially anesthetized extremity remains a controversial practice. Many experts suggest that block supplementation may increase the risk of neurologic complications or other adverse events. However, the ability of ultrasound-guided technology to provide real-time needle and nerve visualization seems ideally suited to minimize potential complications. The following procedural recommendations may *theoretically* enhance block safety during ultrasound-guided block supplementation: 1) ensure complete needle-beam alignment, 2) advance the needle only when completely in view, 3) direct the needle toward the top or bottom or to the right or left of neural targets, 4) slightly withdraw the needle from the nerve before injection to avoid needle-to-nerve contact and inadvertent intraneural injection, and 5) use hydrodissection with local anesthetic or other fluid to improve visualization of the needle tip during advancement toward the nerve.

Clinical Pearls
Needle imaging within patients can be a clinical challenge for even the most experienced ultrasonographer. However, several technical maneuvers and clinical pearls can increase the chance of optimal visualization. It is preferable to visualize the needle tip at all times. However, knowing its precise location through surrogate markers and other

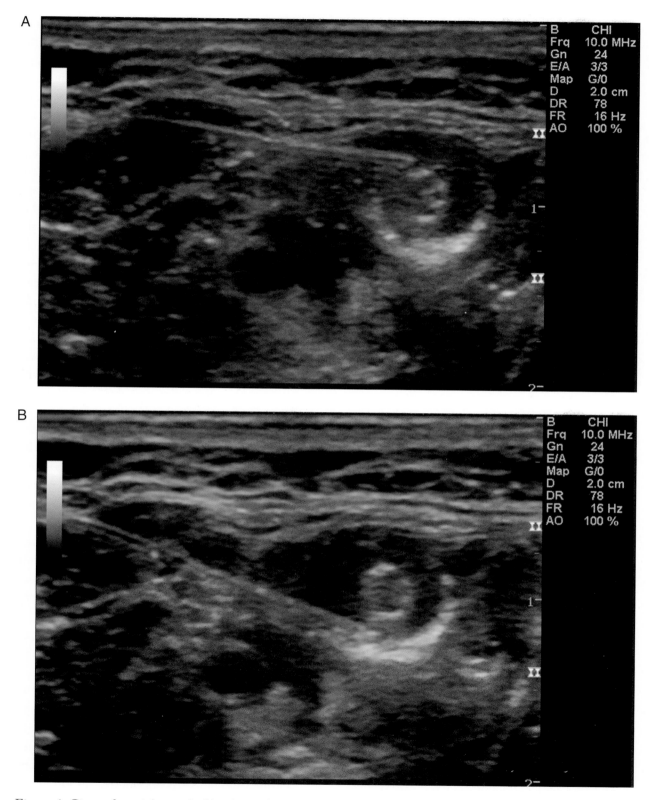

Figure 6. Circumferential spread of local anesthetic. A, Needle trajectory anterior to the nerve. B, Needle trajectory posterior to the nerve.

sources of information may be an acceptable substitute for more experienced ultrasonographers.

- *Needle movement*: Small, rapid movements of the needle (i.e., wiggling), without advancement or withdrawal, produce tissue motion that reveals the location of the needle tip.
- *Elevation of needle tip*: Downward pressure on the hub of the needle elevates the needle shaft and deforms the tissue along its length. The area of tissue deformity can be distinguished from an area of undisturbed tissue—the boundary of which identifies the needle tip. This technique is more appropriate for in-plane needle approaches.
- *Hydrodissection*: The injection of small volumes of local anesthetic, dextrose, or normal saline separates tissue planes and reveals a small, hypoechoic fluid collection at the needle tip. The use of dextrose (a nonconducting solution) preserves the ability to interrogate neural structures with nerve stimulation by decreasing the conductive surface area and increasing the current density at the needle tip. In contrast, the injection of conducting solutions such as local anesthetics or normal saline increases the total conductive surface area at the needle tip, thereby dispersing the current and reducing the current density at the neural target. Hydrodissection is particularly useful for identifying the needle tip during out-of-plane approaches. However, its effectiveness at separating tissue planes is useful with both in-plane and out-of-plane approaches.
- *Color Doppler*: Color Doppler features may be useful for revealing fluid in motion. The highest fluid velocity during injection occurs at the tip of the needle, where the intense color on Doppler reveals the location of the needle tip. The use of color Doppler is particularly useful when deeper imaging (and poor needle visualization) is required.
- *Perpendicular needle-to-beam orientation*: Steep needle trajectories result in low ultrasound signal return to the probe (Figure 7 A). In contrast, shallow needle trajectories are able to maintain a perpendicular needle-to-beam orientation and produce a higher intensity ultrasound signal (Figure 7 B). If a shallow needle path is not feasible because of anatomical

restraints, tilting, or "heeling," the transducer to create a more perpendicular angle of incidence can substantially improve needle viewing. Tilting requires placing pressure on the side of the probe farthest away from the needle hub without losing probe-to-skin contact on the near side. For in-plane approaches, it is advantageous to make the needle insertion site in a location that optimizes a 90° needle-to-beam orientation.

- *Echogenic needles*: Specially designed insulated and noninsulated echogenic needles reflect a higher percentage of the ultrasound beam back to the transducer and thus result in better visualization. The echogenic segment is generally located at the distal tip of the needle (Figure 8 A). As a result, echogenic needles may be particularly useful when steep needle trajectories are required or unavoidable because of clinical circumstances or surrounding anatomical structures. In contrast, nonechogenic needles result in lower signal intensity at similar angles (Figure 8 B).
- *Practice*: The safety and success of ultrasound-guided regional anesthesia is highly dependent on direct observation of both the needle tip and the neural target(s) throughout the procedure. Needle visualization is a critical skill in ultrasound-guided regional anesthesia and requires practice and mastery before patient encounters. Needle imaging can be practiced with artificial gel pads or other forms of simulation media.
- *Assumptions*: When performing ultrasound-guided regional techniques, an important assumption to avoid is that "what is visible on the monitor is all that is there." This is a poor assumption for several reasons. First, ultrasound may fail to provide adequate resolution to delineate small structures. For example, the phrenic nerve is rarely seen during ultrasound imaging despite its predictable anatomical location superficial to the anterior scalene muscle. Clinicians performing an in-plane interscalene block from a medial to lateral direction may unknowingly bring the needle in proximity to the phrenic nerve and increase the risk of traumatic nerve injury. Second, clinicians must remain cognizant that the ultrasound beam is only 1 mm wide. Because this narrow "window" is capable of depicting only a two-dimensional

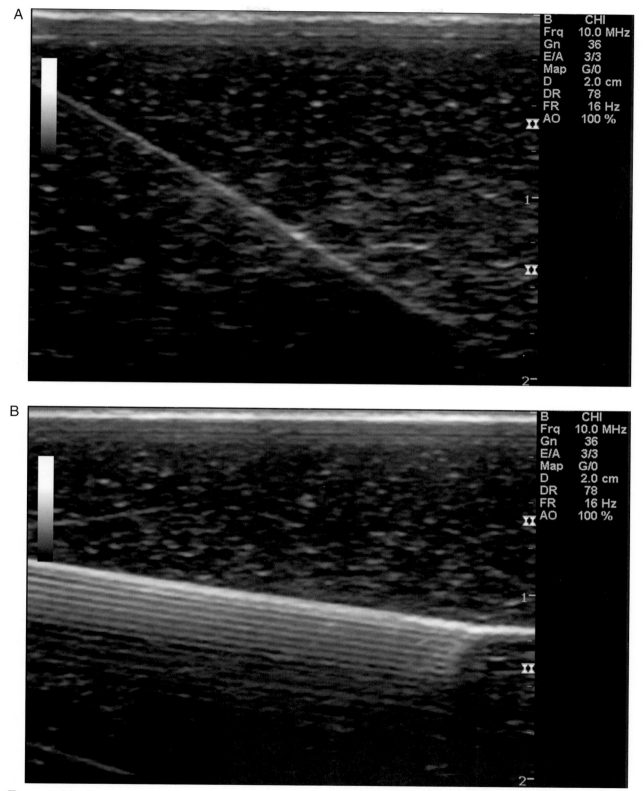

Figure 7. Needle trajectory and signal intensity. A, Steep needle trajectory. B, Shallow needle trajectory with reverberation artifact.

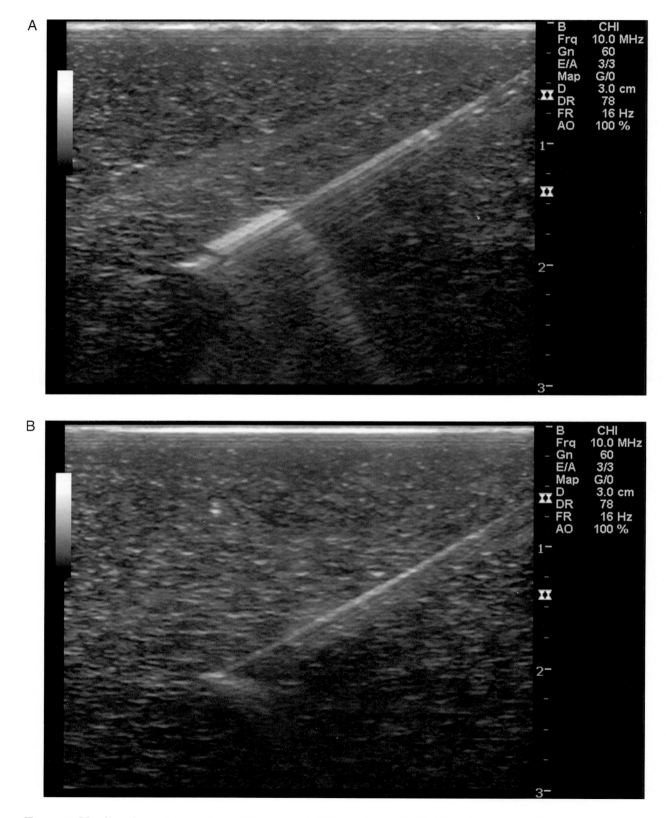

Figure 8. Needle echogenicity and signal intensity. A, Echogenic needle. B, Nonechogenic needle.

image of a three-dimensional object, anatomical structures may travel through the tissue on either side of the ultrasound beam and not appear on the monitor. However, these structures can easily be encountered by needles that wander outside of alignment with the ultrasound beam. Finally, various artifacts can easily distort the ultrasound image and disguise the true location of anatomical structures. Most clinicians agree that ultrasound-guided regional anesthesia is a potentially useful technologic advancement. However, recognizing its limitations may be equally important for understanding its usefulness and unique application.

Common Errors and Pitfalls

Two potential complications associated with regional anesthesia include nerve injury from intraneural injection and local anesthetic toxicity from intravascular injection. Both of these complications may occur during ultrasound-guided regional anesthesia. For example, the risk of intraneural injection may be increased when proceduralists fail to maintain complete needle visualization during an in-plane approach. This loss of visualization may occur when the ultrasound beam is obliquely oriented to the needle, resulting in a partial or incomplete view of the needle (Figure 9).

A second potential complication is intravascular injection. During an ultrasound-guided regional technique, failure to observe local anesthetic spread should be an indication to stop the injection. Witnessing local anesthetic (a hypoechoic solution) spread and the subsequent separation of tissues away from the needle tip confirms an *extravascular* needle location. Conversely, intravascular injection of local anesthetic during ultrasonography appears similar to intravascular dye injection during fluoroscopy. Failure to see local anesthetic spread should prompt clinicians to stop injecting and reassess needle location. Minimal volumes of local anesthetic or other injectable solutions are required to cause tissue separation and the classic hypoechoic appearance (1-2 mL). If doubt persists about needle location and the proximity to vessels, dextrose or saline solution can be substituted and fluid spread

demonstrated before local anesthetic injection. However, incremental injection of local anesthetic and querying patients for early signs and symptoms of central nervous system excitation remain part of prudent practice for the identification of unrecognized intravascular injection or systemic vascular uptake.

Another common mistake of experienced regional anesthesia providers (but novice ultrasonographers) is to use ultrasound as an adjunct to landmark-based or traditional regional anesthetic techniques. Although it may be appealing to "add" direct visualization to a technique familiar to the provider, this approach commonly results in poor clinical outcomes and provider dissatisfaction. Traditional needle trajectories and cross-sectional ultrasound views rarely coincide. Therefore, the goal of the provider should be to acquire an optimal ultrasound image of the relevant neuroanatomy, regardless of classic surface landmarks used during traditional techniques. Once the ideal image has been acquired, the provider need only determine the needle approach (in-plane versus out-of-plane) and site of insertion. Needle insertion sites for ultrasound-guided regional techniques are typically different from those used during conventional methods and should not be determined before ultrasound scanning and image acquisition.

Ultrasound-Guided Continuous Regional Anesthesia

The use of ultrasound-guided technology for the placement of perineural catheters has been described for both upper and lower extremity surgery. Although the fundamental principles and technical aspects of ultrasound are relevant during the sonographic placement of peripheral nerve catheters, several distinguishing features require comment. First, single-injection techniques require only that local anesthetic distribution encapsulate the neural target. The needle trajectory used to accomplish this may be highly variable and dependent on anatomical site, patient body habitus, and provider preference. In contrast, needle trajectories used to place perineural catheters adjacent to peripheral nerves may be restricted. Consequently, out-of-plane techniques may offer some utility in that

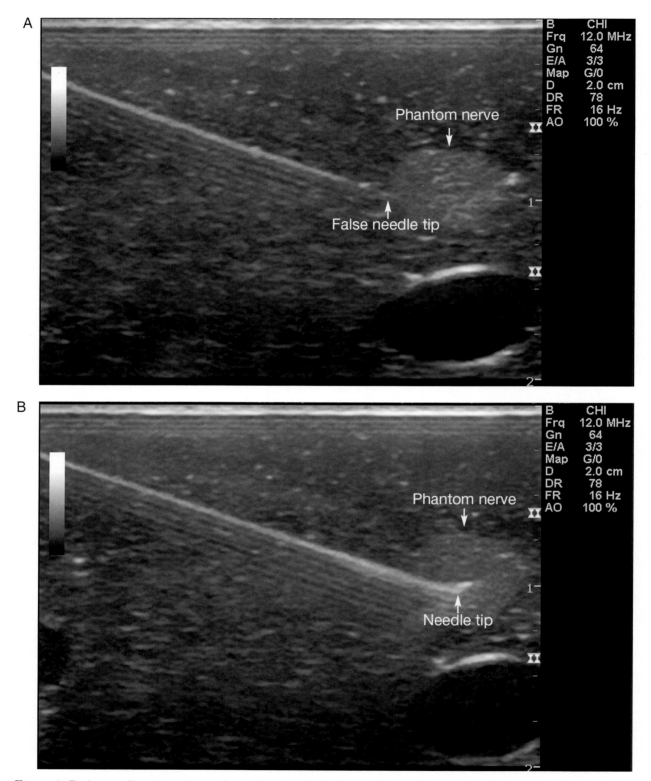

Figure 9. Probe-needle orientation and visualization. A, Probe-needle misalignment results in incomplete visualization and false identification of extraneuronal needle placement. B, Proper needle-probe alignment results in complete needle visualization and correct identification of intraneuronal needle placement.

the nerves can still be well visualized in cross-section while the needle and catheter are inserted along the longitudinal axis of the nerve. Dextrose-containing solutions can be incrementally injected to provide hydrodissection and to identify the needle tip location during needle approximation.

Another difficulty commonly encountered during the placement of perineural catheters is the challenge of having both of the proceduralist's hands available during catheter insertion. This typically requires setting the ultrasound probe down to insert or advance the catheter, a step that results in the temporary loss of visualization of both the needle and the catheter. A potential solution to this problem is the use of a device designed to hold the ultrasound probe in a fixed location, allowing continuous real-time visualization while freeing the provider's hands for catheter placement (Figure 10).

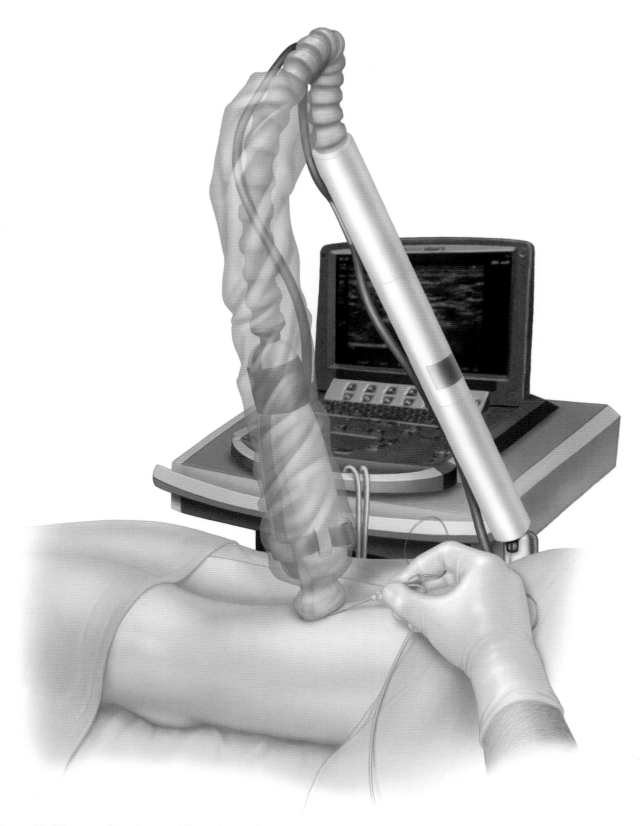

Figure 10. Ultrasound-probe stand for catheter placement.

Suggested Reading

Brull R, McCartney CJ, Chan VW. A novel approach to infraclavicular brachial plexus block: the ultrasound experience. Anesth Analg. 2004 Sep;99(3):950.

Chan VW, Perlas A, Rawson R, Odukoya O. Ultrasound-guided supraclavicular brachial plexus block. Anesth Analg. 2003 Nov;97(5):1514-7.

Perlas A, Chan VW, Simons M. Brachial plexus examination and localization using ultrasound and electrical stimulation: a volunteer study. Anesthesiology. 2003 Aug;99(2):429-35.

Sites BD, Gallagher JD, Cravero J, Lundberg J, Blike G. The learning curve associated with a simulated ultrasound-guided interventional task by inexperienced anesthesia residents. Reg Anesth Pain Med. 2004 Nov-Dec;29(6):544-8.

Urmey WF, Stanton J. Inability to consistently elicit a motor response following sensory paresthesia during interscalene block administration. Anesthesiology. 2002 Mar;96(3):552-4.

Upper Extremity Peripheral Nerve Block Techniques

CHAPTER

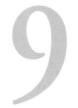

Cervical Plexus Blockade

Laurence C. Torsher, M.D.

James R. Hebl, M.D.

Cervical plexus blockade produces anesthesia of the neck, shoulder, and upper pectoral and occipital regions. The cervical plexus is divided into a deep and a superficial plexus. Each plexus has its own unique innervation, clinical applications, anatomical landmarks, and regional techniques.

Relevant Anatomy

The anterior primary rami of the first four cervical nerves (C1-C4) unite to form the cervical plexus.

The cervical nerves exit from the cervical vertebrae through a gutter in the transverse process immediately posterior to the vertebral artery (Figure 1). The plexus contributes to four primary neurologic entities: 1) the superficial cervical plexus, 2) the ansa cervicalis, 3) the spinal accessory nerve, and 4) the phrenic nerve. The superficial cervical plexus includes four cutaneous nerves that supply the skin of the head and neck from the area of the posterior aspect of the scalp to the supraclavicular fossa. The nerves of the superficial cervical plexus include 1) the lesser occipital,

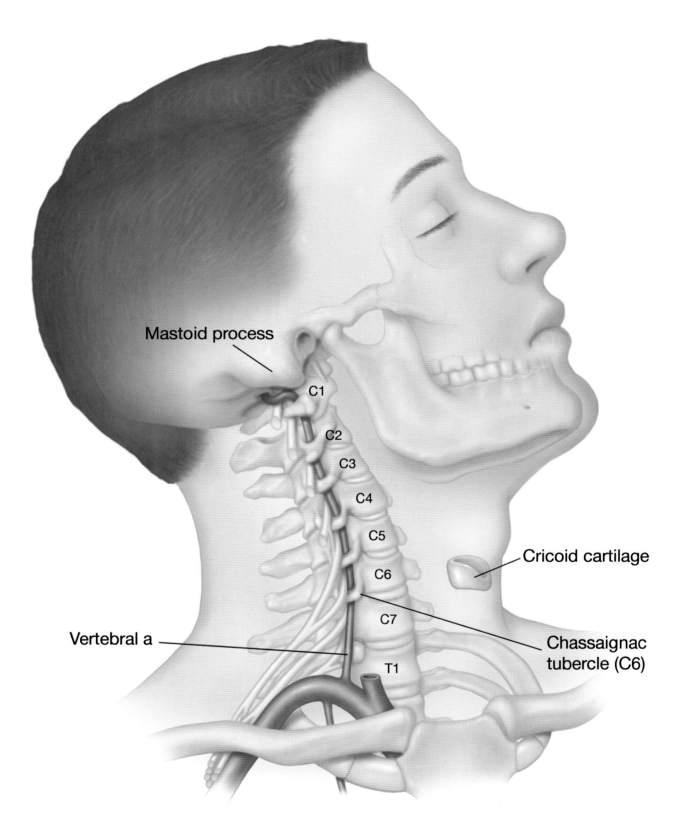

Figure 1. Cervical plexus neuroanatomy.

2) the great auricular, 3) the transverse cervical, and 4) the supraclavicular nerves (Figure 2). The first three of these nerves contain segments from C2 and C3. The supraclavicular nerve contains neural fibers from the C3 and C4 nerve roots. The motor nerves of the ansa cervicalis provide innervation to the suprahyoid (thyrohyoid and geniohyoid muscles) and infrahyoid (sternohyoid, sternothyroid, and omohyoid) musculature. C1 fibers descend the neck to form the superior root of the ansa (branch of cranial nerve XII), and fibers from C2 and C3 form the inferior root. The spinal accessory nerve is formed from the lateral aspect of the anterior horns of the five upper cervical segments. The nerve descends in the neck beneath the posterior belly of the digastric muscle, receiving branches from the anterior primary rami of C2, C3, and C4 before branching to innervate the sternocleidomastoid muscle. From this point, the spinal accessory nerve exits the posterior aspect of the muscle to descend further to innervate the superior aspect of the trapezius muscle. Finally, fibers from C3, C4, and C5 unite to form the phrenic nerve, which courses along the lateral border of the anterior scalene muscle before descending vertically over the ventral surface of this muscle to enter the chest along its medial border (Figure 3).

In conjunction with the superficial cervical plexus, blockade of the deep cervical plexus provides analgesia from the posterior occiput unilaterally to the angle of the jaw (C2 dermatome), down the neck (C3 dermatome) to the supraclavicular fossa (C4 dermatome) (Figure 4). It also provides analgesia to the deep facial layers and motor relaxation of all major muscles of the neck.

Deep Cervical Plexus Block .

Clinical Applications
The deep cervical plexus block is essentially a high cervical paravertebral block and is commonly used for unilateral neck procedures such as carotid endarterectomies, cervical node dissections, or plastic surgical procedures. Bilateral cervical plexus blockade has been described for thyroid surgery and elective tracheostomy. However, patients undergoing bilateral blockade are at risk for bilateral phrenic nerve paralysis and respiratory insufficiency (see "Side Effects and Complications" below).

Patient Position
The patient is positioned supine with the head slightly extended and rotated away from the side to be blocked (Figure 5).

Surface Anatomy and Landmarks
Important landmarks are the cervical transverse processes of C2, C3, and C4. The Chassaignac tubercle (the transverse process of C6) is identified by palpation of the cervical process at the level of the cricoid cartilage. A line is drawn from the mastoid process to the Chassaignac tubercle, and another line is drawn 1.5 cm posterior and parallel to the first line (Figure 5). The puncture site for C2 is approximately 1.5 cm caudad to the mastoid process along the second line. The C3 puncture site is 1.5 cm caudad from C2. Similarly, the C4 needle insertion site is 1.5 cm caudad to the puncture site of C3 along the second line (Figures 5 and 6).

Technique
At each of the three puncture sites (C2, C3, and C4), a 22-gauge 1.5-inch (3.8-cm) needle is advanced medially and slightly caudad to avoid entering the foramen of the cervical vertebra (Figures 5 and 6). The cervical transverse process should be contacted at a depth of 1.5 to 3.0 cm. A paresthesia should be elicited by moving the needle in an anteroposterior plane. All three needles (C2, C3, and C4) are placed before local anesthetic is injected. Before injection, aspiration is done to ensure that neither blood nor cerebrospinal fluid is withdrawn. Three to four milliliters of local anesthetic is injected at each site. Alternatively, a single injection of 10 to 12 mL of local anesthetic at the C4 needle insertion site may successfully anesthetize all three nerve roots (C2, C3, and C4). Anatomical communication beneath the deep cervical fascia, along the paravertebral space, makes this an attractive alternative to the multiple-injection technique.

Needle Redirection Cues
If the anterior tubercle of the transverse process is not contacted, the needle is redirected medially, slightly

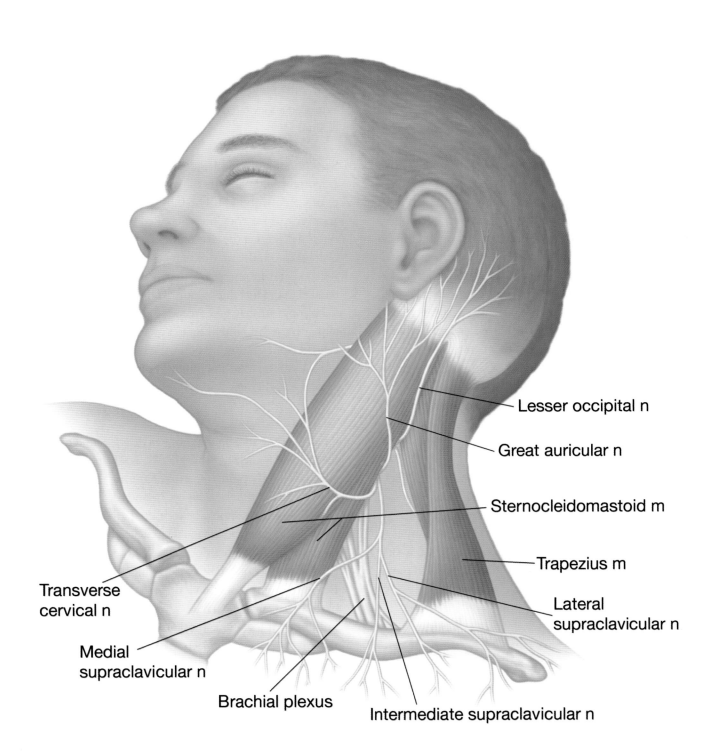

Figure 2. Superficial cervical plexus.

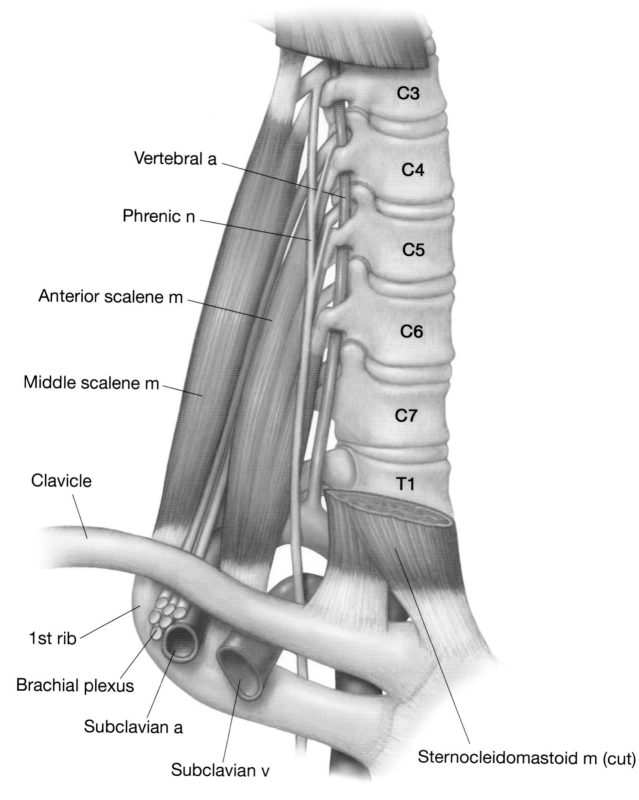

Figure 3. Phrenic nerve anatomy.

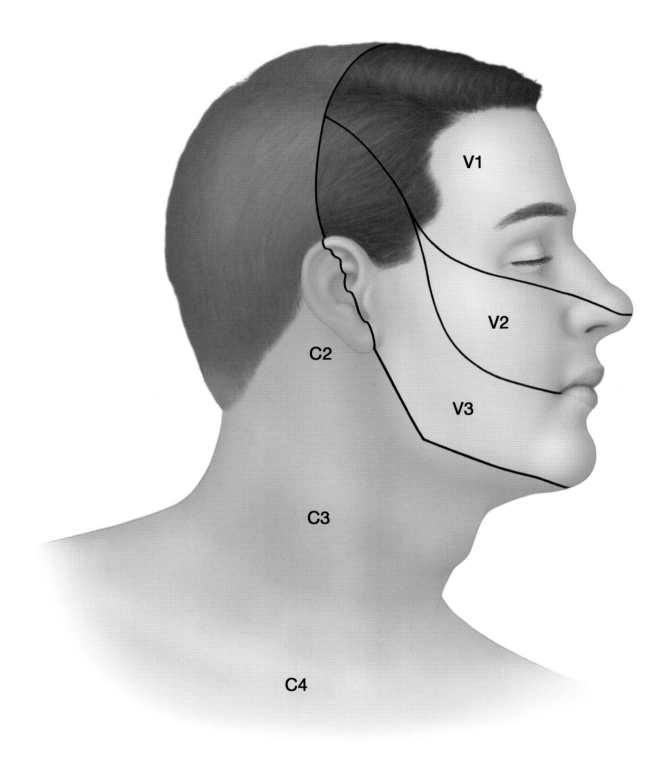

Figure 4. Cutaneous innervation of the deep cervical plexus.

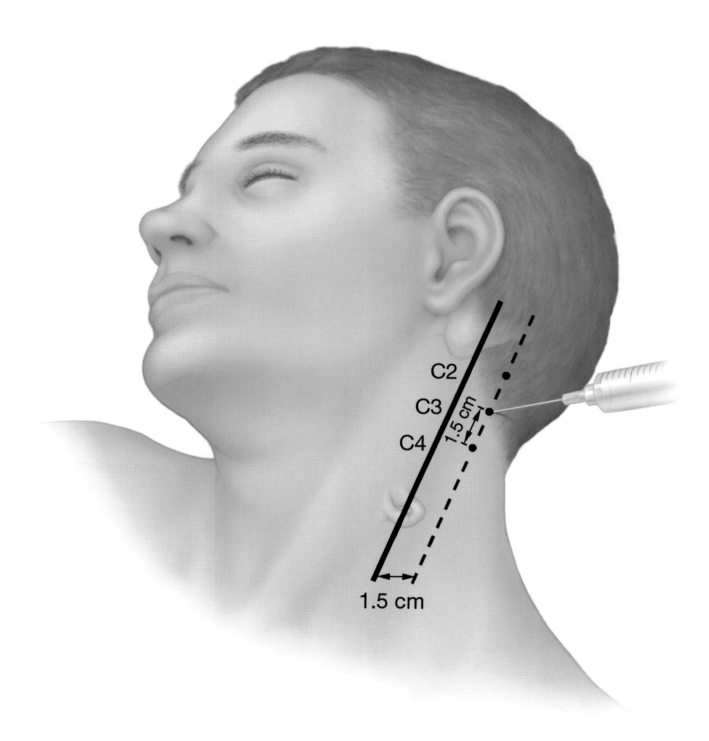

Figure 5. Patient position and surface landmarks for deep cervical plexus blockade.

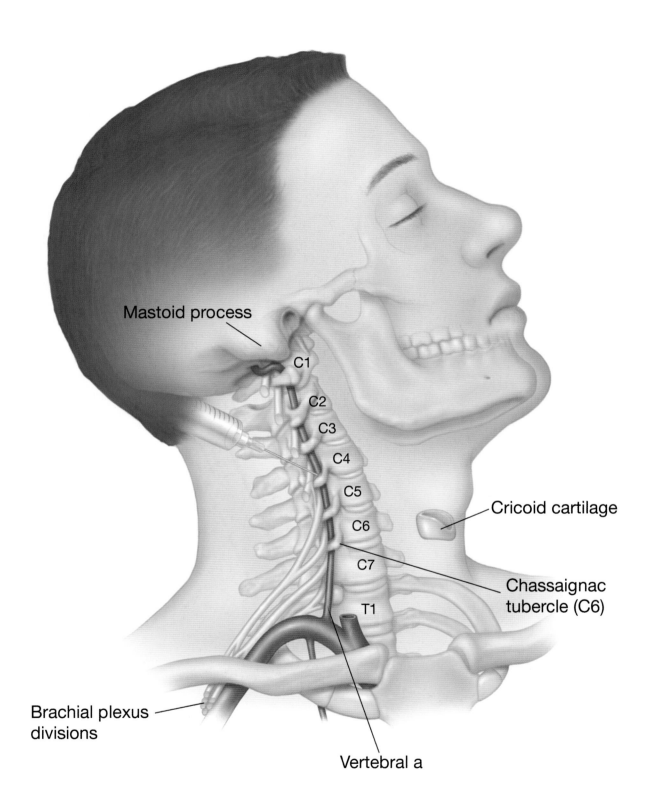

Figure 6. Deep cervical plexus blockade.

caudad, and "walked" in a vertical plane in 10° to 15° increments either inferiorly or superiorly. If the needle is advanced cephalad, it may enter the intervertebral foramen. Proper head position should be reconfirmed, all landmarks reassessed by direct palpation of the mastoid and transverse processes, and relative line projections confirmed. The insertion site is infiltrated intradermally and subcutaneously, blocking the cervical branches of the facial nerve, which innervate the platysma muscle. The patient may better tolerate the surgical procedure with a midline subcutaneous injection from the thyroid cartilage extending distally to the suprasternal notch (blocking the cervical nerve branches from the contralateral side). For carotid endarterectomy, the surgeon should infiltrate a small volume of local anesthetic in the carotid sheath, blocking the sinus carotid body complex.

Side Effects and Complications

Intravascular injection into the vertebral artery and the intrathecal spread of local anesthetic are two potential complications of deep cervical plexus blockade. Frequent aspiration and slow incremental injection of local anesthetic may minimize this risk. Furthermore, directing the needle in a slightly caudad direction reduces the likelihood of the needle tip entering the intervertebral foramen and producing epidural or spinal blockade. Transient phrenic nerve paralysis is also a common side effect of deep cervical plexus blockade. Therefore, this technique should be used with caution in patients with considerable respiratory impairment. Although the sympathetic chain is outside the deep cervical fascia, local anesthetic spread may result in a transient Horner syndrome. Inadvertent blockade of the recurrent laryngeal nerve is also a possibility and can lead to airway obstruction in patients with a preexisting palsy of the contralateral vocal cord.

Superficial Cervical Plexus Block

Clinical Applications

The superficial cervical plexus block is commonly used as an adjunct to either a deep cervical plexus or an interscalene block for procedures requiring thorough coverage over the anterior portions of the neck (e.g., carotid endarterectomy, lymph node biopsies, plastic surgical procedures), top of the shoulder, or anterior aspect of the chest. Although it has been suggested that superficial cervical plexus block alone may be sufficient for carotid surgery or other procedures involving the deep structures of the neck, it is more commonly performed in conjunction with a deep cervical plexus block. Superficial cervical plexus blockade provides comprehensive analgesia to the superficial cutaneous branches of the C2, C3, and C4 nerve roots (Figure 7).

Patient Position

Similar to the deep cervical plexus block, the patient should be supine with the head slightly extended and rotated away from the side to be blocked.

Surface Anatomy and Technique

The posterior border of the sternocleidomastoid muscle is identified, and a line is drawn from the mastoid process to its insertion on the clavicle. The line is divided into thirds. A 25-gauge 2-inch (5-cm) needle is introduced through a skin wheal (over C3), and 10 to 15 mL of local anesthetic is injected for 1.5 inches (3.8 cm) both cephalad and caudad subcutaneously and slightly deep to the investing fascia along the middle third of the line that marks the posterior border of the sternocleidomastoid muscle (Figure 8). This injection produces a field block of the lesser occipital, great auricular, transverse cervical, and supraclavicular nerves as they exit from behind the sternocleidomastoid muscle. Once the nerves pass below the investing fascia of the neck, there is communication with the deep cervical space.

Needle Redirection Cues

Proper head position and surface landmarks should be reconfirmed. Local anesthetic is injected in a fanlike manner subcutaneously and behind the posterior border of the sternocleidomastoid muscle. An injection deeper than the posterior, inferior border of the sternocleidomastoid muscle may anesthetize the recurrent laryngeal nerve.

Side Effects and Complications

Side effects from the superficial cervical plexus block are rare because of the superficial deposition of local anesthetic. The most common complication is incomplete anesthesia due to errors in technique or anatomical variation.

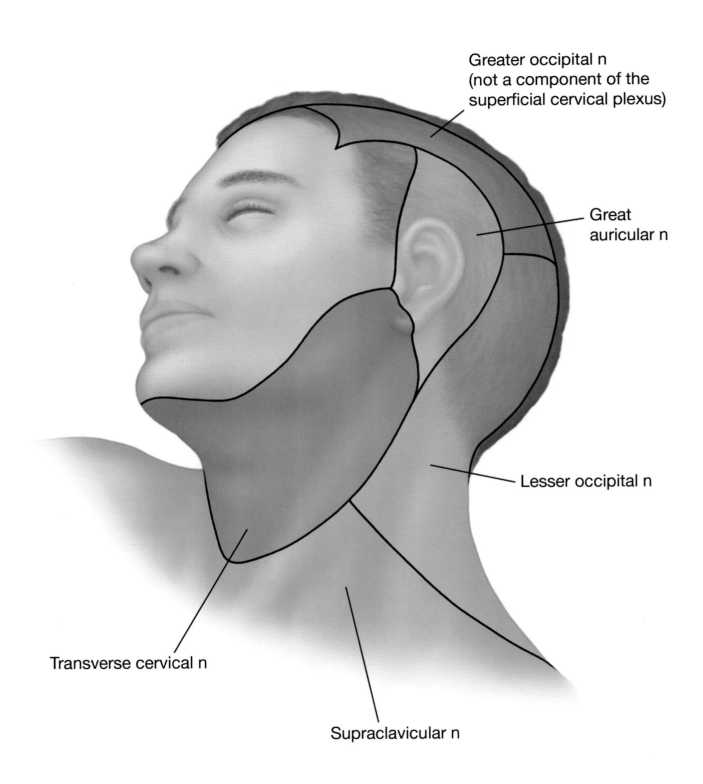

Figure 7. Cutaneous innervation of the superficial cervical plexus.

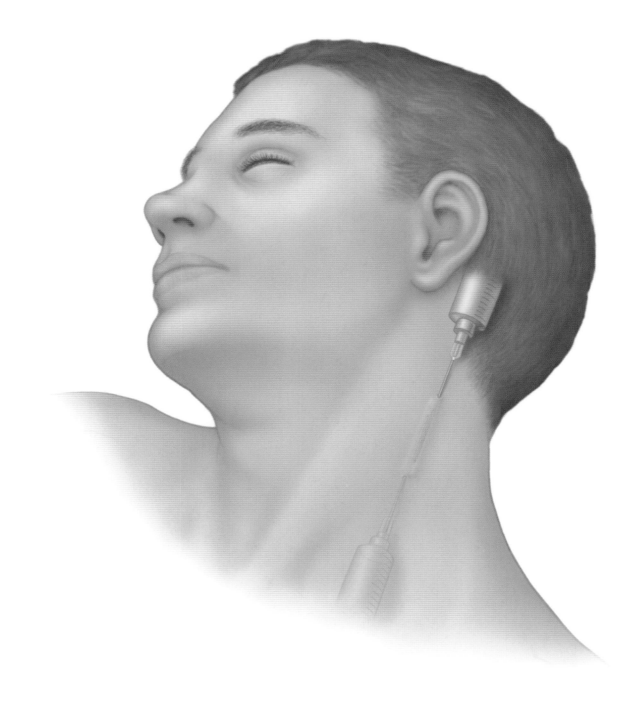

Figure 8. Superficial cervical plexus blockade.

Suggested Reading

de Sousa AA, Filho MA, Faglione W Jr, Carvalho GT. Superficial vs combined cervical plexus block for carotid endarterectomy: a prospective, randomized study. Surg Neurol. 2005;63 Suppl 1:S22-5.

Nash L, Nicholson HD, Zhang M. Does the investing layer of the deep cervical fascia exist? Anesthesiology. 2005 Nov;103(5):962-8.

Pandit JJ, Dutta D, Morris JF. Spread of injectate with superficial cervical plexus block in humans: an anatomical study. Br J Anaesth. 2003 Nov;91(5):733-5.

Stoneham MD, Doyle AR, Knighton JD, Dorje P, Stanley JC. Prospective, randomized comparison of deep or superficial cervical plexus block for carotid endarterectomy surgery. Anesthesiology. 1998 Oct;89(4):907-12.

Weiss A, Isselhorst C, Gahlen J, Freudenberg S, Roth H, Hammerschmitt N, et al. Acute respiratory failure after deep cervical plexus block for carotid endarterectomy as a result of bilateral recurrent laryngeal nerve paralysis. Acta Anaesthesiol Scand. 2005 May;49(5):715-9.

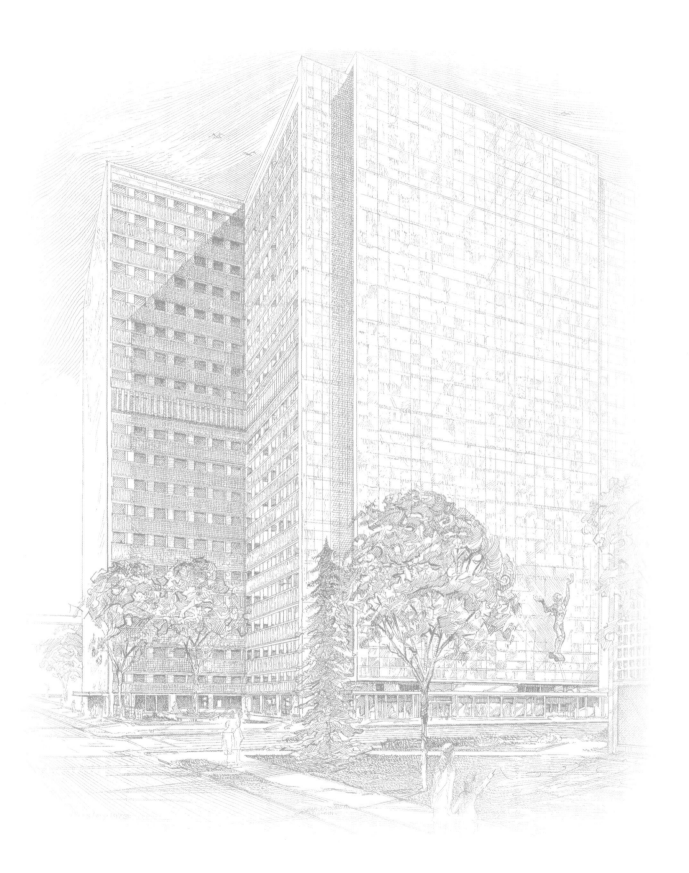

CHAPTER
10

Interscalene Blockade

Laurence C. Torsher, M.D.

Hugh M. Smith, M.D., Ph.D.

Adam K. Jacob, M.D.

Clinical Applications

The interscalene approach to the brachial plexus was first described by Etienne in 1925 and later modified by Winnie in 1970. As the most proximal approach to the brachial plexus, interscalene block is performed as the spinal nerve roots converge to form the trunks of the brachial plexus (Figure 1). The technique provides surgical anesthesia and postoperative analgesia for procedures of the shoulder and proximal aspect of the arm. Concurrent blockade of the superficial cervical plexus extends anesthetic coverage to the shoulder girdle and anterior aspect of the neck. A substantial limitation of the block includes unreliable blockade of the caudal nerve roots of the brachial plexus—the eighth cervical nerve and first thoracic nerve (C8, T1). Incomplete anesthesia of the C8 and T1 nerve roots may result in cutaneous sparing within the ulnar distribution of the upper extremity (Figure 2). This limitation makes the block an unreliable technique for surgery involving the distal extremity.

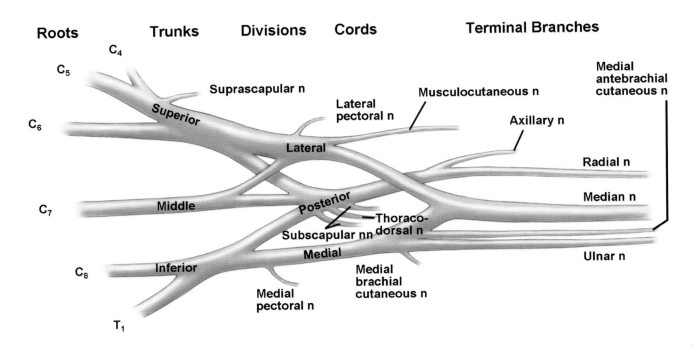

Figure 1. Brachial plexus anatomy.

Relevant Anatomy

The five roots of the brachial plexus (C5-T1) exit their respective neural foramina and pass between the anterior and middle scalene muscles (Figures 3 and 4). The C5 and C6 nerve roots combine to form the superior trunk, the C7 nerve root the middle trunk, and the C8 and T1 nerve roots the inferior trunk of the brachial plexus (Figure 1). As the three trunks approach the first rib, they divide into anterior and posterior divisions, which then fuse into lateral, posterior, and medial cords. The subclavian artery also passes between the anterior and middle scalene muscles at the level of the first rib. At this location, the divisions of the brachial plexus lie posterior, cephalad, and lateral to the subclavian artery. The vertebral artery is derived from the subclavian artery and travels cephalad before entering a bony canal formed by the transverse processes at the level of C6 (Figure 4). As the cervical roots of the brachial plexus leave the transverse processes, they course immediately posterior to the vertebral artery. This close relationship may increase the risk of intravascular injection during interscalene

blockade (Figure 3). The subclavian vein exits the thorax over the first rib anterior to the anterior scalene muscle. The phrenic nerve, derived from the C3, C4, and C5 nerve roots, crosses the plexus as it travels along the anterior surface of the anterior scalene muscle (Figure 4).

Surface Anatomy

The classic approach to the interscalene block is performed at the intersection of the interscalene groove and a line projected laterally from the cricoid cartilage (C6). The interscalene groove is located between the anterior and middle scalene muscles and is palpated immediately posterior to the lateral border of the sternocleidomastoid muscle (Figure 5). Although the interscalene groove may be difficult to palpate in select patients, the muscular borders of the relevant anatomy can be accentuated by having the patient lift his or her head off the pillow or procedural table against gravity. This maneuver allows easy identification of the posterior

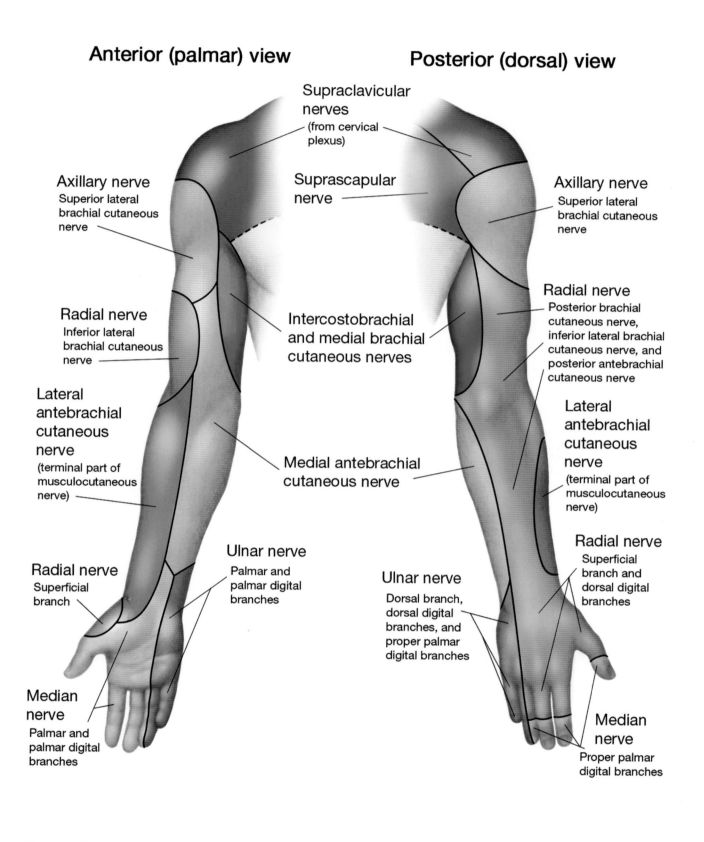

Figure 2. Cutaneous innervation of the upper extremity.

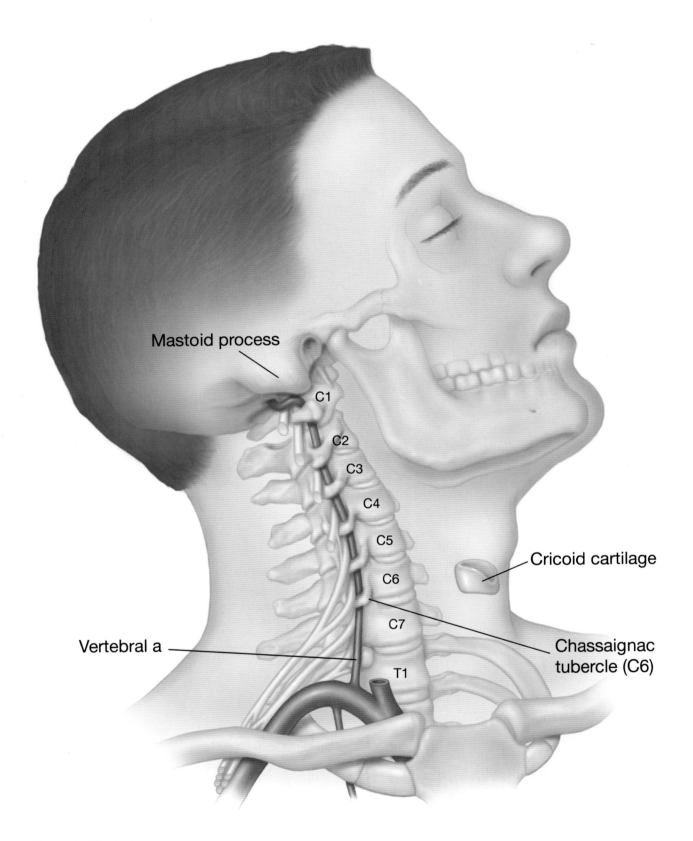

Figure 3. Cervical neuroanatomy.

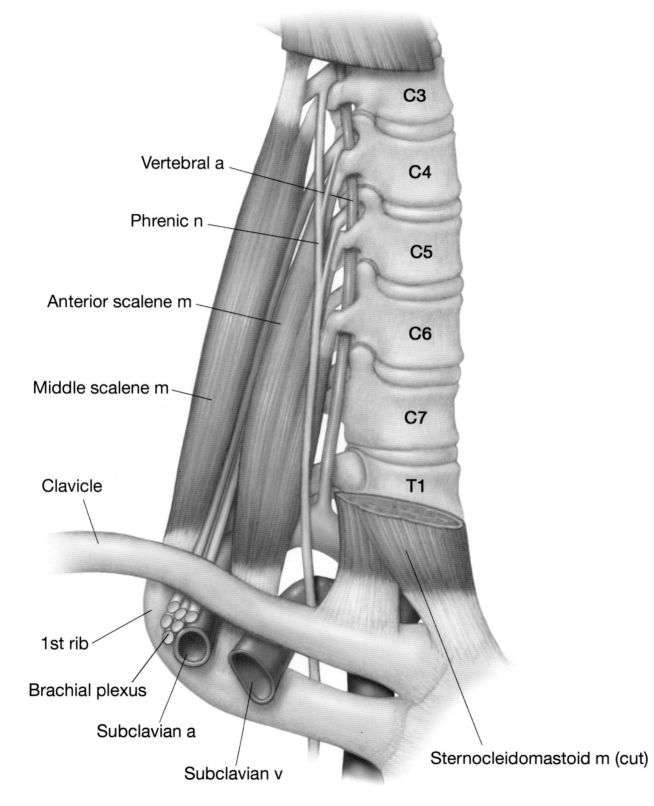

Figure 4. Neurovascular and muscular anatomy of the neck.

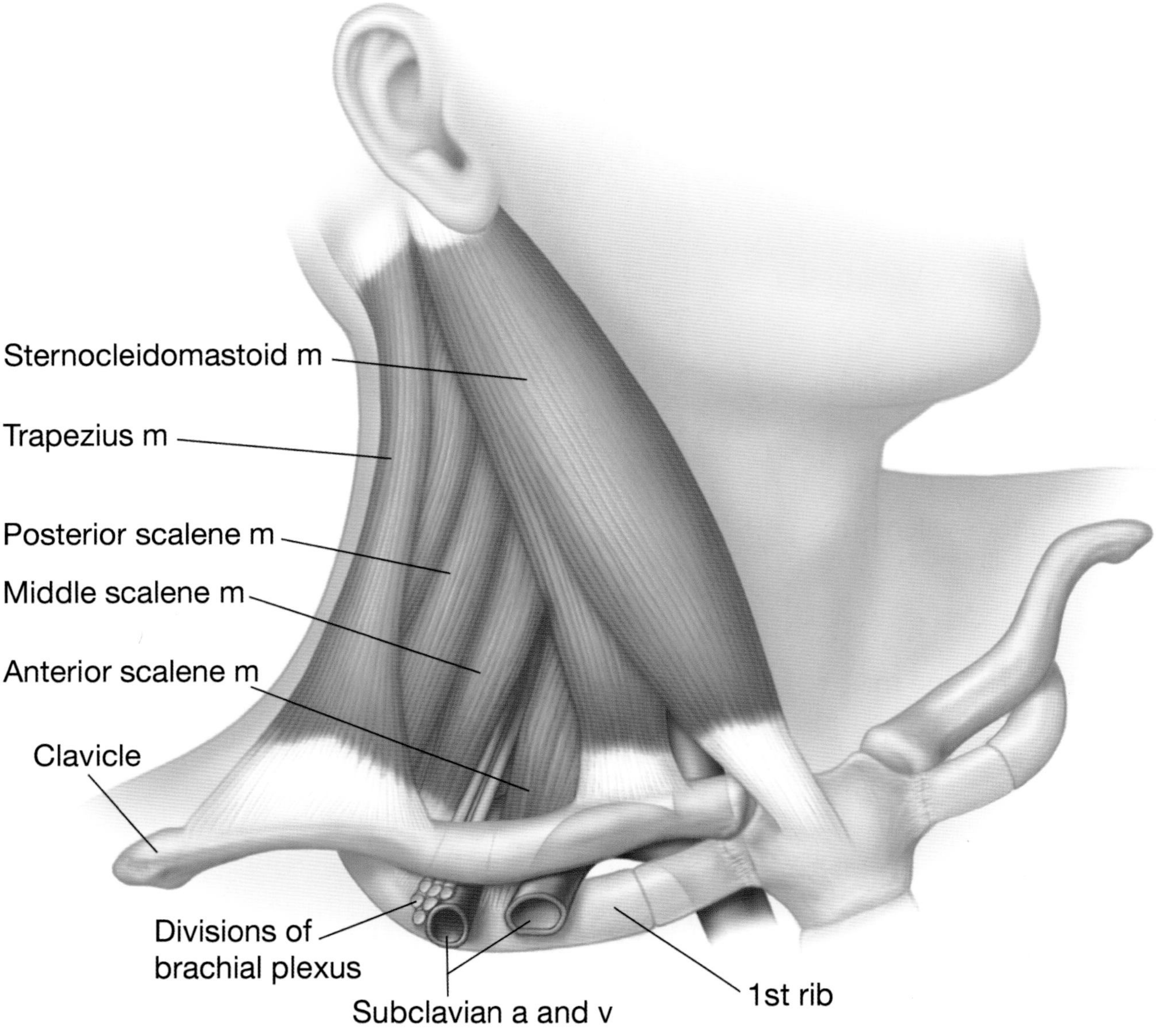

Figure 5. Muscular anatomy surrounding the interscalene groove.

border of the sternocleidomastoid muscle and increases the ability to accurately identify the interscalene groove. The external jugular vein is another surface landmark that may aid in the identification of the interscalene groove. At the level of C6, the external jugular vein is located directly over the groove in approximately 85% of patients.

Patient Position

The patient is positioned supine with the neck slightly extended and the head rotated away from the side to be blocked (Figure 6). The ipsilateral arm is adducted and placed in a comfortable position with adequate exposure to allow visualization of motor responses from nerve stimulation.

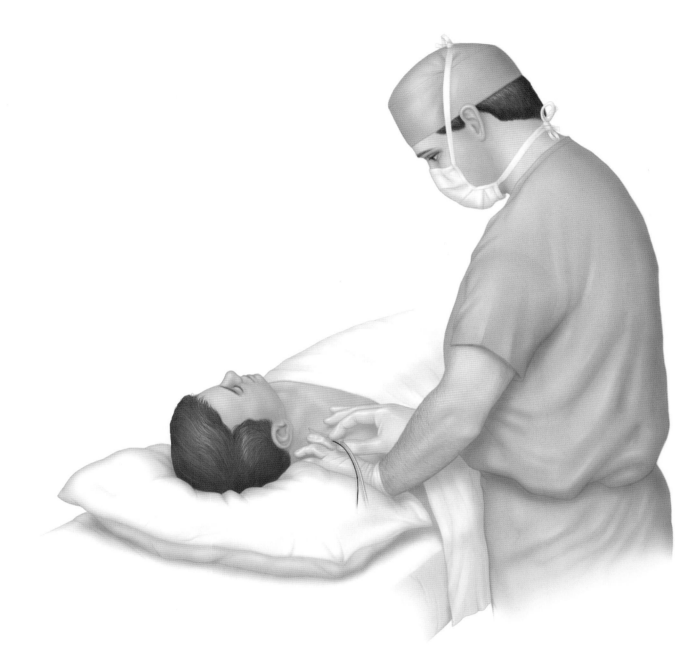

Figure 6. Patient-provider orientation during interscalene blockade.

Technique

Neural Localization Techniques
Nerve stimulation is the most common technique used to locate the brachial plexus during interscalene blockade. Alternative methods include paresthesia-seeking techniques and ultrasound guidance. Recently, ultrasound-guided interscalene blockade has been shown to accurately and reliably identify the brachial plexus within the interscalene groove. The superficial location of the brachial plexus and the

clearly identifiable borders of the scalene muscles provide excellent imaging conditions and a reliable means of localizing neural targets.

Needle Insertion Site

A 22-gauge 2-inch (5-cm) insulated needle is inserted within the interscalene groove at a point directly lateral from the cricoid cartilage (C6). The needle is inserted perpendicular to the skin and advanced in a medial,

caudal, and slightly posterior direction (Figure 7). The posterior needle trajectory should approximate a 60° angle to the sagittal plane to most reliably approach the brachial plexus. A caudal needle direction toward the contralateral nipple minimizes the risk of advancing the needle between adjacent transverse processes and entering the neural foramen. A paresthesia or evoked motor response should be elicited at a depth of 1 to 2 cm. Needle advancement beyond 2 cm may increase the risk of neural trauma,

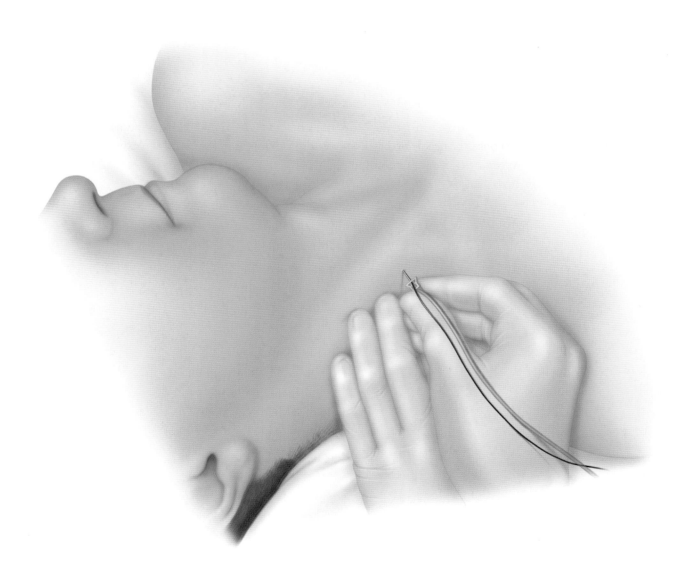

Figure 7. Needle insertion site and trajectory during interscalene blockade.

intrathecal injection, or the epidural spread of local anesthetic. Anatomical studies have shown that the minimum distance between the skin and the C6 neural foramen is approximately 2.3 cm.

The optimal evoked motor response during interscalene blockade has been debated. However, successful interscalene blockade can be achieved after the elicitation of a deltoid or biceps motor response. A distal motor response of the hand or forearm is not required if the technique is being used for shoulder or proximal upper extremity surgery. After an acceptable motor response at a current of 0.5 mA or less is elicited, 20 to 40 mL of local anesthetic is slowly injected with incremental aspiration to minimize the risk of unrecognized intravascular or intrathecal injection.

Needle Redirection Cues

If bony contact occurs at a shallow depth (<2 cm) in the absence of an elicited motor response, the needle tip has likely encountered the transverse cervical process either anterior or posterior to the neural target. Under these conditions, the needle should be redirected in a stepwise manner in an anterior-posterior plane along the line projected from the cricoid cartilage. If bone is contacted at a deeper level, the vertebral body anterior to the plane of the nerve trunks has been contacted and posterior needle redirection is necessary. Inadvertent stimulation of the phrenic nerve will result in diaphragmatic contractions. When this occurs, a more posterior needle redirection is necessary. Finally, contraction of the trapezius muscle posteriorly indicates stimulation of the accessory nerve and the need to redirect the needle more anteriorly.

Ultrasound-Guided Interscalene Blockade

Scanning Technique

Despite the superficial location of the brachial plexus, interscalene imaging can be difficult—particularly when compared with more distal regions of the brachial plexus. The ultrasound probe is positioned on the lateral aspect of the neck at the level of the cricoid cartilage, perpendicular to the plexus and centered over the interscalene

groove (Figure 8). Because the plexus travels from a medial to lateral direction and from a deep to superficial location, the beam of the ultrasound probe needs to be rotated slightly laterally and tilted caudad to optimally image the plexus in cross-section.

Inexperienced ultrasonographers may find it helpful to locate the plexus by initially scanning the supraclavicular fossa. With the probe parallel to the clavicle and the beam directed toward the first rib, the subclavian artery and divisions of the brachial plexus can be easily identified. From this position, the brachial plexus is traced cephalad until the scalene muscles are seen surrounding the trunks within the interscalene groove (Figure 9). Alternatively, scanning can begin near the midline of the neck with identification of the cricoid cartilage. Once identified, the probe is moved laterally over the carotid artery, internal jugular vein, and sternocleidomastoid muscle until the scalene muscles are seen surrounding the trunks or proximal divisions of the brachial plexus.

Sonoanatomy

Sonographically, the trunks of the brachial plexus appear as dark (hypoechoic) circular structures oriented vertically on top of one another and often angled toward the midline (Figure 9). The anterior and middle scalene muscles surround the plexus and appear as dark, heterogeneous muscle tissue with scattered fibrous and hyperechoic septae. In approximately 50% of patients, the tapered posterior margin of the sternocleidomastoid muscle appears directly superficial to (i.e., above) the plexus. Although classic anatomy textbooks depict the brachial plexus as superior, middle, and inferior trunks within this region, the plexus may appear more subdivided when viewed with ultrasound imaging (Figure 10). The distance from the surface of the skin to the superior trunk of the brachial plexus ranges from 0.5 to 2 cm.

Ultrasound Approach

In-plane (IP) and out-of-plane (OOP) needle approaches can be used during ultrasound-guided interscalene blockade. Although in-plane techniques allow visualization of the needle shaft and tip during the block, these approaches may be uncomfortable for patients because

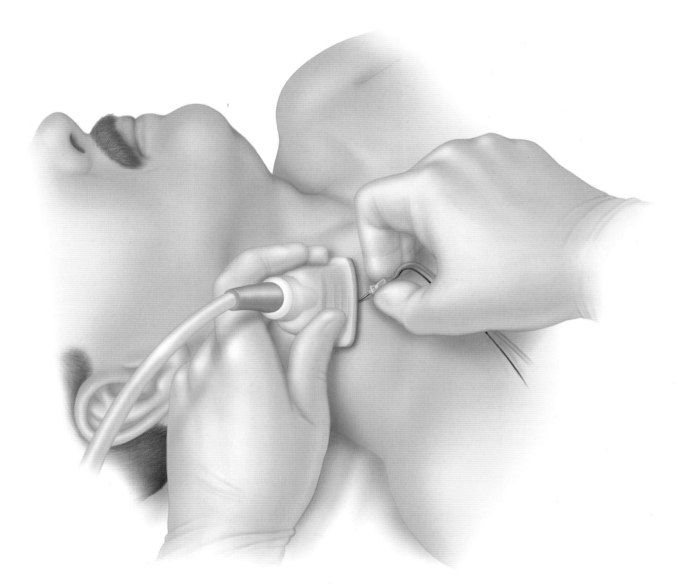

Figure 8. Probe orientation and needle insertion site during ultrasound-guided interscalene blockade.

the needle must travel a greater distance before reaching the brachial plexus. In contrast, out-of-plane needle approaches do not allow continuous imaging of the needle shaft and tip during the block. However, downward tissue displacement observed during the technique closely approximates needle position, direction, and depth. Out-of-plane needle approaches generally provide a shorter, more direct path to neural targets.

When an out-of-plane needle approach is used, the probe should be oriented so that the most superficial portion of the brachial plexus is centered within the ultrasound image. The needle is inserted perpendicular to the skin at the midpoint of the probe and slowly advanced to a point just medial or lateral to the brachial plexus (Figure 8). Hydrodissection can be useful to identify the position and direction of the needle tip. Nerve stimulation can be

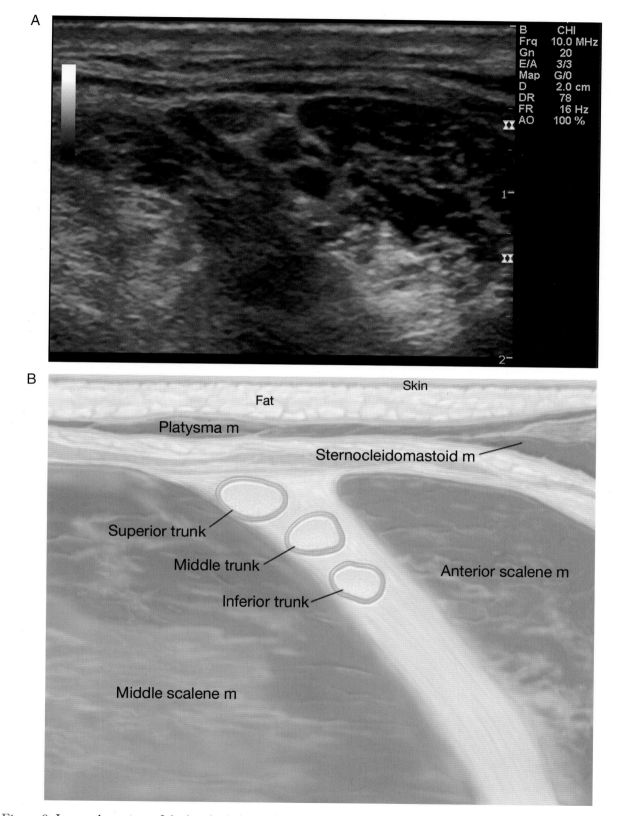

Figure 9. Interscalene view of the brachial plexus. A, Ultrasound image. B, Corresponding anatomical illustration.

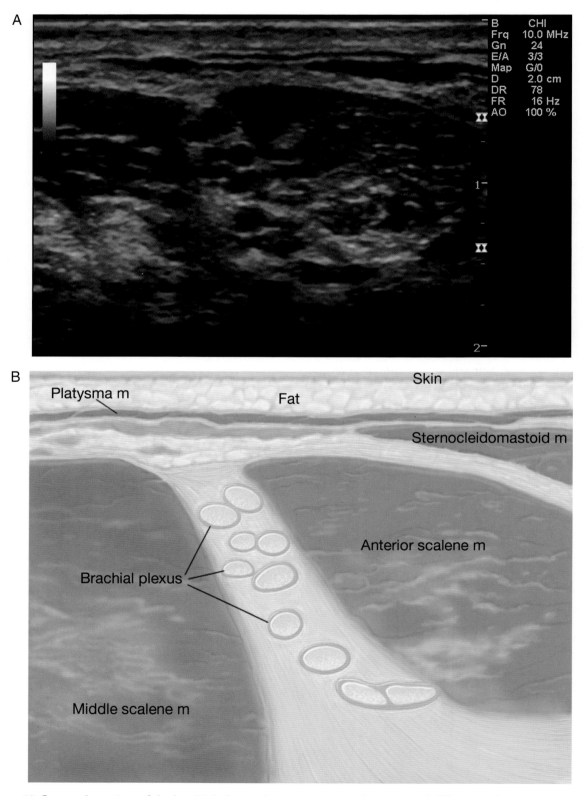

Figure 10. Interscalene view of the brachial plexus, showing anatomical variation. A, Ultrasound image. B, Corresponding anatomical illustration.

used to confirm neural localization once the needle tip has approached the brachial plexus. However, this is rarely performed among experienced ultrasonographers. Once the needle tip has approached the superior trunk of the plexus, 10 to 15 mL of local anesthetic is injected slowly with incremental aspiration (Figure 11). The needle may need to be withdrawn and redirected to the opposite side of the plexus to ensure circumferential spread of local anesthetic. If required, an additional 10 to 15 mL of local anesthetic is injected slowly with incremental aspiration.

Continuous Peripheral Nerve Catheters

Continuous peripheral nerve catheters are commonly used as an adjunct to intraoperative anesthesia and for postoperative pain management. Both stimulating and nonstimulating interscalene catheters have been shown to provide superior analgesia and improve rehabilitation after shoulder surgery compared with traditional intravenous opioids. Although ultrasound technology can be used to accurately guide catheter placement, there is insufficient evidence to suggest that this technique is superior to more conventional methods of nerve stimulation.

Neural localization using peripheral nerve stimulation is similar for both continuous and single-injection techniques. During interscalene catheter placement, an 18-gauge 2-inch (5-cm) insulated Tuohy needle is inserted with the bevel directed caudally toward the first rib and along the path of the brachial plexus. After an appropriate motor response is elicited at a current of 0.5 mA or less, a 20-gauge catheter is advanced 2 to 3 cm beyond the needle tip and secured on the lateral aspect of the neck or proximal aspect of the shoulder.

Ultrasound-guided interscalene catheter placement is similar to that described for out-of-plane single-injection techniques. Under direct visualization, an 18-gauge 2-inch (5-cm) insulated Tuohy needle is inserted and advanced toward the middle trunk of the brachial plexus with the bevel directed either anterior or posterior to the plexus. The location of the needle tip can be confirmed by injecting either saline or a dextrose-containing solution.

After optimal needle placement, a 20-gauge catheter is advanced 1 to 2 cm beyond the needle tip. Ideally, the catheter tip should remain near the middle trunk of the brachial plexus. The distribution of local anesthetic spread is confirmed using real-time ultrasound imaging. If circumferential spread of local anesthetic does not occur, catheter manipulation may be required with direct visualization.

Once the catheter location has been optimized, it is secured using a liquid adhesive, Steri-Strips, and a sterile transparent dressing. Alternatively, the catheter may be tunneled subcutaneously to a location remote from the initial insertion site and covered with a protective dressing. A limitation of continuous interscalene blockade is the relative ease of catheter dislodgment due to the superficial location of the plexus. Subcutaneous tunneling may reduce the risk of catheter dislodgment and help prevent catheter-related infection.

Side Effects and Complications

The most common side effect associated with interscalene block is ipsilateral phrenic nerve blockade. Transient phrenic nerve paresis reduces pulmonary reserve and causes some patients to experience mild dyspnea for the duration of the block. The frequency of phrenic nerve blockade approaches 100%—particularly when high volumes of local anesthetic are used during the block. Therefore, interscalene block may not be a suitable technique for patients with respiratory compromise (e.g., chronic obstructive pulmonary disease). Additional neural structures at risk of inadvertent blockade include the vagus and recurrent laryngeal nerves and the cervical sympathetic chain.

Horner syndrome is another side effect commonly associated with interscalene blockade. It occurs in 70% to 90% of patients and is most common when large volumes of local anesthetic are used. The syndrome is characterized by the classic triad of ptosis, miosis, and anhydrosis and is caused by inadvertent blockade of the stellate ganglion. Clinical symptoms persist for the duration of the block. No intervention is required with the exception

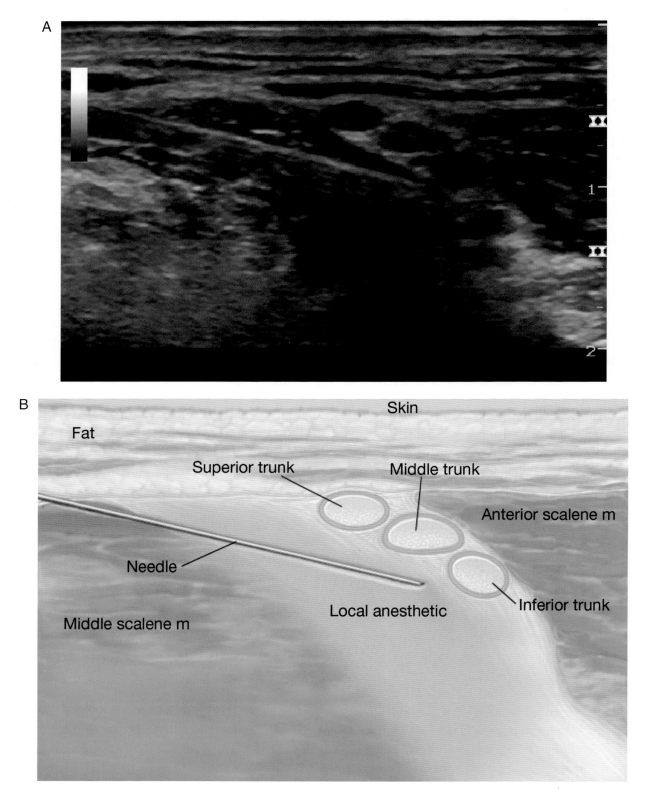

Figure 11. Ultrasound-guided interscalene blockade using an in-plane needle approach. A, Ultrasound image. B, Corresponding anatomical illustration.

of reassuring patients that the clinical symptoms are transient and self-limited.

The proximity of the brachial plexus to major vascular structures within the neck (e.g., vertebral and carotid arteries) increases the risk of intravascular injection and systemic local anesthetic toxicity. Similarly, the proximity to the central neuraxis increases the risk of intrathecal injection and epidural spread of local anesthetic. Cervical spinal cord injuries have also been reported after interscalene blockade. However, the risk of these and other complications can be minimized by ensuring that the patient is awake and responsive during the block, that the depth of needle insertion is limited to 2 cm, and that a caudal needle trajectory is maintained to avoid traversing the neural foramen. Finally, if a perineural catheter is inserted for continuous peripheral nerve blockade, local anesthetic dosing should be modified to minimize the risk of toxic serum drug levels.

Suggested Reading

Bennani SE, Vandenabele-Teneur F, Nyarwaya JB, Delecroix M, Krivosic-Horber R. An attempt to prevent spread of local anaesthetic to the phrenic nerve by compression above the injection site during the interscalene brachial plexus block. Eur J Anaesthesiol. 1998 Jul;15(4):453-6.

Boezaart AP. Continuous interscalene block for ambulatory shoulder surgery. Best Pract Res Clin Anaesthesiol. 2002 Jun;16(2):295-310.

Candido KD, Sukhani R, Doty R Jr, Nader A, Kendall MC, Yaghmour E, et al. Neurologic sequelae after interscalene brachial plexus block for shoulder/upper arm surgery: the association of patient, anesthetic, and surgical factors to the incidence and clinical course. Anesth Analg. 2005 May;100(5):1489-95.

Chan VW. Applying ultrasound imaging to interscalene brachial plexus block. Reg Anesth Pain Med. 2003 Jul-Aug;28(4):340-3.

Long TR, Wass CT, Burkle CM. Perioperative interscalene blockade: an overview of its history and current clinical use. J Clin Anesth. 2002 Nov;14(7):546-56.

Sardesai AM, Patel R, Denny NM, Menon DK, Dixon AK, Herrick MJ, et al. Interscalene brachial plexus block: can the risk of entering the spinal canal be reduced? A study of needle angles in volunteers undergoing magnetic resonance imaging. Anesthesiology. 2006 Jul; 105(1):9-13.

Silverstein WB, Saiyed MU, Brown AR. Interscalene block with a nerve stimulator: a deltoid motor response is a satisfactory endpoint for successful block. Reg Anesth Pain Med. 2000 Jul-Aug;25(4):356-9.

Tonidandel WL, Mayfield JB. Successful interscalene block with a nerve stimulator may also result after a pectoralis major motor response. Reg Anesth Pain Med. 2002 Sep-Oct;27(5):491-3.

Urmey WF, Talts KH, Sharrock NE. One hundred percent incidence of hemidiaphragmatic paresis associated with interscalene brachial plexus anesthesia as diagnosed by ultrasonography. Anesth Analg. 1991 Apr;72(4):498-503.

Wong GY, Brown DL, Miller GM, Cahill DR. Defining the cross-sectional anatomy important to interscalene brachial plexus block with magnetic resonance imaging. Reg Anesth Pain Med. 1998 Jan-Feb;23(1):77-80.

CHAPTER
11

Suprascapular Blockade

Thomas J. Jurrens, M.D.

Clinical Applications

Suprascapular nerve blockade was first described by Wertheim and Rovenstine in 1941. Although the suprascapular nerve represents a single terminal branch of the brachial plexus, its sensorimotor innervation warrants consideration under various clinical conditions. For example, suprascapular nerve blockade may provide analgesia in patients experiencing adhesive capsulitis, rheumatoid arthritis, myofascial pain syndrome, pain from malignancy, rotator cuff lesions, and pain after shoulder surgery. Unlike interscalene blockade, suprascapular blockade provides analgesia of the shoulder joint, capsule, and skin without anesthetizing the phrenic nerve. The avoidance of phrenic nerve blockade may be of benefit in patients with compromised pulmonary mechanics (e.g., chronic obstructive pulmonary disease). Suprascapular blockade has also been used to diagnose and differentiate shoulder pain of unclear etiology.

Relevant Anatomy

The suprascapular nerve, a branch of the superior trunk of the brachial plexus, arises from the fifth (C5), sixth (C6), and occasionally fourth (C4) cervical nerve roots (Figure 1). It passes behind the brachial plexus parallel to the omohyoid muscle, travels beneath the upper trapezius muscle to the superior edge of the scapula, and then traverses the suprascapular notch. Within the suprascapular notch, the suprascapular artery and vein pass above the transverse scapular ligament and the nerve passes below and into the supraspinous fossa. The suprascapular nerve provides sensory innervation to approximately 70% of the shoulder joint (including the superior and posterior-superior regions), capsule, and overlying skin (Figure 2). After innervating the supraspinatus muscle (arm abduction), it courses around the lateral border of the scapular spine and provides sensory innervation to the acromioclavicular and glenohumeral joints, subacromial bursa, and coracoclavicular ligament. The suprascapular nerve terminates in the infraspinous fossa, where it supplies motor innervation to the infraspinatus muscle (external rotation) (Figure 3).

Surface Anatomy

The most important anatomical surface landmark is the scapular spine, located on the posterior aspect of the shoulder girdle. This bony prominence, extending from the medial margin of the scapula to the tip of the acromion process, divides the posterior surface of the scapula into the supraspinous and infraspinous fossae. The scapular spine is relatively superficial and easily palpated, even in muscular or obese patients.

Patient Position

The patient should be placed in the sitting position with the neck slightly flexed. The ipsilateral hand should be placed on the contralateral shoulder to rotate the posterior shoulder girdle away from the chest wall (Figure 4).

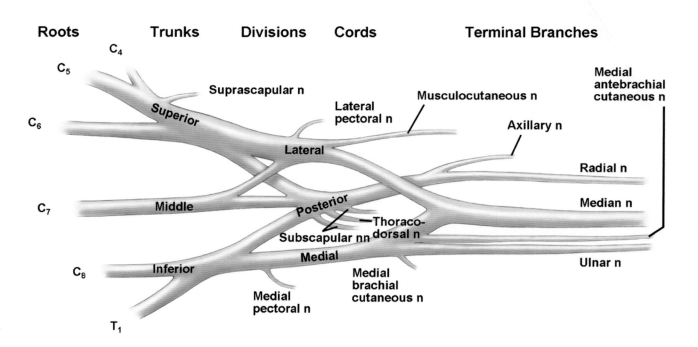

Figure 1. Brachial plexus anatomy.

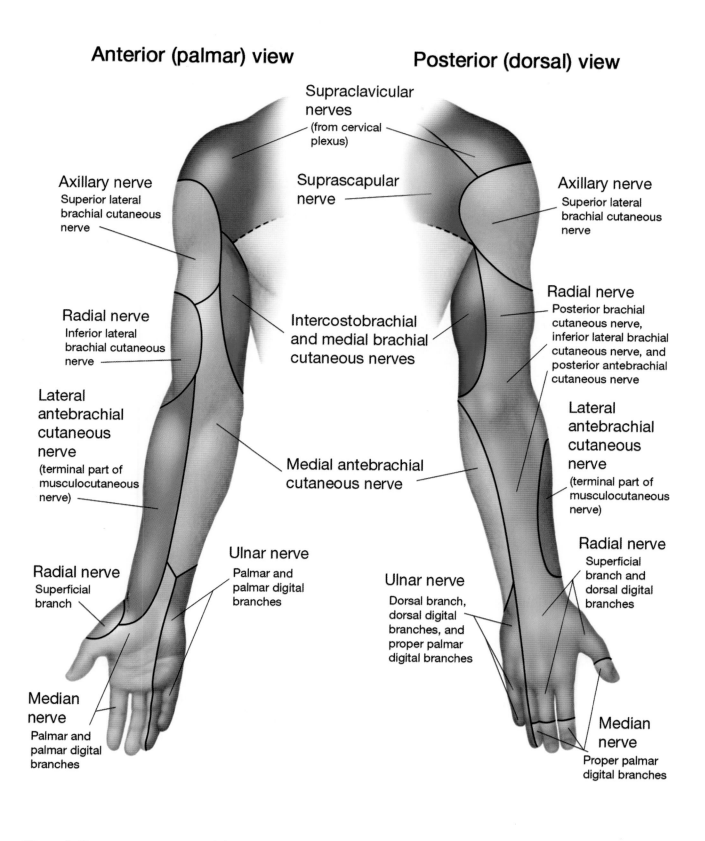

Anterior (palmar) view

Posterior (dorsal) view

Supraclavicular nerves
(from cervical plexus)

Suprascapular nerve

Axillary nerve
Superior lateral brachial cutaneous nerve

Axillary nerve
Superior lateral brachial cutaneous nerve

Radial nerve
Inferior lateral brachial cutaneous nerve

Intercostobrachial and medial brachial cutaneous nerves

Radial nerve
Posterior brachial cutaneous nerve, inferior lateral brachial cutaneous nerve, and posterior antebrachial cutaneous nerve

Lateral antebrachial cutaneous nerve
(terminal part of musculocutaneous nerve)

Lateral antebrachial cutaneous nerve
(terminal part of musculocutaneous nerve)

Medial antebrachial cutaneous nerve

Radial nerve
Superficial branch and dorsal digital branches

Radial nerve
Superficial branch

Ulnar nerve
Palmar and palmar digital branches

Ulnar nerve
Dorsal branch, dorsal digital branches, and proper palmar digital branches

Median nerve
Palmar and palmar digital branches

Median nerve
Proper palmar digital branches

Figure 2. Cutaneous innervation of the suprascapular nerve.

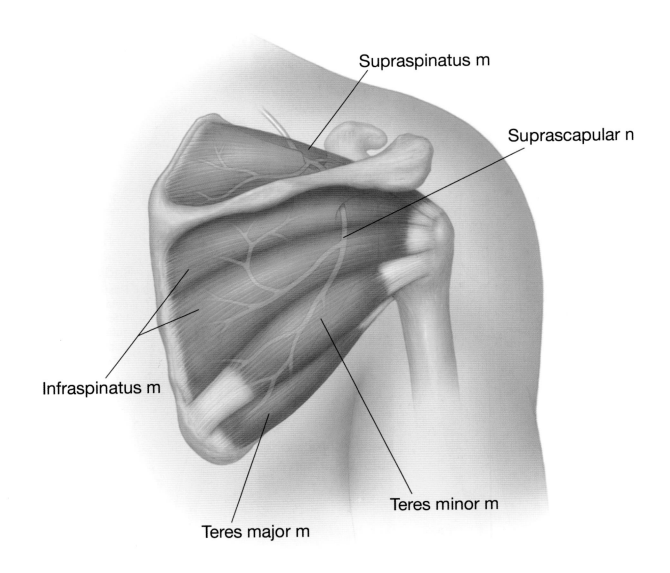

Figure 3. Motor innervation of the suprascapular nerve.

Technique

Neural Localization Techniques

The suprascapular nerve may be identified using nerve stimulation or paresthesia-seeking techniques. Alternatively, a field block of the suprascapular nerve may be performed within the supraspinous fossa.

Needle Insertion Site

Two approaches to the suprascapular nerve have been described. The classic approach described by Wertheim and Rovenstine uses a line drawn along the length of the superior border of the scapular spine. This line is then bisected with a perpendicular line, thereby creating four quadrants. Finally, a third line is drawn that diagonally bisects the upper outer quadrant, and a point is marked 1.5 to 2.0 cm along this line. A 22-gauge 2-inch (5-cm) insulated needle is inserted perpendicular to the skin and advanced until the scapula is contacted or the needle tip is felt slipping into the suprascapular notch (Figure 5). Maximal needle depth is approximately 1.5 to 3 cm. If nerve stimulation is used, shoulder abduction or

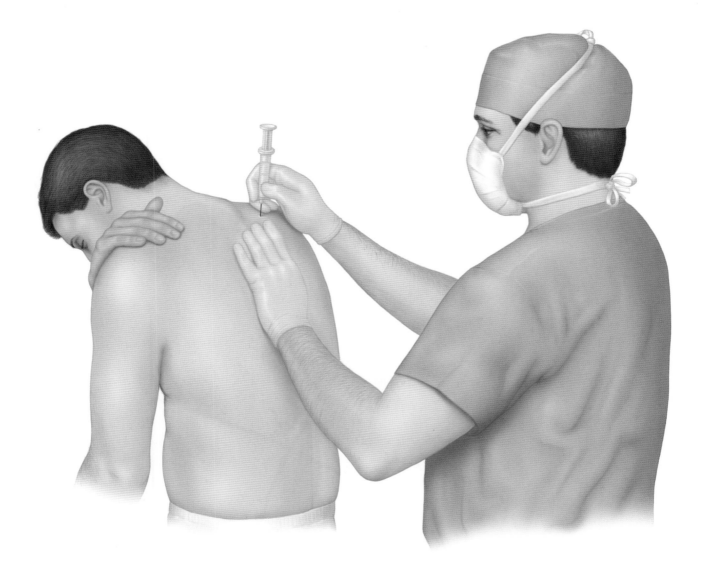

Figure 4. Patient positioning during suprascapular blockade.

external rotation reflects stimulation of the suprascapular nerve. However, severe rotator cuff injuries may restrict the degree of motor response acquired with nerve stimulation. Five to 10 mL of local anesthetic solution is injected to anesthetize the nerve.

A second approach was described by Dangoisse and colleagues in 1994. Similar to the classic approach, the scapular spine is palpated and marked with a line drawn along its superior border. A second perpendicular line is drawn that bisects the line of the scapular spine. Needle insertion is performed 1 cm above the point of intersection (i.e., 1 cm above the scapular spine midway along its length). The needle is advanced directly downward (i.e., perpendicular to the floor) until the bony floor of the supraspinous fossa is reached (Figure 4). After negative aspiration, 10 mL of local anesthetic solution is injected into the floor of the supraspinous fossa.

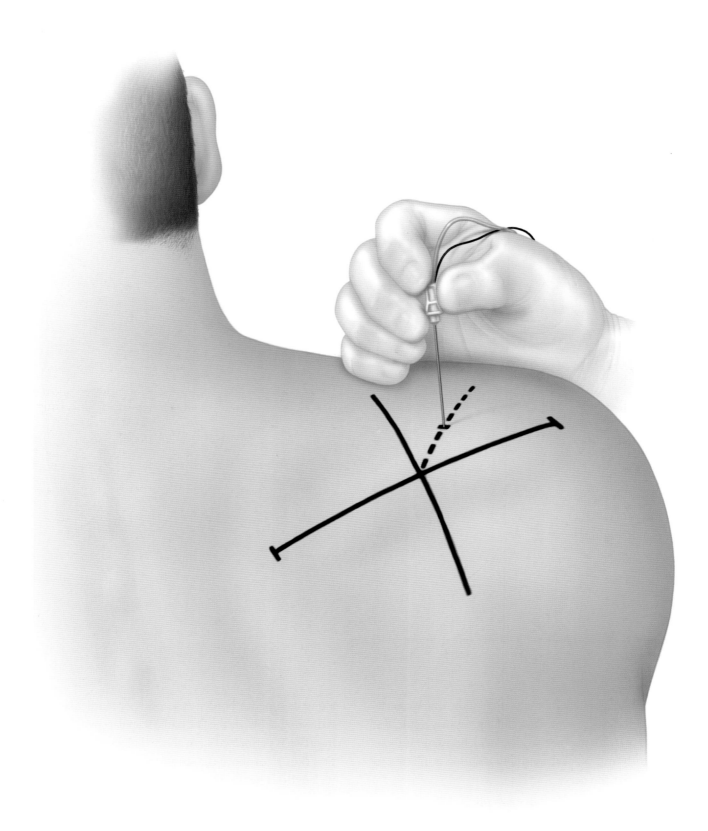

Figure 5. Surface landmarks and needle insertion site for suprascapular blockade.

Needle Redirection Cues

When the classic approach is used, medial, lateral, or superior needle redirection may be necessary to avoid superficial contact with bone. Small, incremental needle redirections are continued until the needle slides into the suprascapular notch at a depth of approximately 1.5 to 3 cm.

Side Effects and Complications

The most serious complication of suprascapular blockade is pneumothorax. Advancing the needle beyond the suprascapular notch may result in penetration of the pleura. The Dangoisse technique may theoretically reduce this risk by advancing the needle parallel to the blade of the scapula (i.e., perpendicular to the floor) and away from the chest wall. Careful aspiration is also necessary as the suprascapular artery and vein travel in proximity to the nerve. Nerve damage has been reported, but persistent paresthesias are usually self-limited.

Suggested Reading

Aszmann OC, Dellon AL, Birely BT, McFarland EG. Innervation of the human shoulder joint and its implications for surgery. Clin Orthop Relat Res. 1996 Sep;(330):202-7.

Dangoisse MJ, Wilson DJ, Glynn CJ. MRI and clinical study of an easy and safe technique of suprascapular nerve blockade. Acta Anaesthesiol Belg. 1994;45(2):49-54.

Karatas GK, Meray J. Suprascapular nerve block for pain relief in adhesive capsulitis: comparison of 2 different techniques. Arch Phys Med Rehabil. 2002 May; 83(5):593-7.

Neal JM, McDonald SB, Larkin KL, Polissar NL. Suprascapular nerve block prolongs analgesia after nonarthroscopic shoulder surgery but does not improve outcome. Anesth Analg. 2003 Apr;96(4): 982-6.

Raj PP, Lou L, Erdine S, Staats PS. Radiographic imaging for regional anesthesia and pain management. New York: Churchill Livingstone; 2003. Chapter 21, Suprascapular nerve block; p. 128-31.

Ritchie ED, Tong D, Chung F, Norris AM, Miniaci A, Vairavanathan SD. Suprascapular nerve block for postoperative pain relief in arthroscopic shoulder surgery: a new modality? Anesth Analg. 1997 Jun;84(6):1306-12.

Singelyn FJ, Lhotel L, Fabre B. Pain relief after arthroscopic shoulder surgery: a comparison of intraarticular analgesia, suprascapular nerve block, and interscalene brachial plexus block. Anesth Analg. 2004 Aug;99 (2):589-92.

Wertheim HM, Rovenstine EA. Suprascapular nerve block. Anesthesiology. 1941 Sept;2:541-5.

CHAPTER 12

Intersternocleidomastoid Blockade

Michelle A. O. Kinney, M.D.

Clinical Applications

The intersternocleidomastoid approach to the brachial plexus was first described by Pham-Dang and colleagues in 1997. The block is a variation of the classic supraclavicular approach, with considerable modifications from more contemporary approaches to the brachial plexus (e.g., interscalene, parascalene, subclavian perivascular). As with the supraclavicular approach, the intersternocleidomastoid block is indicated for surgical procedures of

the shoulder, upper arm, and forearm. However, given the possibility of inadequate blockade of the eighth cervical (C8) and first thoracic (T1) nerves, the approach may not provide sufficient anesthesia for surgery on the distal forearm or hand.

Proponents of the intersternocleidomastoid approach describe four distinct advantages of the block. First, the approach uses simple, easily identified surface landmarks. Second, the risk of an inadvertent vertebral artery or neuraxial injection may be lower than with traditional interscalene techniques. This advantage is postulated on the intersternocleidomastoid's lateral approach to the brachial plexus. Third, the approach may have a lower risk of pneumothorax than traditional supraclavicular techniques. Finally, the block is easily amenable to the placement and maintenance of a perineural catheter because of its tangential relationship to the brachial plexus. Furthermore, this region of the neck (i.e., between the clavicular and sternal heads of the sternocleidomastoid muscle) may be associated with limited movement and thereby reduce the risk of catheter dislodgment.

Relevant Anatomy

After the five roots of the brachial plexus (C5-T1) exit their respective neural foramina and begin coursing between the anterior and middle scalene muscles, the C5 and C6 nerve roots combine to form the superior trunk, the C7 nerve root the middle trunk, and the C8

and T1 nerve roots the inferior trunk of the brachial plexus (Figure 1). The three trunks, which lie within the lower portion of the posterior cervical triangle, continue to course laterally and inferiorly toward the first rib (Figure 2). At the lateral border of the first rib and just above or behind the middle third of the clavicle, the trunks undergo a primary anatomical division into anterior and posterior divisions. After passing over the first rib, the neurovascular bundle courses beneath the middle third of the clavicle at or near its midpoint and continues on to the axilla.

The intersternocleidomastoid approach anesthetizes the brachial plexus at the level of the trunks or proximal divisions. The technique is dependent on identifying the anatomical landmarks associated with the two triangles of the cervical region. The first triangle defines the surface anatomy and is formed by the clavicular and sternal heads of the sternocleidomastoid muscle and the medial third of the clavicle. The second triangle defines

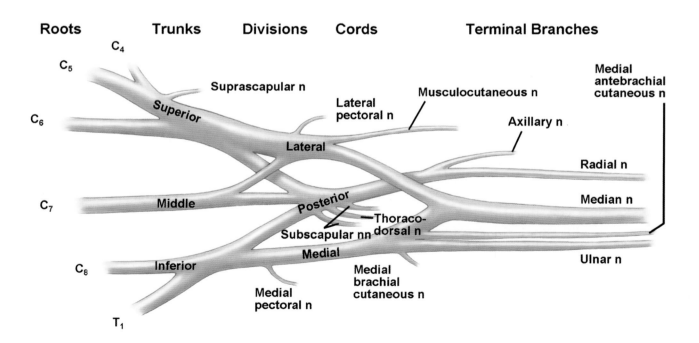

Figure 1. Brachial plexus anatomy.

the supraclavicular space and is formed by the sterno-cleidomastoid and omohyoid muscles and the clavicle. It is covered by a pretracheal layer of cervical fascia (the middle cervical fascia) that lies superficial and lateral to the anterior scalene muscle. The phrenic nerve lies beneath this cervical fascia on the anterior surface of the anterior scalene muscle. The trunks of the brachial plexus emerge next to the scalene muscles and course laterally toward the midpoint of the clavicle (Figure 2).

Surface Anatomy

Primary surface landmarks include the suprasternal notch, the midpoint of the clavicle, and the triangle formed by the sternal and clavicular heads of the sterno-cleidomastoid muscle and the medial third of the clavicle (Figure 3). The muscular borders of the triangle can be easily identified and readily palpated when the patient raises his or her head against gravity off the surgical bed or pillow.

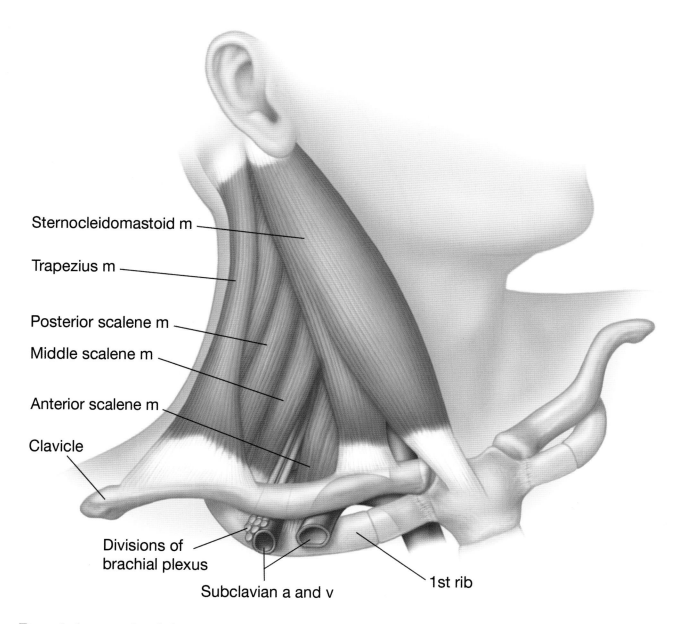

Figure 2. Anatomical neck dissection of the posterior cervical triangle.

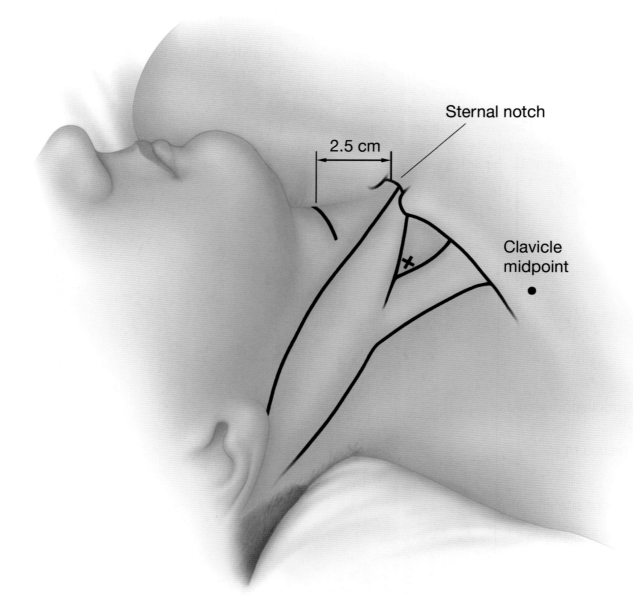

Figure 3. Surface landmarks for intersternocleidomastoid blockade.

Patient Position

The patient is positioned supine with the head slightly rotated away from the side to be blocked. The ipsilateral arm is at the patient's side with the elbow flexed and hand resting on the abdomen. The proceduralist should stand at the patient's head, contralateral to the surgical site or side to be blocked (Figure 4).

Technique

Neural Localization Techniques

The intersternocleidomastoid approach to the brachial plexus is typically performed using peripheral nerve stimulation. Elbow flexion or diaphragmatic contractions are often the first elicited motor responses because

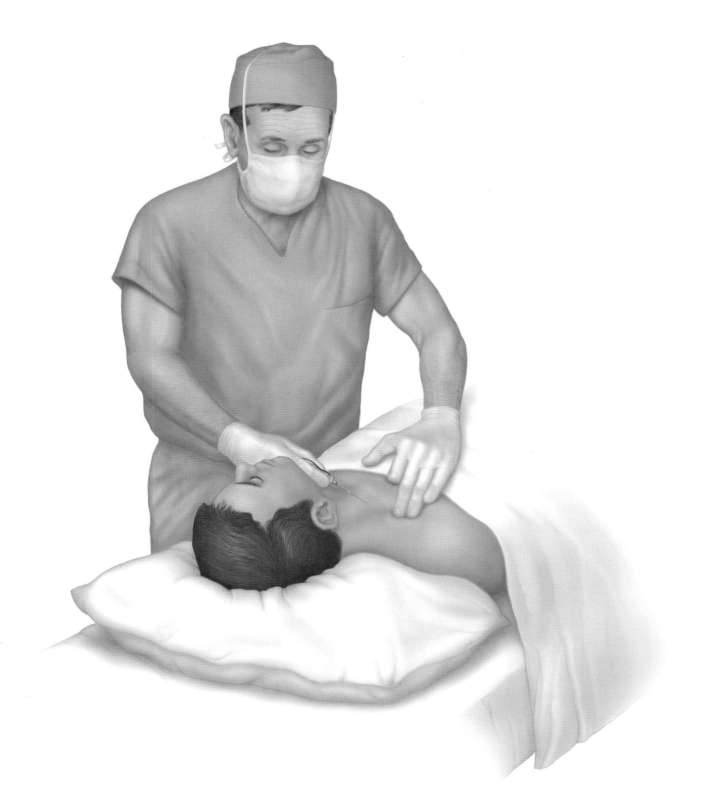

Figure 4. Patient-provider positioning during intersternocleidomastoid blockade.

the superior trunk of the brachial plexus and the phrenic nerve appear early in the course of the needle trajectory. As with the interscalene approach, the optimal motor response is somewhat controversial. In general, successful blockade for shoulder surgery requires a motor response of the elbow. However, optimal neural localization for hand surgery includes finger flexion, shoulder contractions, and concurrent paresthesias radiating to the fingers.

Needle Insertion Site

The block needle is inserted at the medial border of the clavicular head of the sternocleidomastoid muscle 2 fingerbreadths (2-3 cm) above the superior margin of the clavicle (the original description recommends a level 2 fingerbreadths above the sternal notch) (Figure 5). A 22-gauge 2-inch (5-cm) stimulating needle is recommended for slender patients (neck circumference, 32-38 cm). However, a 21-gauge 4-inch (10-cm) needle may be necessary for patients with broader necks (neck circumference, 38-48 cm). Before needle insertion, the index finger should press on the hollow between the two heads of the sternocleidomastoid muscle to elevate the clavicular head so that the needle can easily pass just medial and posterior to this muscle belly and avoid the internal jugular vein (Figure 5). The needle is then advanced in a lateral, caudal, and slightly posterior direction toward a point 1 cm lateral to the midpoint of the clavicle. This trajectory passes the needle immediately posterior to the clavicular head of the sternocleidomastoid muscle and forms a 45° angle with the plane of the operating table. Alternatively, the needle may be advanced along a path directed toward the coracoid process. Regardless, the needle trajectory courses through the middle cervical fascia, passes immediately lateral to the phrenic nerve, and continues through the anterior scalene muscle before coming into contact with the brachial plexus. The brachial plexus commonly is located at a depth of less than 5 cm in slender patients (neck circumference, 32-38 cm) and 6 or 7 cm in patients with broader necks (neck circumference, 38-48 cm).

The needle should never be advanced beyond a depth of 7 cm nor angled in a caudal direction toward the dome of the pleura. After an acceptable motor response is elicited, 20 to 40 mL of local anesthetic is injected incrementally with frequent aspiration to minimize the risk of inadvertent intravascular injection.

Needle Redirection Cues

Stimulation of the phrenic nerve (i.e., diaphragmatic contractions) may suggest that the needle trajectory is too medial or posterior. When this occurs, the needle should be redirected more laterally to avoid direct contact and potential injury to the phrenic nerve. The needle should not continue to be advanced if a phrenic motor response is elicited. If no motor response is elicited after a depth of 5 to 7 cm, the needle should be withdrawn to the skin and redirected medially and slightly more caudal in small incremental maneuvers.

Side Effects and Complications

The two most serious complications of the intersternocleidomastoid approach are phrenic nerve paralysis and inadvertent pleural puncture. Although relatively uncommon, permanent phrenic nerve injuries and clinically significant pneumothoraces have been reported with this technique. The risk of the latter may be minimized by inserting the needle lateral to a line representing the lateral and superior aspect of the chest wall and avoiding needle directions greater than 45° to the coronal plane. However, the potentially devastating sequelae of these two complications may prevent this technique from becoming a common approach to the brachial plexus.

Additional side effects and potential complications of the block include transient phrenic nerve paralysis and hemidiaphragm elevation (60%), Horner syndrome, internal jugular or subclavian vein puncture, subclavian artery puncture, recurrent laryngeal nerve blockade with or without dysphonia, local anesthetic toxicity (seizure-related events), and neural injury.

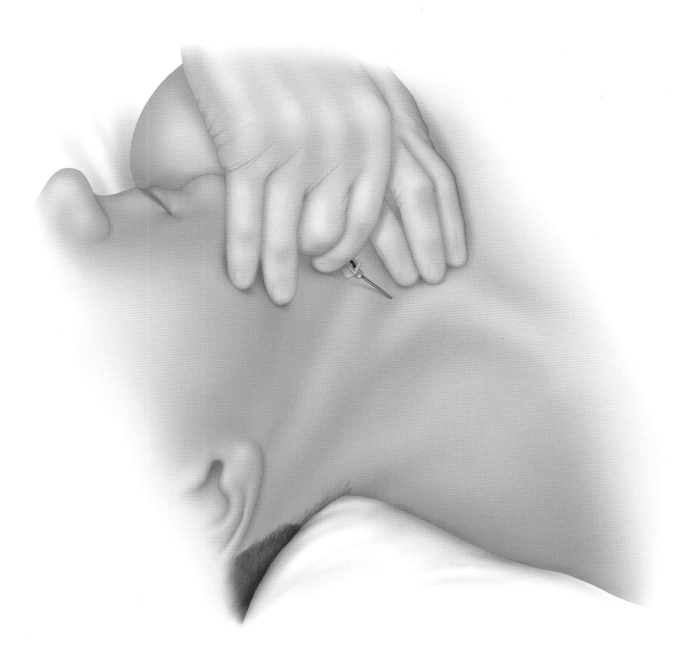

Figure 5. Needle insertion site for intersternocleidomastoid blockade.

Suggested Reading

Brachial plexus intersternocleidomastoid approach. ASRA News. 2001 Nov:2-3.

Dewees JL, Schultz CT, Wilkerson FK, Kelly JA, Biegner AR, Pellegrini JE. Comparison of two approaches to brachial plexus anesthesia for proximal upper extremity surgery: interscalene and intersternocleidomastoid. AANA J. 2006 Jun;74(3):201-6.

Pham-Dang C. Correct needle direction in the intersternocleidomastoid approach to the brachial plexus.

Reg Anesth Pain Med. 2005 Nov-Dec;30(6): 595-6.

Pham-Dang C, Gunst JP, Gouin F, Poirier P, Touchais S, Meunier JF, et al. A novel supraclavicular approach to brachial plexus block. Anesth Analg. 1997 Jul;85(1):111-6.

Pham-Dang C, Kick O, Collet T, Gouin F, Pinaud M. Continuous peripheral nerve blocks with stimulating catheters. Reg Anesth Pain Med. 2003 Mar-Apr; 28(2):83-8.

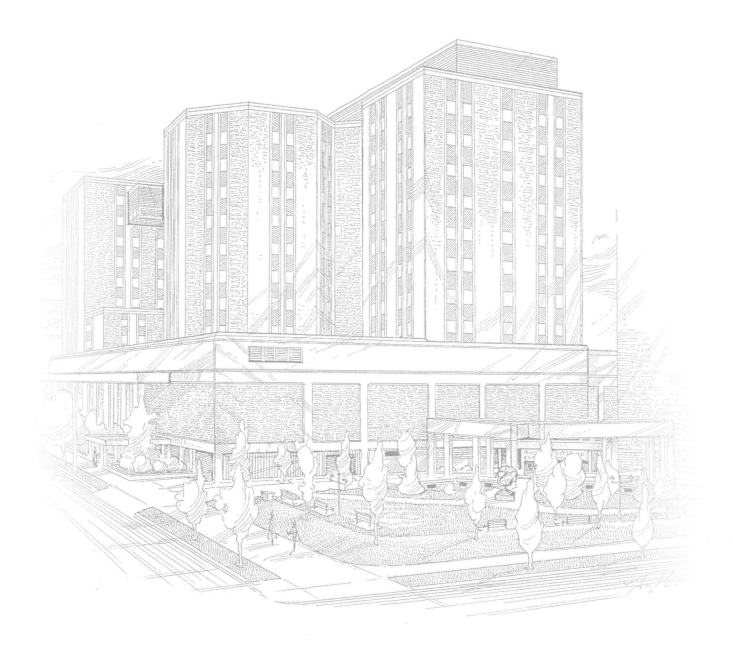

CHAPTER 13

Supraclavicular Blockade

Adam K. Jacob, M.D.

Kenneth P. Scott, M.D.

Clinical Applications

The supraclavicular block was first introduced into clinical practice by Kulenkampff in 1911. The approach followed a surgical description of the brachial plexus at the level of the subclavian artery. The block is performed at the level of the divisions where the majority of the innervation to the upper extremity is contained within six nerves. The proximity of the six divisions at this level allows a dense and comprehensive block to be performed at this location. The technique is optimal for surgical procedures of the upper extremity distal to the shoulder, including the elbow, forearm, and hand. However, because of anatomical variations of the cervical plexus and proximal branches of the brachial plexus, the block may provide inadequate anesthesia for surgical procedures of the shoulder.

Relevant Anatomy

After the five roots of the brachial plexus—cervical nerve 5 (C5) through the first thoracic nerve (T1)—exit their respective neural foramina and pass between the anterior and middle scalene muscles, the C5 and C6 nerve roots combine to form the superior trunk, the C7 nerve root the middle trunk, and the C8 and T1 nerve roots the inferior trunk of the brachial plexus (Figure 1). As the three trunks approach the first rib, they divide into anterior and posterior divisions, which then fuse into lateral, posterior, and medial cords. The divisions are located posterior and lateral to the subclavian artery and are commonly surrounded by a fascial sheath, which is considered to be a continuation of the prevertebral and anterior and middle scalene muscle fascia (Figure 2). After passing over the first rib, the neurovascular bundle courses beneath the middle third of the clavicle at or near its midpoint and continues on to the axilla.

Surface Anatomy

Surface structures of importance can be found within the supraclavicular triangle and fossa (a depression overlying the triangle). The triangle is bordered medially by the lateral margin of the clavicular head of the sternoclei-domastoid muscle, superiorly by the inferior belly of the omohyoid muscle (rarely palpable except in thin patients),

and inferiorly by the middle third of the clavicle. In select patients, the caudal portion of the interscalene groove may be palpated within the supraclavicular triangle. The pulse of the subclavian artery may also be an important landmark when palpable within the supraclavicular fossa.

Patient Position

The patient is supine or in a semi-sitting position with the head rotated slightly away from the side to be blocked. The ipsilateral extremity should be positioned at the patient's side with the arm adducted, elbow flexed, and forearm resting on the abdomen. The shoulder should be dropped to facilitate identification of the brachial plexus at this level. This maneuver is accomplished by placing a small towel roll along the midline between the scapulae.

Technique

Neural Localization Techniques

Historically, the brachial plexus has been identified using a paresthesia or nerve stimulation technique

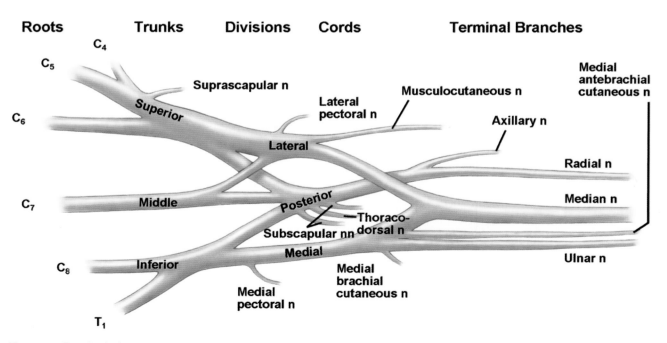

Figure 1. Brachial plexus anatomy.

when performing the classic supraclavicular approach. However, a concern about these techniques has always been the risk of procedure-related pneumothorax. In an effort to address these concerns, newer techniques to supraclavicular blockade have been developed, including modifications of the classic approach and the use of ultrasound-guided technology. Several studies have examined the use of ultrasound guidance for supraclavicular blockade. Advocates of this technique suggest that real-time anatomical visualization may lessen the risk of pneumothorax compared with traditional techniques. Confirmation of circumferential spread of local anesthetic may also improve block success. However, evidence within the literature is currently insufficient to definitively support or refute these claims.

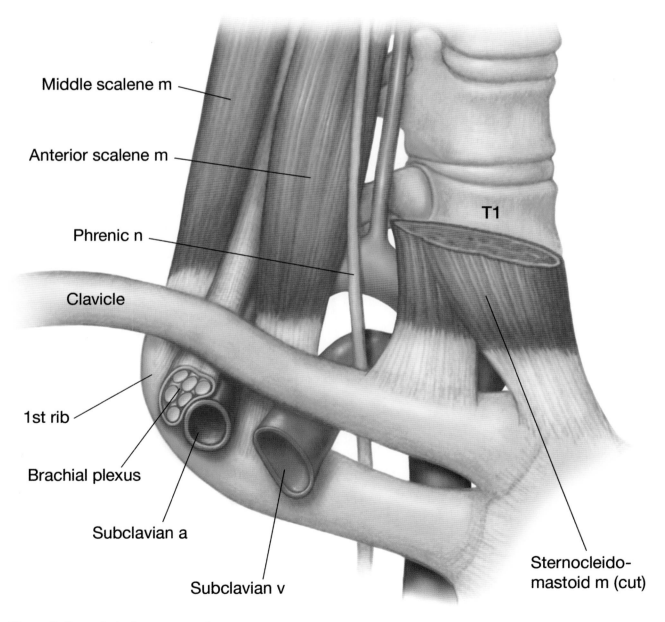

Figure 2. Supraclavicular neurovascular anatomy.

Needle Insertion Site

A modification of the classic supraclavicular approach identifies a point 2.5 cm lateral to the lateral border of the clavicular head of the sternocleidomastoid muscle (Figure 3). In many patients, this approximates the midpoint of the clavicle. The site of needle insertion is marked 1 cm superior (approximately 1 fingerbreadth) to the clavicle at its midpoint. This point should roughly coincide with the intersection of the projected interscalene groove. A 22-gauge 2-inch (5-cm) insulated needle is inserted perpendicular to the skin and advanced in a parasagittal (caudal) plane parallel to the patient's midline until an

appropriate motor response (i.e., flexion or extension of the fingers or wrist) is elicited at a current of 0.5 to 0.8 mA (Figure 3). However, the needle should *not* be advanced more than 2.5 to 3 cm on the first pass in the absence of an appropriate motor response. After an acceptable motor response is elicited, 30 to 40 mL of local anesthetic is injected incrementally with frequent aspiration to minimize the risk of inadvertent intravascular injection.

Needle Redirection Cues

If no paresthesia or nerve stimulation is obtained and the first rib is not encountered, the needle should be

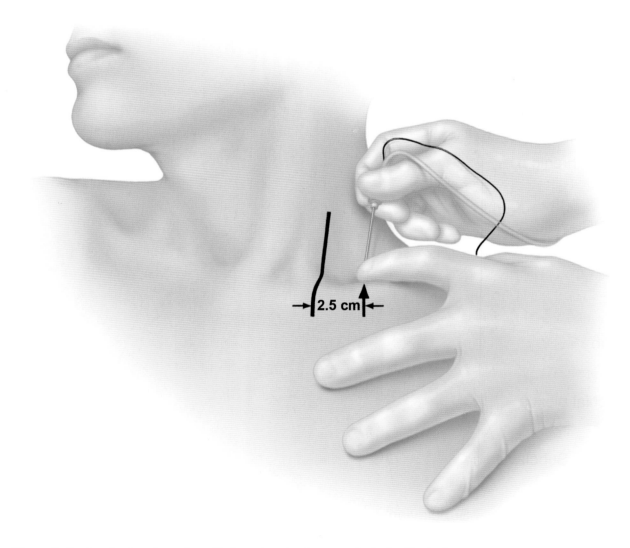

Figure 3. Surface landmarks and needle insertion site for supraclavicular blockade.

redirected slightly laterally in small increments until the rib is contacted. Once the rib is contacted (assuming no paresthesia or nerve stimulation was obtained), the needle should be redirected posteriorly in small increments through an arc of approximately 15°. If there is still no paresthesia or nerve stimulation, the original needle pathway where the rib was first contacted is returned to, and the needle is redirected anteriorly in small increments through an arc of approximately 15°. The tip of the needle should *always* be kept above the clavicle. If the subclavian artery is contacted, the needle should be redirected in a more lateral and posterior direction.

Ultrasound-Guided Supraclavicular Blockade

The advent of ultrasound guidance has renewed interest in the supraclavicular approach to the brachial plexus. Continuous, real-time visualization of the needle tip has the potential to reduce the risk of inadvertently entering the pleura or adjacent vascular structures.

Scanning Technique

To visualize the neurovascular arrangement, the ultrasound probe should be placed in the supraclavicular fossa, parallel to the clavicle, with the beam directed caudally toward the first rib (Figures 4 and 5). Optimization of

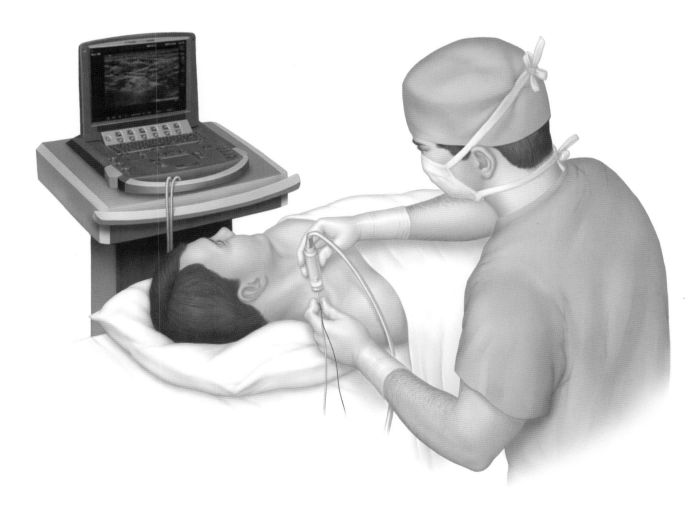

Figure 4. Patient-provider orientation for ultrasound-guided supraclavicular blockade.

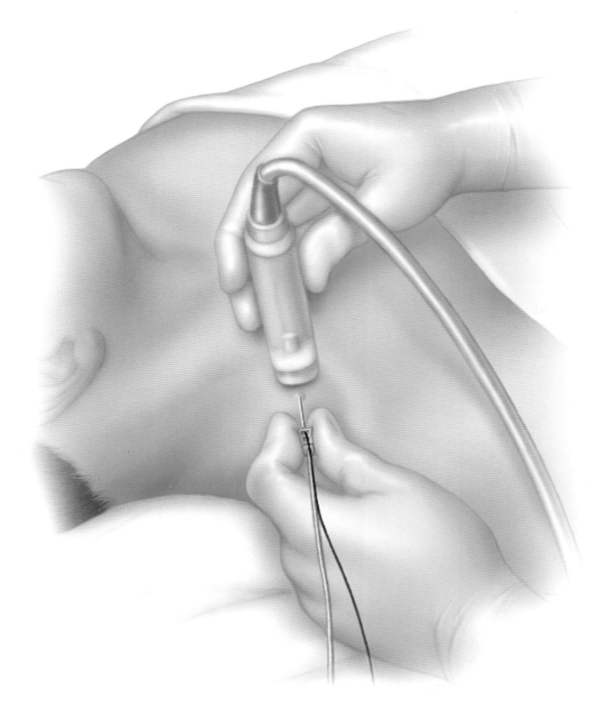

Figure 5. Probe and needle position for supraclavicular blockade.

the ultrasound image may require minor adjustments of probe rotation, pitch, and tilt. The ideal image captures the divisions of the brachial plexus, the subclavian artery, and the subclavian vein in perfect cross-section (i.e., appearing as circular structures) resting superficial to the first rib.

Sonoanatomy

As with any ultrasound-guided technique, accurate visualization of the neurovascular structure(s) is critical. Sonographically, the plexus appears as a group of four to six or more hypoechoic (dark) circular structures contained within a relatively hyperechoic (bright) surrounding layer (Figure 6). This arrangement of the proximal divisions of the brachial plexus within a neurofascial sheath is commonly described as a "bag of grapes." The subclavian artery can be confirmed with color Doppler and is identified as a circular, hypoechoic, pulsatile structure located immediately medial to the plexus. The subclavian vein also appears as a circular, hypoechoic, nonpulsatile structure that can be readily distinguished from the artery by its ability to be compressed. The position of the vein can vary, but it is typically located medial to the artery.

Ultrasound Approach

An in-plane approach is preferred during ultrasound-guided supraclavicular blockade. The in-plane approach allows optimal visualization of the needle throughout the entire procedure. A 22-gauge 2-inch (5-cm) insulated needle should be inserted immediately lateral to the probe and advanced slowly in a lateral to medial direction in plane with the ultrasound beam to allow complete visualization of the needle shaft (Figures 5 and 7). The inherent safety in this approach depends entirely on continuous visualization of the needle tip during advancement.

The needle should enter the skin posterolateral to the plexus and advance anteromedially (and slightly caudal) toward the divisions of the brachial plexus. Once the needle tip is within the sheath, 20 mL of local anesthetic is injected under direct visualization to confirm perineural spread. To ensure a comprehensive block, the needle tip may need to be redirected several times within the sheath to ensure that all divisions are bathed in local anesthetic and that local anesthetic spread has extended inferiorly to the subclavian artery.

Side Effects and Complications

The most common side effects of the supraclavicular block are phrenic nerve blockade with hemidiaphragmatic paralysis and sympathetic nerve block resulting in Horner syndrome (ipsilateral eye ptosis, miosis, and anhydrosis). Both have been estimated to occur in 30% to 50% of patients. Other complications common to most regional anesthesia techniques, including intravascular injection, neuronal injury, infection, and hematoma, have also been reported. However, these complications are considered uncommon in the setting of proper nerve block technique.

The most serious complication of the supraclavicular approach to the brachial plexus is pneumothorax. The incidence of pneumothorax has been estimated between 0.5% and 5%. However, proceduralists experienced with the technique tend to have complication rates less than the lowest range reported. This complication can best be avoided by limiting needle redirection strictly in the anteroposterior direction, avoiding medial redirection, and maintaining the needle tip above the level of the clavicle.

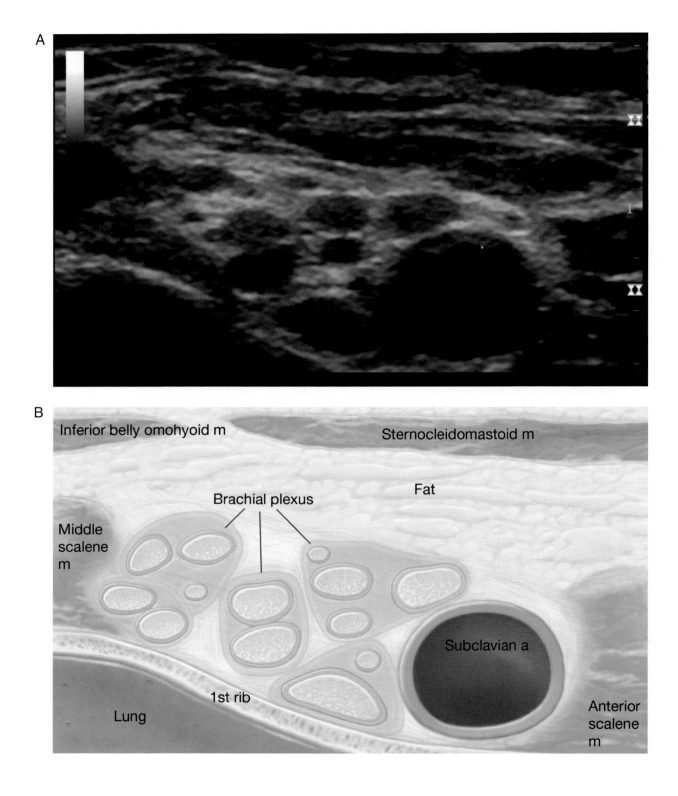

Figure 6. Supraclavicular view of the brachial plexus. A, Ultrasound image. B, Corresponding anatomical illustration.

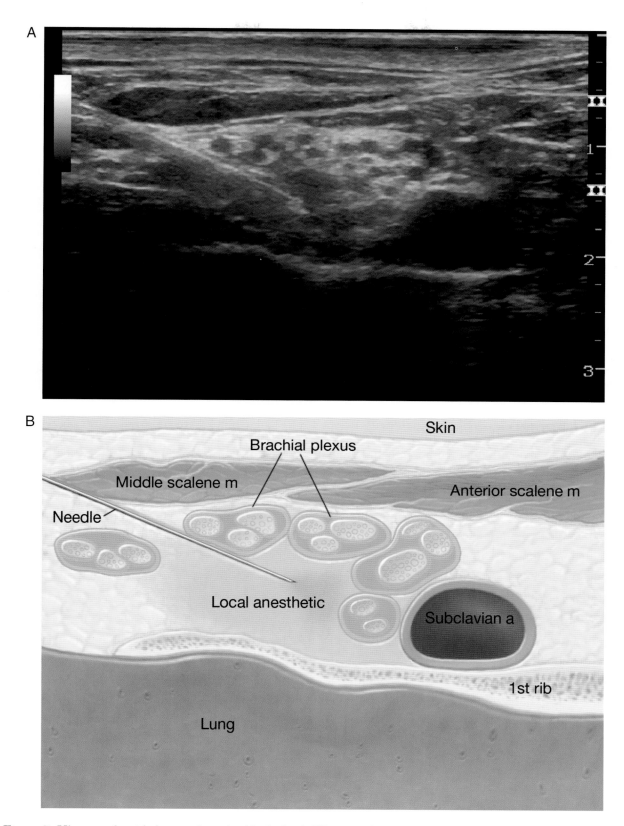

Figure 7. Ultrasound-guided supraclavicular blockade. A, Ultrasound image. B, Corresponding anatomical illustration.

Suggested Reading

Arcand G, Williams SR, Chouinard P, Boudreault D, Harris P, Ruel M, et al. Ultrasound-guided infraclavicular versus supraclavicular block. Anesth Analg. 2005 Sep;101(3):886-90.

Brown DL. Atlas of regional anesthesia. 2nd ed. Philadelphia: W. B. Saunders Company; c1999. Chapter 4, Supraclavicular block; p. 31-40.

Chan VW, Perlas A, Rawson R, Odukoya O. Ultrasound-guided supraclavicular brachial plexus block. Anesth Analg. 2003 Nov;97(5):1514-7.

Dupre LJ, Danel V, Legrand JJ, Stieglitz P. Surface landmarks for supraclavicular block of the brachial plexus. Anesth Analg. 1982 Jan;61(1):28-31.

Franco CD. The subclavian perivascular block. Tech Reg Anesth Pain Mgmt. 1999;3:212-6.

Franco CD. Brachial plexus blocks. In: Chelly JE, editor. Peripheral nerve blocks: a color atlas. 2nd ed. Philadelphia: Lippincott Williams & Wilkins; c2004. p. 44-5.

Franco CD, Domashevich V, Voronov G, Rafizad AB, Jelev TJ. The supraclavicular block with a nerve stimulator: to decrease or not to decrease, that is the question. Anesth Analg. 2004 Apr;98(4):1167-71.

Franco CD, Gloss FJ, Voronov G, Tyler SG, Stojiljkovic LS. Supraclavicular block in the obese population: an analysis of 2020 blocks. Anesth Analg. 2006 Apr;102(4):1252-4.

Thompson AM, Newman RJ, Semple JC. Brachial plexus anaesthesia for upper limb surgery: a review of eight years' experience. J Hand Surg [Br]. 1988 May;13(2):195-8.

Williams SR, Chouinard P, Arcand G, Harris P, Ruel M, Boudreault D, et al. Ultrasound guidance speeds execution and improves the quality of supraclavicular block. Anesth Analg. 2003 Nov;97(5):1518-23.

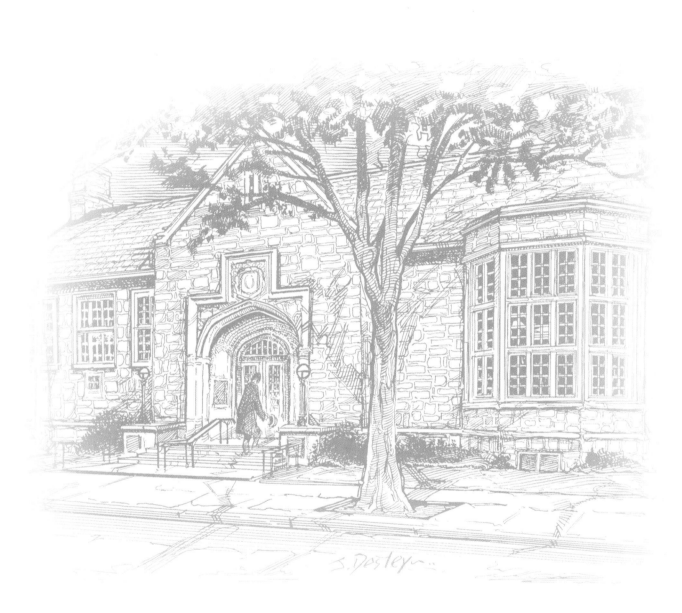

CHAPTER 14

Infraclavicular Blockade

Jack L. Wilson, M.D.

Adam K. Jacob, M.D.

Hugh M. Smith, M.D., Ph.D.

Clinical Applications

The infraclavicular approach to brachial plexus blockade was first described by Gaston Labat in 1922. The initial technique of Labat was later modified by both Raj and colleagues (1973) and Sims (1977), who tried to improve reproducibility and safety by redefining surface landmarks and needle trajectories. In 1998, Wilson and colleagues described yet another modification of the technique using the coracoid process as a pivotal landmark (i.e., the coracoid approach). This most recent description, which emphasizes a more lateral needle insertion point, prompted a renewed interest in the infraclavicular approach. Infraclavicular blockade is best suited for patients undergoing surgery of the elbow, forearm, wrist, or hand. An advantage of the infraclavicular approach is the relatively neutral, adducted arm position used during block placement. This arm position is beneficial for patients with upper extremity injuries or those with severe osteoarthritic pain that may limit full range of motion.

Relevant Anatomy

Important anatomical boundaries of the infraclavicular fossa include the major and minor pectoralis muscles anteriorly, the ribs inferomedially, the coracoid process and clavicle superiorly, and the humerus laterally. At the lateral border of the first rib, the subclavian artery becomes the axillary artery, an important vascular structure within the infraclavicular fossa. Within the fossa, the brachial plexus consists of the lateral, posterior, and medial cords that are distributed around the superior, posterior, and inferior aspects of the artery, respectively (Figure 1). This neurovascular bundle is beneath the pectoralis major and minor muscles and immediately deep to the pectoralis fascia. As visualized on an anterior-posterior chest radiograph, the parietal pleura and lung lie several centimeters inferomedially from the infraclavicular fossa (Figure 1).

Surface Anatomy

Surface landmarks for the coracoid approach to the brachial plexus include the head of the humerus, the clavicle, the coracoid process, and the acromioclavicular joint. The coracoid process is identified by palpating deep and

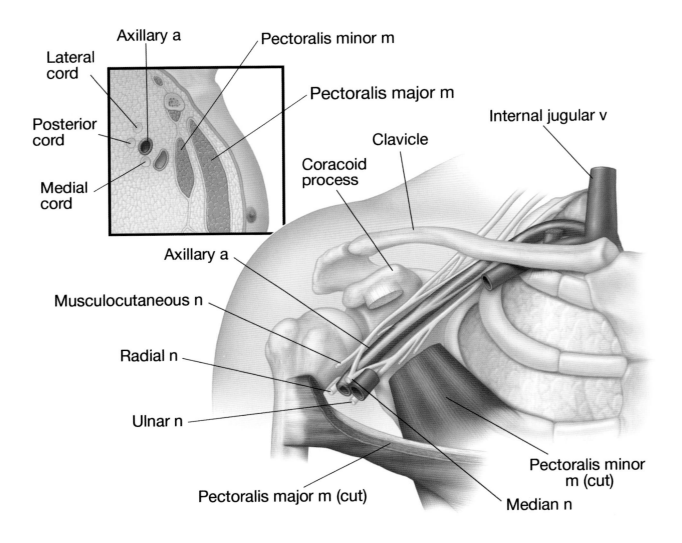

Figure 1. Infraclavicular neurovascular anatomy with cross-sectional view.

medial to the head of the humerus and acromioclavicular joint just inferior to the clavicle. In most patients, direct pressure on the coracoid process produces discomfort. The brachial plexus travels in a slight inferolateral direction, directly beneath the pectoralis muscles, at a point 2 cm inferior and 2 cm medial to the coracoid process (Figure 2).

Patient Position

The patient should be in a supine position with the head rotated slightly away from the side to be blocked. The arm is commonly adducted with the elbow extended and hand at the patient's side (Figure 3). Alternatively, the block can be performed with the arm abducted, externally rotated, and flexed at the elbow.

Technique

Neural Localization Techniques

Nerve stimulation is most commonly used to facilitate neural localization during the infraclavicular approach. Controversy exists as to which neurostimulatory response(s) best predicts block success. However, a motor response within the distal extremity (i.e., hand and intrinsic finger movement) at a current of 0.3 to 0.5 mA is ideal. Biceps (musculocutaneous nerve) and deltoid (axillary nerve) motor responses are generally not acceptable, because the musculocutaneous and axillary nerves commonly exit the sheath of the brachial plexus proximal to the infraclavicular fossa. The use of real-time ultrasound guidance for infraclavicular blockade, alone or in conjunction with nerve stimulation, is rapidly gaining popularity.

Needle Insertion Site

A 21-gauge 4-inch (10-cm) insulated needle is inserted 2 cm medial and 2 cm inferior to the tip of the coracoid process (Figure 2). The needle is advanced directly posterior in a vertical paramedian plane (Figure 4). The depth of the brachial plexus is highly dependent on body habitus, ranging from 2.5 to 3 cm in slender patients and 6 to 8 cm in obese patients. The infraclavicular approach

requires a relatively high volume of local anesthetic to achieve complete anesthesia of the plexus. After an acceptable motor response is acquired (i.e., hand and intrinsic finger movement), 30 to 40 mL of local anesthetic is injected incrementally with frequent aspiration to minimize the risk of inadvertent intravascular injection.

Needle Redirection Cues

If the plexus is not encountered on the first needle pass, redirection in a cephalad/caudad paramedian plane should identify the appropriate neurostimulation response. The needle should *not* be directed medially or laterally from the plane of insertion. Medial redirection may increase the risk of pneumothorax. Lateral redirection may place the needle tip lateral to the cords, a position that will likely result in incomplete anesthesia from insufficient spread of local anesthetic.

Alternative Techniques

Several alternative techniques have been described for the infraclavicular approach. Among the most common are the lateral and medial modifications. The clavicle and coracoid process are convenient landmarks to guide needle placement. Kapral and colleagues described a lateral infraclavicular approach that is performed with the needle inserted posteriorly in a sagittal plane and directed toward the coracoid process. Once the coracoid process is contacted, the needle is slightly withdrawn and redirected inferiorly 2 to 3 cm as guided by neurostimulation.

In 1995, Kilka and colleagues described a more medial infraclavicular approach to the brachial plexus. The technique directs the needle posteriorly at a point immediately below the mid-clavicle. The proposed benefit of this midclavicular approach is that the width of the brachial plexus in this region is at its most narrow point—facilitating a single injection technique with comprehensive spread of local anesthetic. The mid clavicle is defined as half the distance between the acromion and midsuprasternal notch. Alternatively, the midpoint between the acromioclavicular joint and the sternoclavicular joint has been used as an anatomical landmark. Regardless of technique, anatomical variation within the infraclavicular fossa and the acceptance of proximal

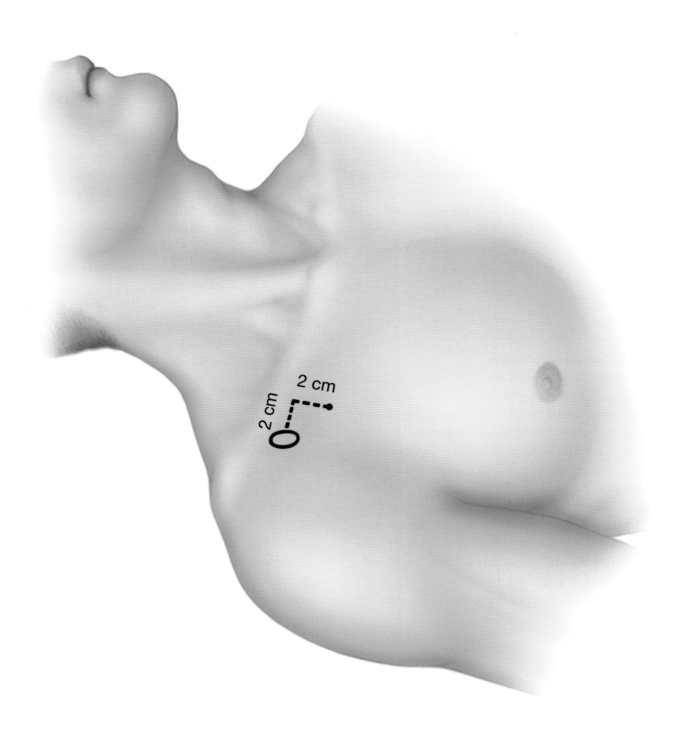

2 cm

2 cm

Figure 2. Surface landmarks for infraclavicular blockade (coracoid approach).

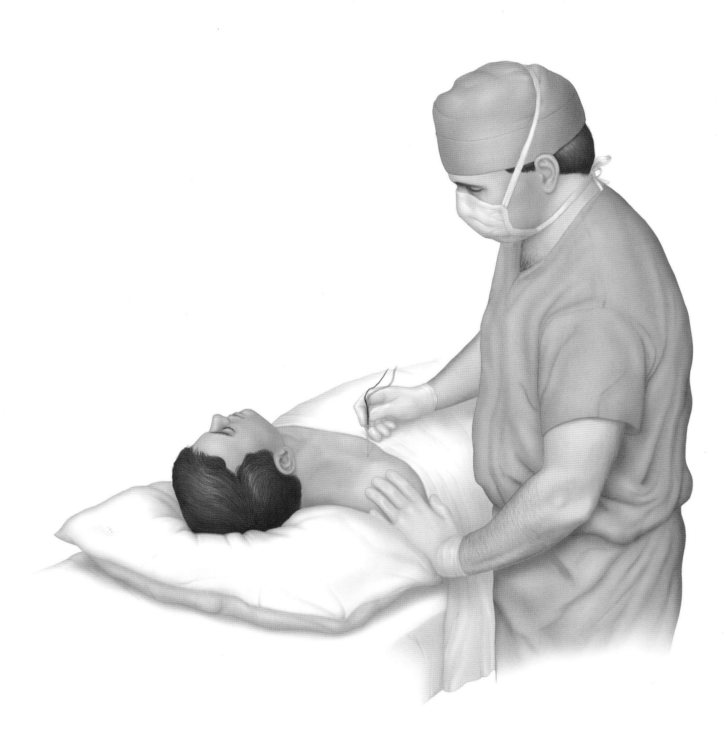

Figure 3. Patient-provider orientation during infraclavicular blockade.

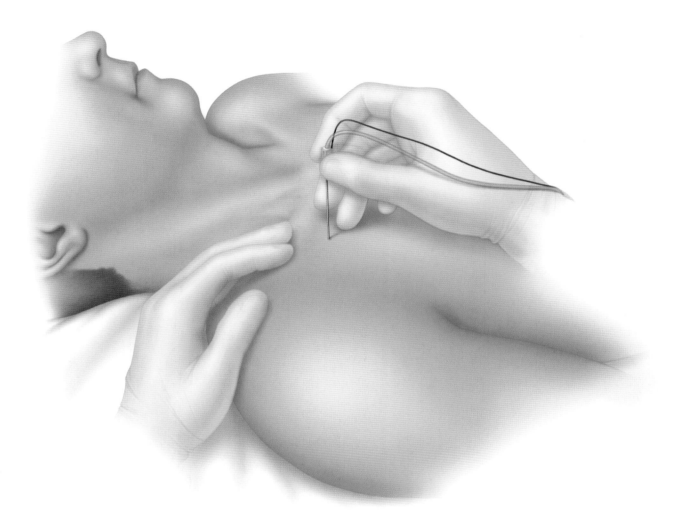

Figure 4. Needle trajectory during infraclavicular blockade (coracoid approach).

motor responses may significantly increase the rate of block failure. However, the use of real-time ultrasound guidance, alone or in conjunction with nerve stimulation, may facilitate comprehensive and circumferential spread of local anesthetic around the brachial plexus within this region.

Ultrasound-Guided Infraclavicular Blockade

Scanning Technique

To visualize the neurovascular arrangement, the ultrasound probe should be oriented perpendicular and inferior to the clavicle along the lateral segment in the infraclavicular fossa (Figure 5). Optimization of the ultrasound image may require minor adjustments of probe rotation, pitch, and tilt. If the axillary artery is not readily visualized, the probe has been positioned too medially and requires lateral advancement. Low-frequency ultrasound (6-8 MHz) may be necessary to optimize imaging if the neurovascular structures are deeper than 4 cm.

Sonoanatomy

The ideal sonographic image of the infraclavicular fossa captures both the axillary artery and the three cords of the brachial plexus in perfect cross-section,

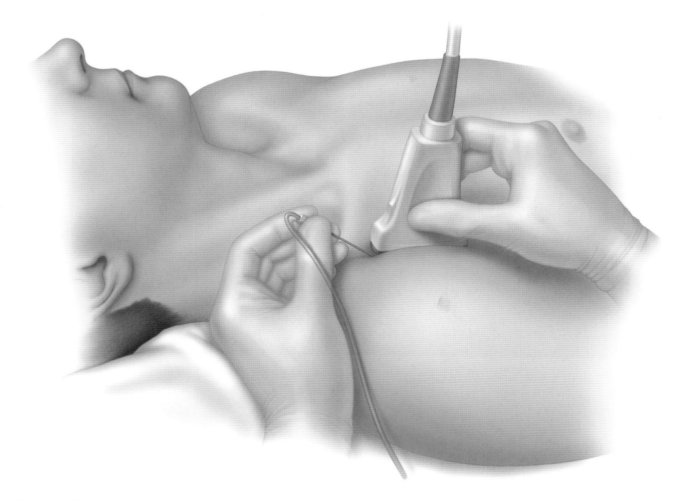

Figure 5. Probe and needle orientation during ultrasound-guided infraclavicular blockade.

resting immediately deep to the pectoralis minor muscle (Figure 6). The plexus and vessels are typically located 2 to 4 cm below the surface of the skin. However, depth of the neurovascular structures may vary, depending on the thickness of the pectoralis musculature. Unfortunately, complete imaging of the plexus is often inconsistent—particularly when compared with interscalene and supra-clavicular views. Sonographically, the plexus should appear as three hyperechoic, honeycombed structures (medial, posterior, and lateral cords) arranged around the axillary artery at approximately the 3-, 6-, and 9-o'clock positions. However, the position of the cords relative to the axillary artery is variable. The axillary artery is readily identified as a circular, hypoechoic, pulsatile structure (which

can be confirmed with color Doppler) located deep to the pectoralis minor muscle and centered within the cords. The axillary vein also appears as a circular, hypoechoic structure. However, unlike the artery, the axillary vein is nonpulsatile and should be somewhat compressible with deep pressure. The position of the vein can vary, but it is typically located anterior and inferior to the artery.

Ultrasound Approach
Needle insertion is typically immediately inferior to the clavicle and superior to the transducer in plane with the ultrasound beam (Figure 5). To accomplish this, the pro-ceduralist should be positioned on the ipsilateral side of the block, facing the patient (Figure 7). This orientation

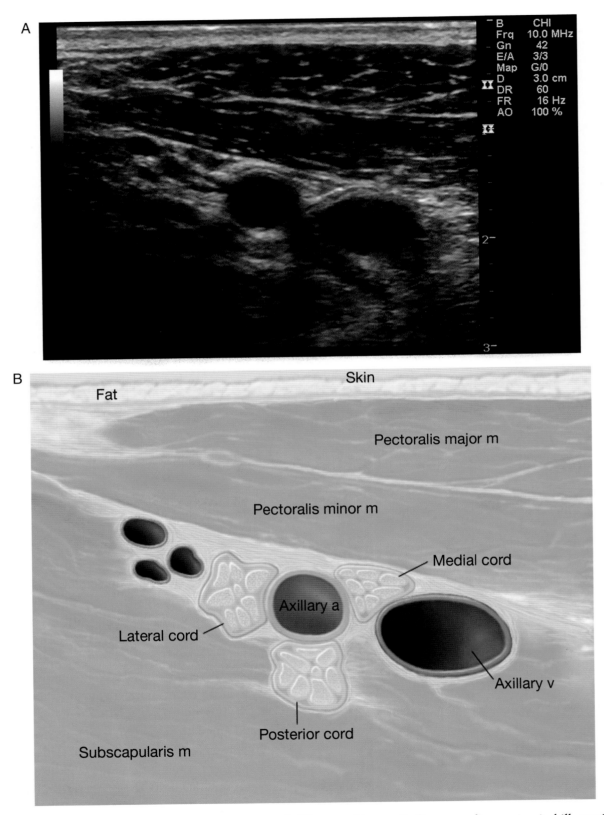

Figure 6. Infraclavicular view of the brachial plexus. A, Ultrasound image. B, Corresponding anatomical illustration.

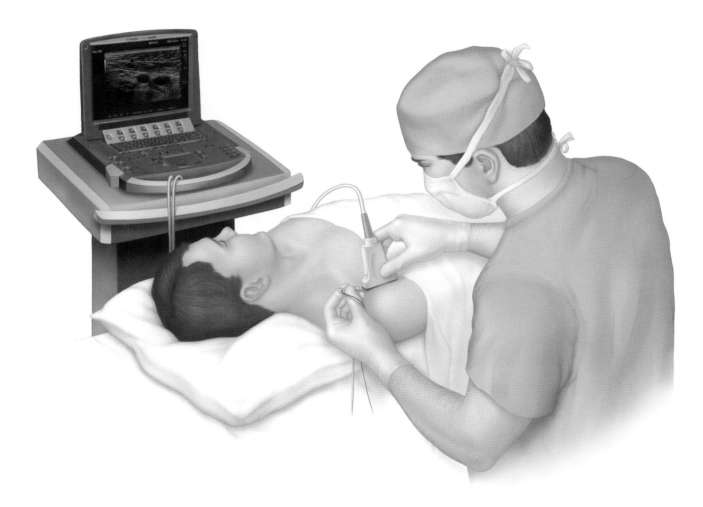

Figure 7. Patient-provider orientation during ultrasound-guided infraclavicular blockade.

allows a stable position for advancing the needle in plane toward the posterior cord, which lies posterior to the axillary artery. Alternatively, the proceduralist may sit at the head of the bed facing the patient's feet.

Continuous visualization of the needle tip during advancement is imperative. Proper identification of the posterior cord can be confirmed with nerve stimulation and may appear as a "radial" twitch (i.e., arm, hand, or finger extension). Once identified, approximately 15 to 20 mL of local anesthetic is injected incrementally around the posterior cord. Ideally, this needle location allows local anesthetic to spread toward the medial cord. The needle can then be slightly withdrawn to deposit

5 to 10 mL of local anesthetic around the lateral cord (Figure 8). Optimally, local anesthetic should encompass the axillary artery from the 3- to the 12-o'clock position.

Continuous Peripheral Nerve Catheters

Perineural catheters are commonly used as an adjunct to anesthesia or for postoperative pain management. Specifically, continuous infraclavicular catheters have been shown to provide exceptional postoperative analgesia for both inpatient and outpatient surgical procedures. Infraclavicular catheters may be placed using stimulating catheters, nonstimulating catheters, or ultrasound-guided techniques.

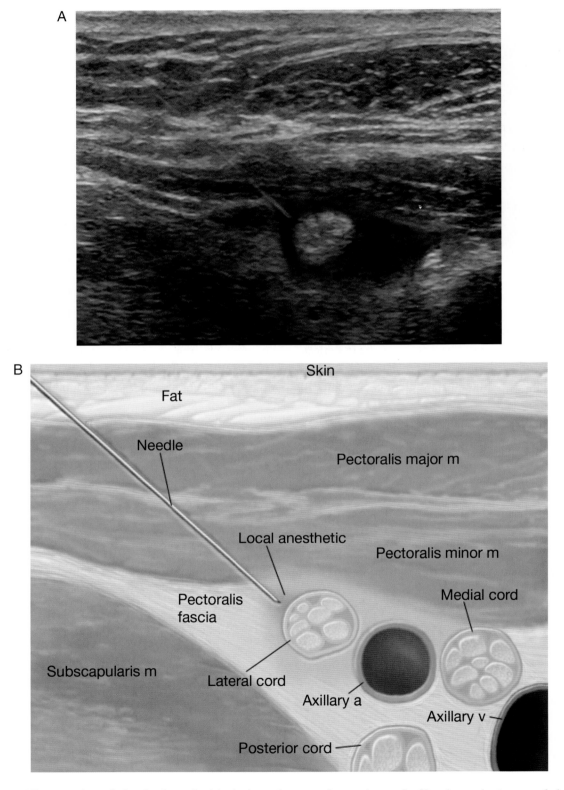

Figure 8. Ultrasound-guided infraclavicular blockade with circumferential spread of local anesthetic around the lateral cord. A, Ultrasound image. B, Corresponding anatomical illustration.

In the absence of ultrasound guidance, neural localization for catheter placement is essentially identical to conventional nerve stimulation techniques. For placement of a perineural catheter, an 18-gauge 4-inch (10-cm) insulated Tuohy needle should be used instead of a traditional 21-gauge (single-injection) stimulating needle. The needle should be inserted and advanced as described above with the bevel directed in a cephalad direction toward the scalene muscles and along the path of the brachial plexus. After satisfactory needle placement (based on an appropriate neurostimulation response), the catheter should be advanced 3 to 5 cm beyond the needle tip and secured on the anterior chest wall.

Ultrasound-guided catheter placement is similar to that described for the ultrasound-guided single-injection technique. An 18-gauge 4-inch (10-cm) insulated Tuohy needle is advanced under direct visualization toward the posterior cord. The location of the posterior cord can be confirmed with neural stimulation. Once the location is identified, the catheter should be advanced 1 to 2 cm beyond the needle tip. Ideally, the catheter tip should remain in proximity to the posterior cord. Next, a test injection with either a dextrose solution (to preserve neurostimulation) or a normal saline solution should be performed to confirm the anticipated spread of local anesthetic. The test solution should migrate in the direction of the medial and lateral cords. If adequate spread occurs, a slow, incremental loading dose of local anesthetic should be injected through the catheter. If insufficient spread occurs, the catheter should be manipulated with serial test injections under direct visualization until adequate spread is observed.

Infraclavicular catheters can be secured to the chest wall with various techniques. Many proceduralists advocate tunneling the catheters subcutaneously to minimize the risk of dislodgment, inadvertent removal, or infectious complications. In contrast, others simply cover the catheter with a sterile, occlusive dressing and secure with tape. Regardless, the catheter site should be examined daily to identify early signs of infection (erythema, induration, discharge) or evidence of catheter dislodgment.

Side Effects and Complications

Infraclavicular blockade has been shown to produce less respiratory compromise than supraclavicular or interscalene techniques. In contrast, incomplete anesthesia may occur at higher rates than with more proximal approaches. In particular, because the musculocutaneous and axillary nerves may depart from the brachial plexus in a proximal location, comprehensive blockade of these nerve distributions is somewhat unreliable. Other complications of infraclavicular blockade may include intravascular injection, infection, hematoma formation, or pneumothorax. The risk of pneumothorax can be minimized by using well-defined anatomical landmarks (e.g., the coracoid process) to identify the point of needle insertion and to avoid needle advancement in a medial or inferomedial direction toward the chest wall. The infraclavicular approach to the brachial plexus should be avoided in patients with significant coagulopathies. Inadvertent puncture of the axillary artery may result in significant bleeding within a poorly confined, noncompressible anatomical site. Horner syndrome and direct neural injury are also potential complications. However, the frequency of these events is unknown. When using a continuous catheter technique, providers should monitor for signs and symptoms of local anesthetic toxicity.

Suggested Reading

Dabu A, Chan VWS. A practical guide to ultrasound imaging for peripheral nerve blocks. c2004. p. 50-5.

Kapral S, Jandrasits O, Schabernig C, Likar R, Reddy B, Mayer N, et al. Lateral infraclavicular plexus block vs. axillary block for hand and forearm surgery. Acta Anaesthesiol Scand. 1999 Nov;43(10):1047-52.

Kilka HG, Geiger P, Mehrkens HH. [Infraclavicular vertical brachial plexus blockade: a new method for anesthesia of the upper extremity. An anatomical and clinical study.] Anaesthesist. 1995 May;44(5):339-44. German.

Ootaki C, Hayashi H, Amano M. Ultrasound-guided infraclavicular brachial plexus block: an alternative technique to anatomical landmark-guided approaches. Reg Anesth Pain Med. 2000 Nov-Dec;25(6):600-4.

Raj PP, Montgomery SJ, Nettles D, Jenkins MT. Infraclavicular brachial plexus block: a new approach. Anesth Analg. 1973 Nov-Dec;52(6):897-904.

Raphael DT, McIntee D, Tsuruda JS, Colletti P, Tatevossian R. Frontal slab composite magnetic resonance neurography of the brachial plexus: implications for infraclavicular block approaches. Anesthesiology. 2005 Dec;103(6):1218-24.

Sandhu NS, Capan LM. Ultrasound-guided infraclavicular brachial plexus block. Br J Anaesth. 2002 Aug;89(2):254-9.

Sims JK. A modification of landmarks for infraclavicular approach to brachial plexus block. Anesth Analg. 1977 Jul-Aug;56(4):554-5.

Wilson JL, Brown DL, Wong GY, Ehman RL, Cahill DR. Infraclavicular brachial plexus block: parasagittal anatomy important to the coracoid technique. Anesth Analg. 1998 Oct;87(4):870-3.

Weller RS, Gerancher JC. Brachial plexus block: "best" approach and "best" evoked response: where are we? Reg Anesth Pain Med. 2004 Nov-Dec;29(6):520-3.

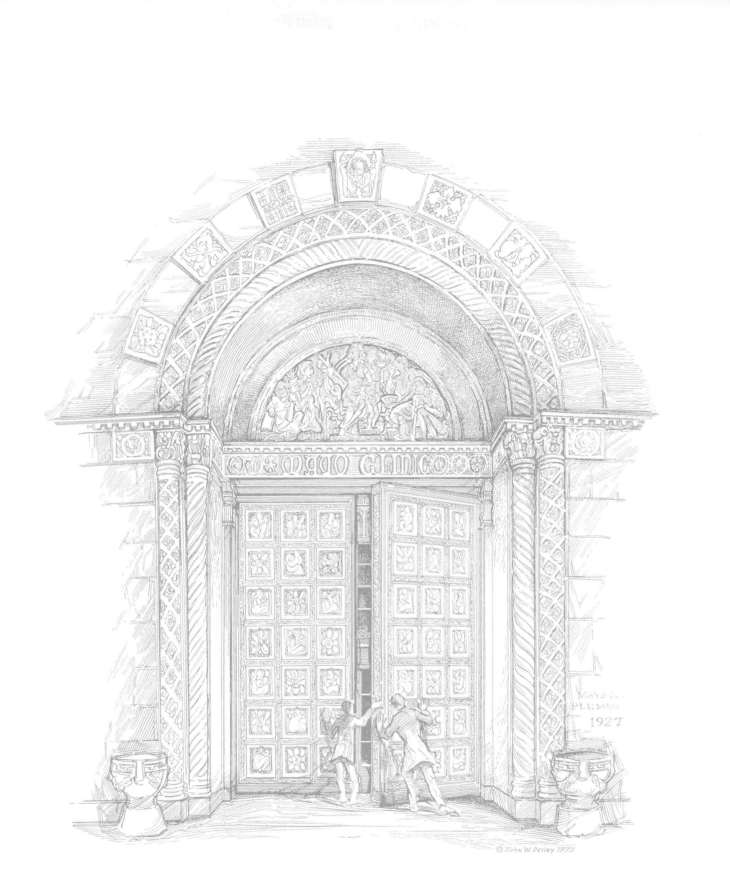

CHAPTER
15

Axillary Blockade

Sandra L. Kopp, M.D.
Hugh M. Smith, M.D., Ph.D.

Clinical Applications

First described in 1911 by Hirschel, the axillary block has become one of the most popular regional anesthetic techniques for upper extremity surgery. In contrast to both supraclavicular and infraclavicular techniques, the axillary approach offers the safest and most superficial access to the brachial plexus. Axillary blockade can reliably anesthetize the three terminal branches of the brachial plexus—the median, radial, and ulnar nerves (Figure 1). In addition, it may provide variable blockade of the musculocutaneous and axillary nerves. Given the potential for inadequate proximal anesthesia, this approach is commonly used for surgical procedures on the elbow, forearm, wrist, and hand. Continuous axillary blockade may provide extended postoperative analgesia that may otherwise require multiple repeat single-injection techniques.

251

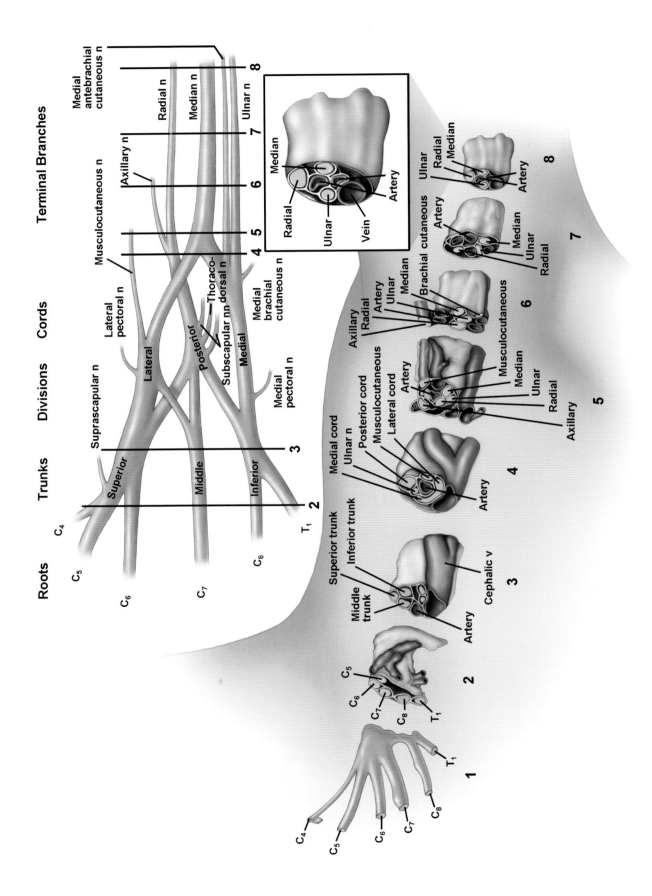

Figure 1. Brachial plexus anatomy.

Relevant Anatomy

Within the axilla, the three terminal branches of the brachial plexus typically surround the axillary artery (Figure 2). Traditional anatomical descriptions suggest that the artery is anterior to the radial nerve, postero-medial to the median nerve, and posterolateral to the ulnar nerve (Figure 3). However, recent anatomical studies and ultrasonography have shown considerable variation of the neurovascular anatomy. More predictably,

the musculocutaneous nerve is separate from the brachial plexus, embedded within the coracobrachialis muscle posterior and cephalad to the artery. The axillary vein varies in both size and position. The intercostobrachial nerve (ICB), a small terminal branch of the second thoracic nerve root, supplies cutaneous innervation to the medial arm and axilla as either a single, discrete nerve or multiple cutaneous branches (Figure 4).

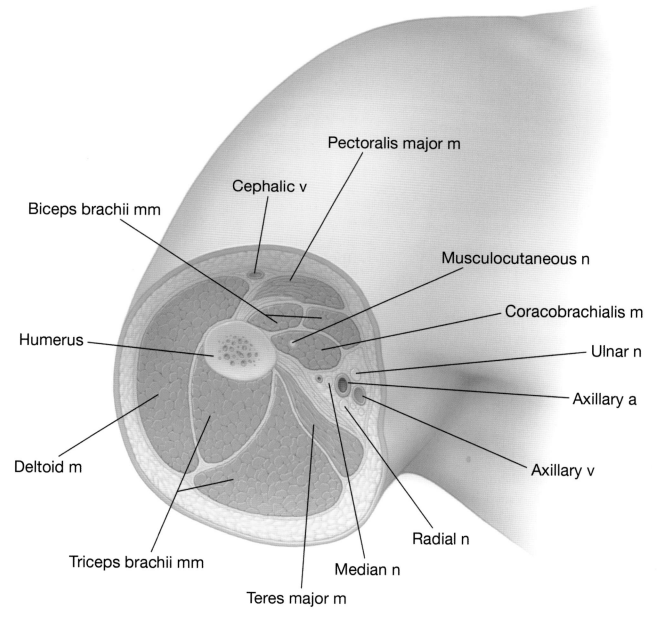

Figure 2. Cross-sectional axillary anatomy.

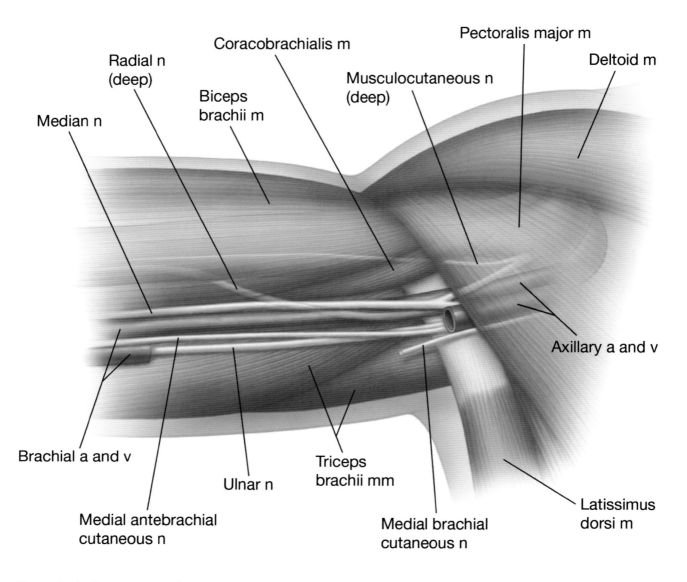

Figure 3. Axillary neurovascular anatomy.

Surface Anatomy

The primary surface landmark for the axillary block is the pulse of the axillary artery. It is commonly located in the groove beneath the coracobrachialis muscle adjacent to the lateral margin of the pectoralis major muscle. If the artery is not easily palpated, arm adduction against resistance tenses the pectoralis and coracobrachialis muscles and enhances the groove between the two muscles. A reference line should be drawn along the course of the axillary artery beginning as proximal as possible within the axilla.

Patient Position

The patient should be supine with the head in the neutral position or rotated slightly away from the side to be blocked. The arm is abducted and the elbow flexed to approximately 90° (Figure 5). It is important to ensure that the arm remains in a neutral anterior-posterior position relative to the trunk of the body. Anterior displacement of the humeral head may impede arterial flow if the arm is extended posterior to the trunk.

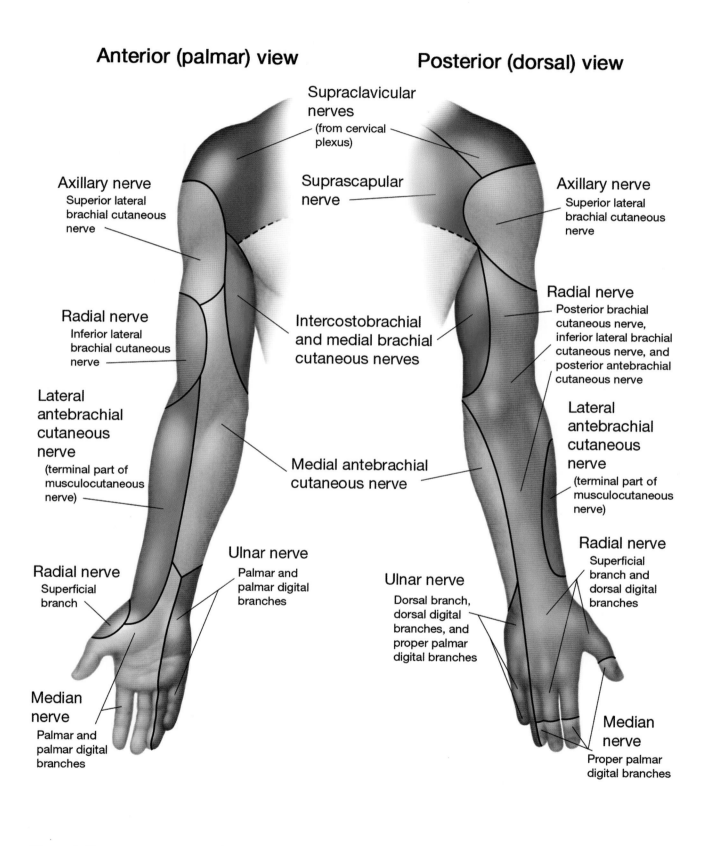

Figure 4. Cutaneous innervation of the upper extremity.

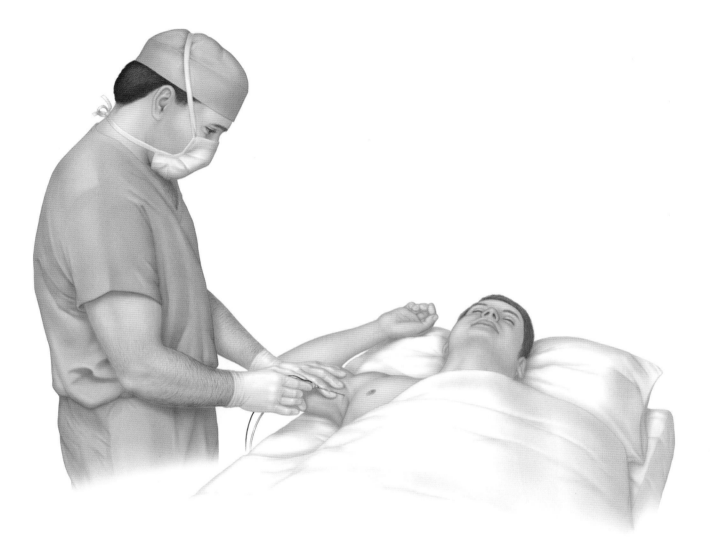

Figure 5. Patient-provider orientation during axillary blockade.

Technique

Neural Localization Techniques
Peripheral nerve stimulation is one of the most common techniques used to identify the terminal nerves of the brachial plexus during axillary blockade. A description of the elicited motor responses for each terminal nerve is listed in Table 1. Motor responses are illustrated in Figures 6-9.

Paresthesia-seeking techniques and transarterial injections are still commonly used by clinicians during axillary blockade. However, the reliability of these techniques may be highly dependent on provider experience, the number of injections (i.e., single or multiple), local anesthetic volumes, and anatomical variation. Ultrasonography performed in conjunction with nerve stimulation is rapidly gaining popularity and has become an effective and reliable technique for the identification of both neural and vascular structures.

Needle Insertion Site
A 25-gauge 2-inch (5-cm) insulated needle is inserted at a proximal point within the axilla superior or inferior

Table 1. Elicited Motor Responses of Terminal Nerves During Peripheral Nerve Stimulation

Nerve	Motor response
Median	Flexion of wrist, second and third digits Opposition of thumb Pronation of forearm
Ulnar	Flexion of wrist, fourth and fifth digits Adduction of thumb
Radial	Extension of all digits Extension of wrist and forearm at the elbow Supination of forearm
Musculocutaneous	Flexion of forearm at the elbow

to the artery. The needle is angled approximately 45° from the skin and parallel to the artery (Figure 10). The needle is slowly advanced until an appropriate motor response is elicited (Figures 6-9). Neural structures are commonly identified at a depth of 1 to 2 cm. Ideally, the terminal branch innervating the surgical site should be identified and anesthetized first.

After the desired motor response is elicited at 0.5 mA or less, local anesthetic is slowly injected in 5-mL increments with intermittent aspiration (10-15 mL). To improve the likelihood of block success, at least two terminal nerves should be identified for local anesthetic injection. Although there is controversy as to precisely which nerves should be identified, it appears that identification of the ulnar nerve may be least important in producing a successful block. A total of 30 to 40 mL of local anesthetic is used to anesthetize the median, ulnar, and radial nerves.

The musculocutaneous nerve may be approached through the same insertion site within the axilla by directing the needle superior to the artery toward the coracobrachialis muscle. Once the musculocutaneous nerve is identified and an appropriate motor response elicited at 0.5 mA or less, 5 to 8 mL of local anesthetic is slowly injected (Figure 9). In the absence of a nerve stimulator, a similar volume of local anesthetic can be deposited in a fanlike manner in a lateral to medial plane through the body of the coracobrachialis muscle (i.e., anterior to the head of the humerus).

Blockade of the intercostobrachial nerve may be necessary to prevent tourniquet-related mechanical or ischemic pain. At the site of needle insertion within the axilla, 5 to 8 mL of local anesthetic is injected subcutaneously across the axilla extending approximately 2 to 3 cm superior and inferior to the artery.

Needle Redirection Cues

If the needle is advanced more than 2 to 3 cm without eliciting a motor response or paresthesia, the needle should be withdrawn and redirected either superiorly or inferiorly in a stepwise manner in a plane perpendicular to the long axis of the plexus. Aspiration of venous blood generally indicates that the needle is inferior (i.e., medial) to the artery.

Alternative Techniques

The paresthesia technique seeks to elicit a distinct paresthesia in one or more of the terminal branches of the brachial plexus. The surface anatomy, patient position, and needle insertion site are identical to those described for peripheral nerve stimulation. However, the paresthesia-seeking technique has two distinct caveats. First, patients should receive minimal or no sedation so that they can immediately and accurately describe the paresthesia and its associated distribution. Second, the needle should be moved *slowly* to immediately identify the paresthesia and prevent inadvertent neural trauma. As with all regional blocks, cautious observation for a painful response to the initial injection of local anesthetic is important to minimize the risk of intrafascicular injection. If arterial blood is aspirated at any point during the paresthesia-seeking technique, conversion to a transarterial approach is widely accepted.

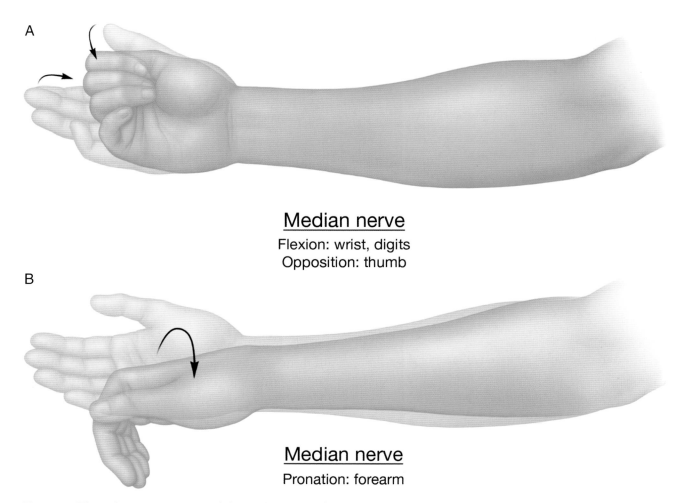

Median nerve
Flexion: wrist, digits
Opposition: thumb

Median nerve
Pronation: forearm

Figure 6. Elicited motor responses of the median nerve. A, Flexion of the wrist and digits. B, Pronation of the forearm.

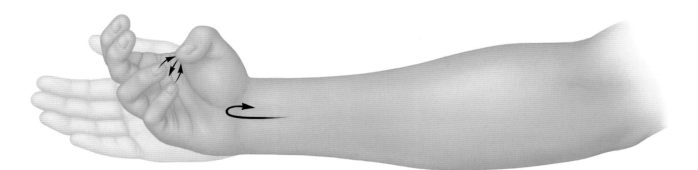

Ulnar nerve
Flexion: wrist, 4th and 5th digits
Adduction: thumb

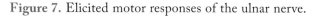

Figure 7. Elicited motor responses of the ulnar nerve.

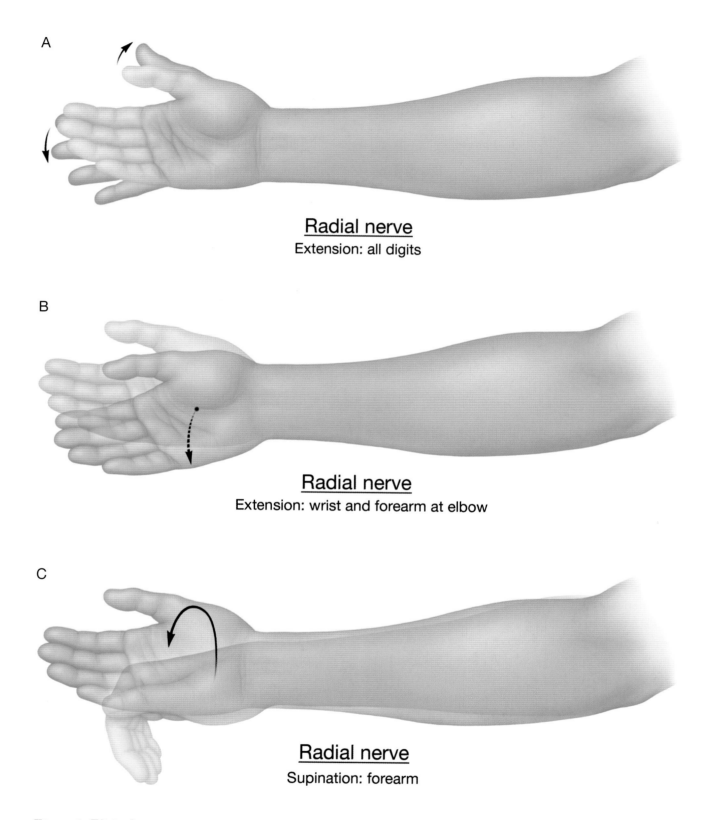

A

Radial nerve
Extension: all digits

B

Radial nerve
Extension: wrist and forearm at elbow

C

Radial nerve
Supination: forearm

Figure 8. Elicited motor responses of the radial nerve. A, Extension of all digits. B, Extension of the wrist and forearm at the elbow. C, Supination of the forearm.

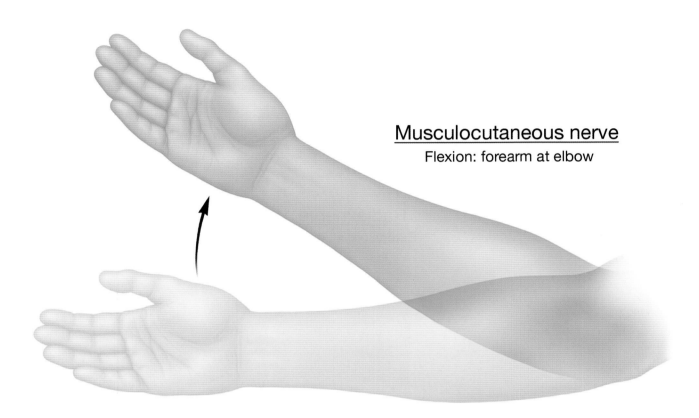

Figure 9. Elicited motor response of the musculocutaneous nerve.

Within the axilla, the median, ulnar, and radial nerves are located in proximity to the axillary artery (Figure 2). The transarterial technique utilizes this relationship and relies on the presence of an axillary sheath. With use of continuous aspiration, a 25-gauge 1.5-inch (3.8-cm) needle is directed toward the axillary artery and advanced through the vessel until blood is no longer aspirated. At this posterior position (i.e., deep to or "behind" the artery), 15 to 20 mL of local anesthetic is injected in 5-mL increments with intermittent aspiration. Once complete, the needle is slowly withdrawn under continuous aspiration, again until blood is no longer aspirated. In this anterior position (i.e., superficial to or "in front of" the artery), an additional 15 to 20 mL of local anesthetic is injected in 5-mL increments. Because of the vascular puncture, the patient should be monitored closely for signs and symptoms of systemic local anesthetic toxicity or hematoma formation.

Ultrasound-Guided Axillary Blockade

Scanning Technique
The ultrasound probe is placed within the axilla perpendicular to the long axis of the arm (Figure 11). This orientation provides a cross-sectional view of the relevant neurovascular anatomy (Figure 12). To further optimize visualization, the probe is positioned to ensure that the axillary artery is centered on the screen of the ultrasound monitor. Simultaneous cross-sectional viewing of all four terminal nerves (median, radial, ulnar, and musculocutaneous) may be difficult with a single probe position. Therefore, proximal and distal scanning is often necessary to acquire ideal imaging of all relevant neuroanatomy. Proximal scanning may improve radial nerve visualization, and more distal scanning may enhance musculocutaneous imaging. Because the plexus is superficial at this location, a high-frequency

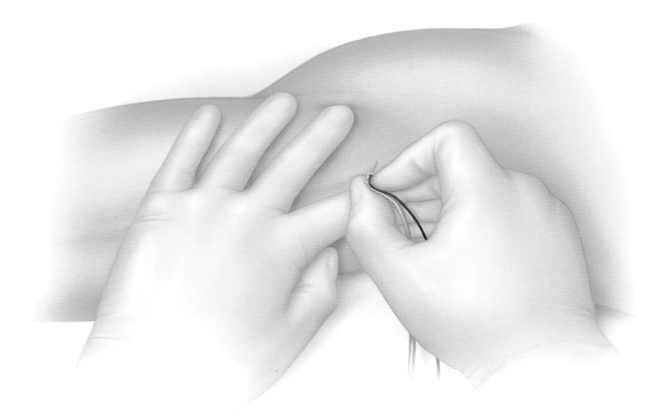

Figure 10. Needle trajectory during axillary blockade.

probe (10-15 MHz) is used to optimally image all neurovascular structures.

Sonoanatomy

The ideal ultrasound image during axillary blockade captures the axillary artery in perfect cross-section surrounded by round, hyperechoic median, ulnar, and radial nerves (Figure 13). The axillary artery is easily identified as a round, noncompressible, pulsatile, hypoechoic structure. In contrast, the terminal branches of the brachial plexus have a honeycomb appearance, representing the fascicular components of the peripheral neuroanatomy (Figure 14). The median nerve is commonly located above and to the left of the artery (approximating the 10-o'clock position) when the ultrasound probe marker has been placed in a lateral anatomical position.

With this same probe orientation, the ulnar nerve commonly is identified above and to the right of the artery, near the axillary vein. The radial nerve is frequently found deep to the ulnar nerve and ranges between the 3- and 6-o'clock positions relative to the artery (Figure 12). However, considerable anatomical variation may occur for all terminal branches of the plexus.

Ultrasound Approach

Ultrasound-guided axillary blockade is commonly performed using an in-plane needle approach. The superficial anatomical location and rounded contour of the arm allow for a needle trajectory that is perpendicular to the ultrasound beam resulting in excellent needle visualization (Figure 15). The needle insertion site is generally located 1 to 2 cm away from the edge of the transducer to improve

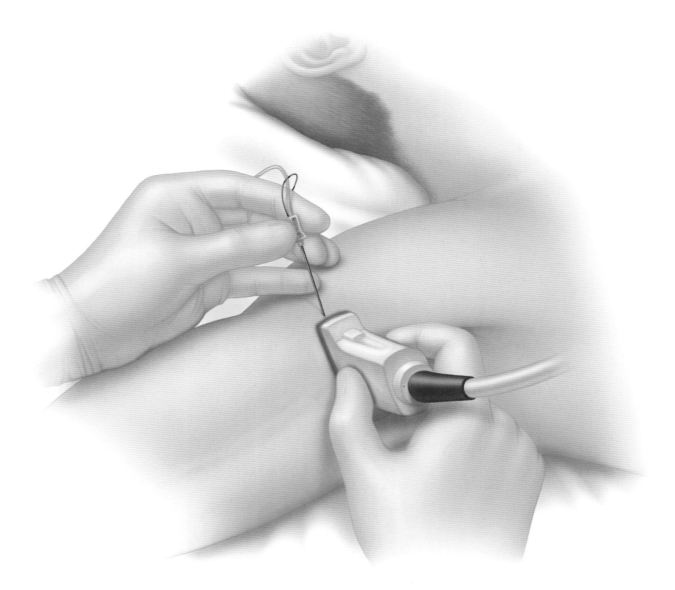

Figure 11. Probe and needle orientation during ultrasound-guided axillary blockade.

the angle of incidence relative to the ultrasound beam. To minimize the risk of unintentional venous puncture, the needle is typically inserted superior (i.e., lateral) to the artery and advanced inferiorly (i.e., medially, Figure 11). With this approach, it may be prudent to anesthetize the deepest and most distant neural structures first (i.e., radial and ulnar nerves) to minimize the risk of injury to partially anesthetized nerves during needle advancement

and redirection. A 22-gauge 2-inch (5-cm) stimulating needle is slowly advanced posterior to the axillary artery toward the radial nerve. The needle should always be directed immediately above or below neural structures to minimize the risk of direct needle trauma should the entire needle not be in view. If nerve stimulation is used to verify neural identity, direct contact between the needle and the nerve is often required to elicit a motor response.

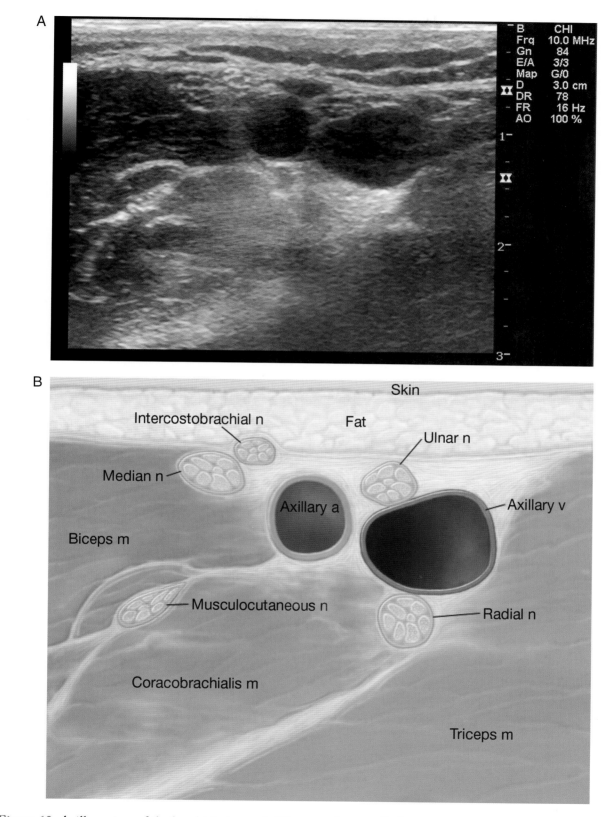

Figure 12. Axillary view of the brachial plexus. A, Ultrasound image. B, Corresponding anatomical illustration.

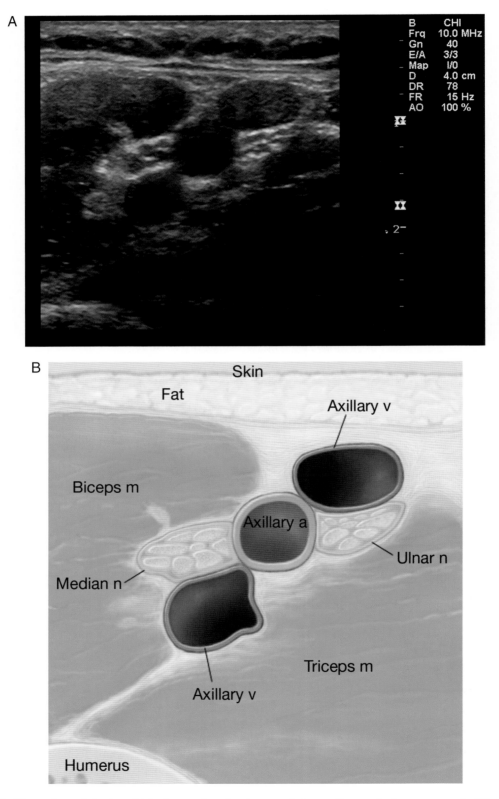

Figure 13. Axillary view of the brachial plexus, showing hyperechoic median and ulnar nerves. A, Ultrasound image. B, Corresponding anatomical illustration.

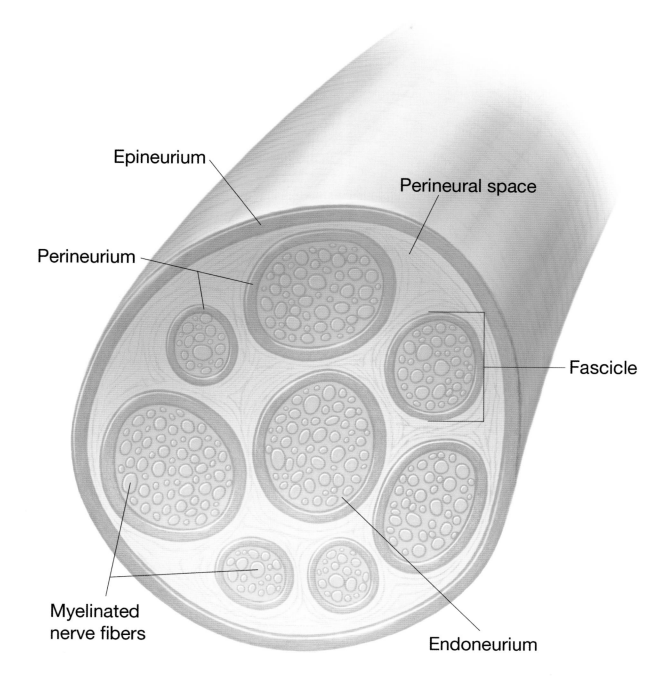

Figure 14. Peripheral nerve anatomy.

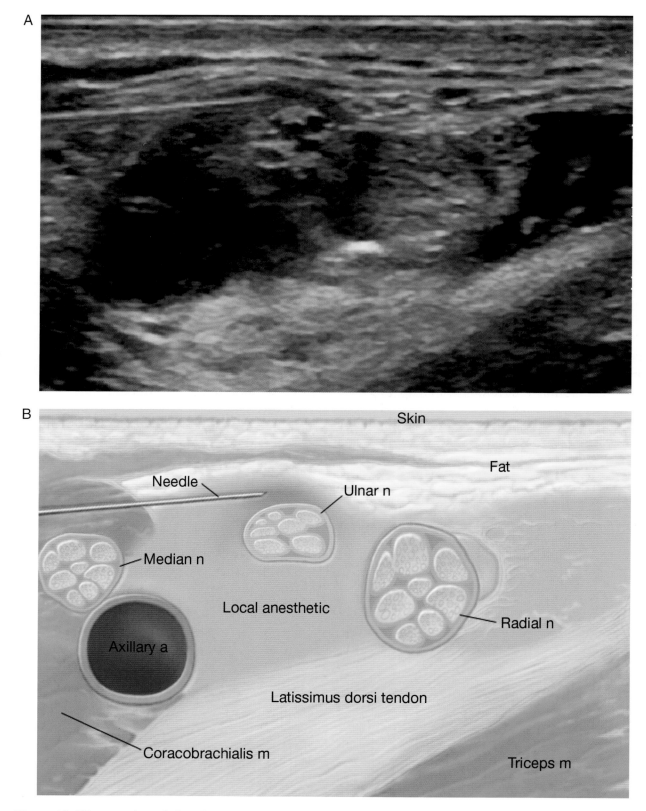

Figure 15. Ultrasound-guided axillary blockade. A, Ultrasound image. B, Corresponding anatomical illustration.

Local anesthetic (8-12 mL) is injected circumferentially around each terminal nerve of the brachial plexus (Figure 15). Complete circumferential spread increases the likelihood of a rapid onset and successful block. It is recommended that deeper neural structures are anesthetized first, because the local anesthetic volume may "force" tissue planes upward and improve visualization. After injection around the radial nerve, the needle is withdrawn to the skin and advanced anterior to the artery toward the median and ulnar nerves. The median nerve is often best visualized and anesthetized after ulnar blockade. Nerve stimulation can be used at any time during the procedure to verify either neural identity or location before local anesthetic injection.

The last terminal branch of the brachial plexus to be anesthetized is the musculocutaneous nerve. To acquire an optimal image of the nerve, the probe may need to be positioned more lateral over the biceps muscle. With an in-plane approach, needle insertion and advancement techniques are similar to those previously described for the radial, ulnar, and median nerves (Figure 16).

Continuous Peripheral Nerve Catheters

Continuous peripheral nerve catheters are commonly used as an adjunct to intraoperative anesthesia or for postoperative pain management. Both stimulating and nonstimulating axillary catheters have been used with success for patients undergoing inpatient and ambulatory surgical procedures. Although ultrasound technology can be used to accurately guide catheter placement, the evidence is insufficient to suggest that this technique is superior to more conventional methods of nerve stimulation.

Neural localization using peripheral nerve stimulation is similar for both continuous and single-injection techniques. During axillary catheter placement, an 18-gauge 2-inch (5-cm) insulated Tuohy needle is inserted superior (i.e., lateral) to the artery and advanced in a cephalad and slightly posterior direction toward the axilla. The intent is to position the needle tip posterior to the axillary artery

near the radial nerve. Needle trajectories inferior to the axillary artery are avoided because of an increased risk of inadvertent venous puncture. Once a radial motor response (Figure 8) is elicited at a current of 0.5 mA or less, a 20-gauge catheter is advanced 3 to 5 cm beyond the tip of the needle.

Ultrasound-guided perineural catheter placement is similar to that described for single-injection ultrasound techniques. Under ultrasound guidance, an 18-gauge 2-inch (5-cm) insulated Tuohy needle is inserted superior (i.e., lateral) to the axillary artery. Optimally, the catheter is advanced to a position between the ulnar and radial nerves. At this location, the catheter is advanced approximately 1 cm beyond the needle tip. The distribution of local anesthetic spread is confirmed using real-time ultrasound imaging (Figure 17). If circumferential spread of local anesthetic does not occur, catheter manipulation may be required with direct visualization.

Once the catheter location has been optimized, the catheter is secured with a liquid adhesive, Steri-Strips, and a sterile transparent dressing. Alternatively, the catheter may be tunneled subcutaneously to a location remote from the initial insertion site and covered with a protective dressing.

Side Effects and Complications

Complications associated with axillary brachial plexus blockade are extremely uncommon. Although localized bruising and tenderness may occur, true hematoma formation occurs much less often. Serious complications such as systemic local anesthetic toxicity and seizure-related events rarely occur when appropriate vigilance and cautious injection techniques are used during the block. Transient postoperative dysesthesias may occur in 0.5% to 4% of cases. However, severe sensorimotor dysfunction or permanent neurologic sequelae are extremely rare. Interestingly, the method of neural localization (paresthesia, transarterial, nerve stimulation, or ultrasound) has not been found to affect the overall rate of nerve-related complications.

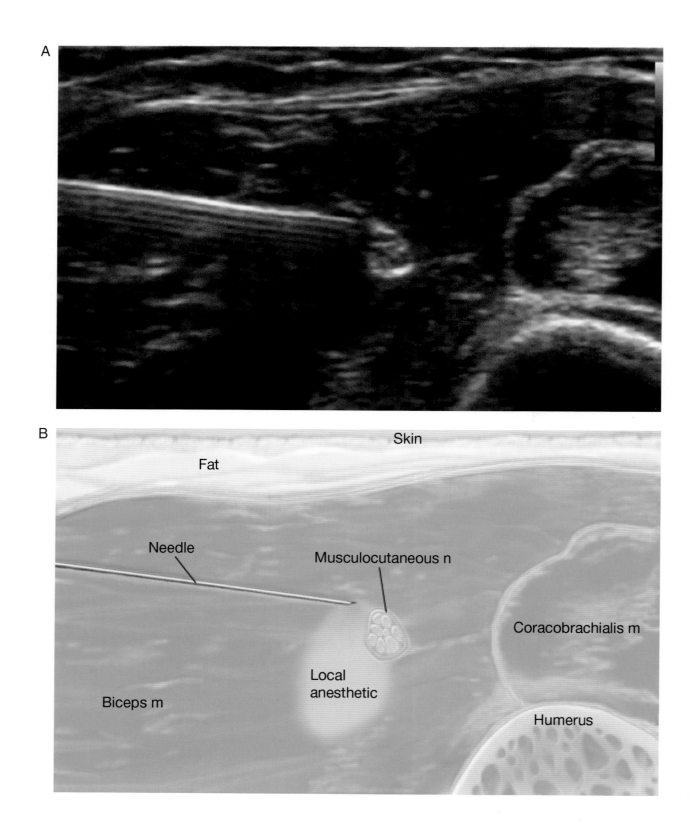

Figure 16. Ultrasound-guided musculocutaneous blockade. A, Ultrasound image. B, Corresponding anatomical illustration.

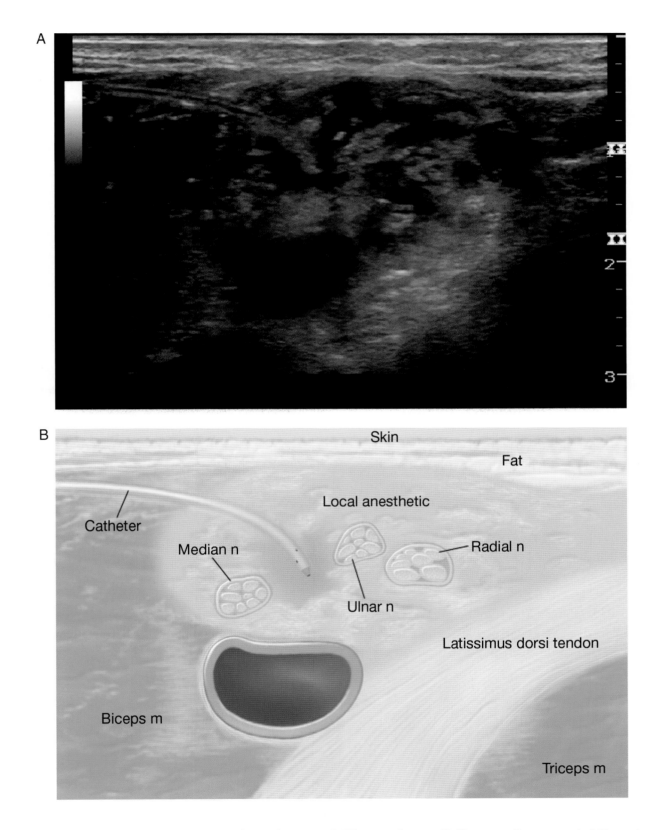

Figure 17. Ultrasound-guided axillary catheter placement. A, Ultrasound image. B, Corresponding anatomical illustration.

Suggested Reading

Aantaa R, Kirvelä O, Lahdenperä A, Nieminen S. Transarterial brachial plexus anesthesia for hand surgery: a retrospective analysis of 346 cases. J Clin Anesth. 1994 May-Jun;6(3):189-92.

Brown DL. Atlas of regional anesthesia. 2nd ed. Philadelphia: W. B. Saunders; c1999.

Brull R, McCartney CJ, Chan VW, El-Beheiry H. Neurological complications after regional anesthesia: contemporary estimates of risk. Anesth Analg. 2007 Apr;104(4):965-74.

De Jong RH. Axillary block of the brachial plexus. Anesthesiology. 1961 Mar-Apr;22:215-25.

Handoll HH, Koscielniak-Nielsen ZJ. Single, double or multiple injection techniques for axillary brachial plexus block for hand, wrist or forearm surgery. Cochrane Database Syst Rev. 2006 Jan 25;(1):CD-003842.

Neal JM, Gerancher JC, Hebl JR, Ilfeld BM, McCartney CJ, Franco CD, et al. Upper extremity regional anesthesia: essentials of our current understanding, 2008. Reg Anesth Pain Med. 2009 Mar-Apr;34(2):134-70.

Schroeder LE, Horlocker TT, Schroeder DR. The efficacy of axillary block for surgical procedures about the elbow. Anesth Analg. 1996 Oct;83(4):747-51.

Selander D, Dhunér KG, Lundborg G. Peripheral nerve injury due to injection needles used for regional anesthesia. An experimental study of the acute effects of needle point trauma. Acta Anaesthesiol Scand. 1977; 21(3):182-8.

Selander D, Edshage S, Wolff T. Paresthesiae or no paresthesiae? Nerve lesions after axillary blocks. Acta Anaesthesiol Scand. 1979 Feb;23(1):27-33.

Sia S, Bartoli M. Selective ulnar nerve localization is not essential for axillary brachial plexus block using a multiple nerve stimulation technique. Reg Anesth Pain Med. 2001 Jan-Feb;26(1):12-6.

Sia S, Bartoli M, Lepri A, Marchini O, Ponsecchi P. Multiple-injection axillary brachial plexus block: a comparison of two methods of nerve localization-nerve stimulation versus paresthesia. Anesth Analg. 2000 Sep;91(3):647-51.

Stan TC, Krantz MA, Solomon DL, Poulos JG, Chaouki K. The incidence of neurovascular complications following axillary brachial plexus block using a transarterial approach: a prospective study of 1,000 consecutive patients. Reg Anesth. 1995 Nov-Dec;20(6):486-92.

Thompson G. The multiple compartment approach to brachial plexus anesthesia. Tech Reg Anesth Pain Management. 1997;1:163-8.

Winnie AP. Does the transarterial technique of axillary block provide a higher success rate and a lower complication rate than a paresthesia technique? New evidence and old. Reg Anesth. 1995 Nov-Dec;20(6):482-5.

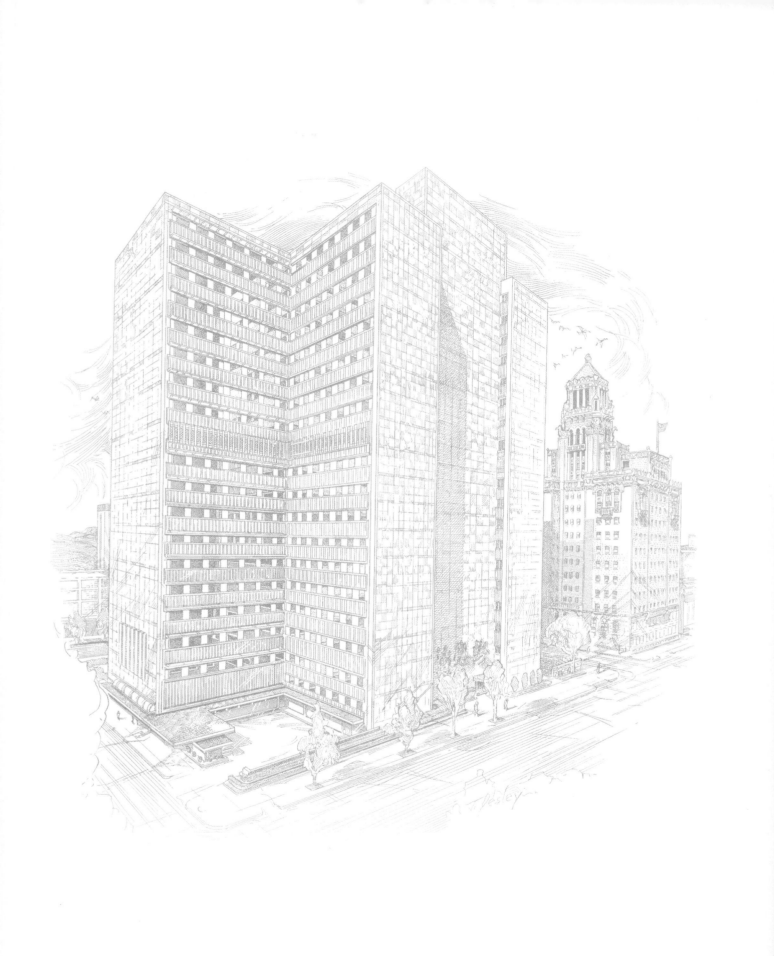

CHAPTER 16

Midhumeral Blockade

Sandra L. Kopp, M.D.

Clinical Applications

In 1994, Dupré described anesthetizing the four terminal branches of the brachial plexus (median, ulnar, radial, and musculocutaneous nerves) at the midhumeral level of the arm. Midhumeral blockade is commonly used for surgical procedures involving the hand, wrist, and forearm. The technique was initially developed to minimize the theoretical risk of nerve injury associated with multiple stimulations during axillary block techniques and to allow "differential blockade" of the brachial plexus. Differential blockade refers to anesthetizing individual peripheral nerves with different local anesthetic solutions depending on the clinical circumstances. The approach allows clinicians to selectively block individual nerves when limited anesthetic duration or distribution is needed for surgery. A detailed knowledge of the surgical site and the cutaneous innervation of the upper extremity is required to successfully incorporate differential blockade into the plan of care (Figure 1).

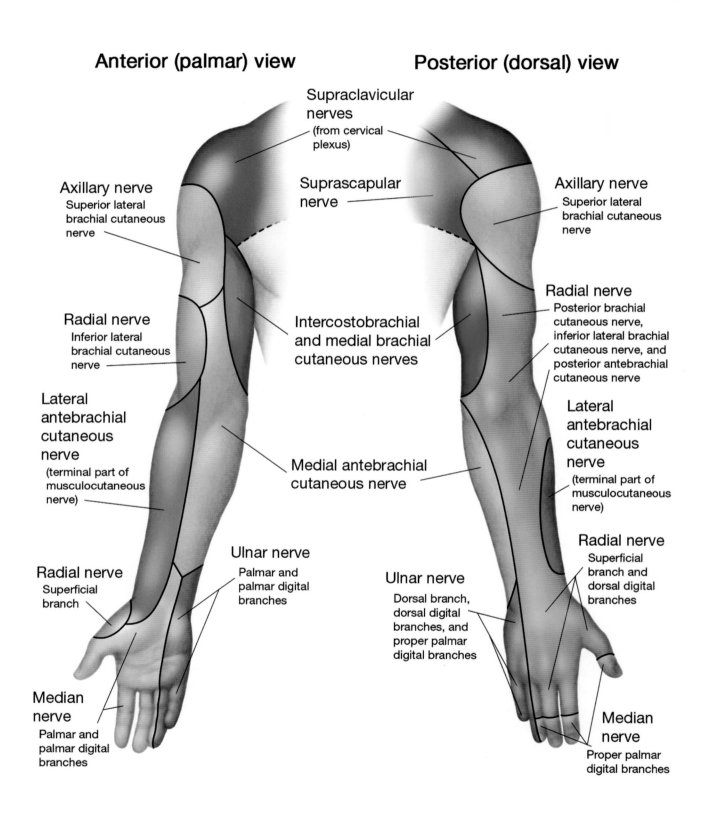

Figure 1. Cutaneous innervation of the upper extremity.

Finally, midhumeral blockade can be used to supplement specific nerves after failed or incomplete proximal approaches to the brachial plexus.

Relevant Anatomy

The brachial, or humeral, canal is located on the medial aspect of the arm. It is bordered superiorly by the biceps muscle, inferiorly by the triceps muscle, laterally by the coracobrachialis muscle, and medially by skin and subcutaneous tissue (Figure 2). The brachial artery and vein travel through this canal and serve as the primary superficial landmarks for the midhumeral technique. The median nerve is located anterior and medial to the artery, and the ulnar nerve is more superficial and inferior to the artery (Figure 2). However, tremendous anatomical variation may exist. The radial nerve is also located inferior to the artery, but immediately posterior to the humerus (Figure 3). After passing through the coracobrachialis musculature, the musculocutaneous nerve

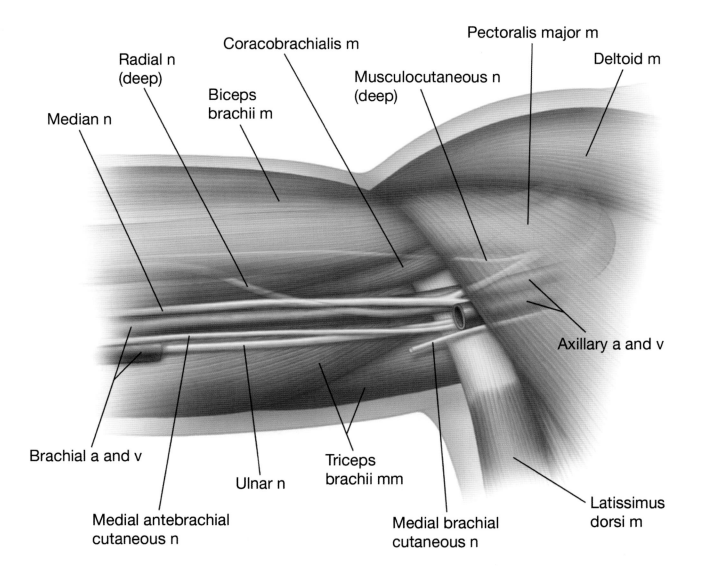

Figure 2. Neurovascular and muscular anatomy of the proximal aspect of the arm.

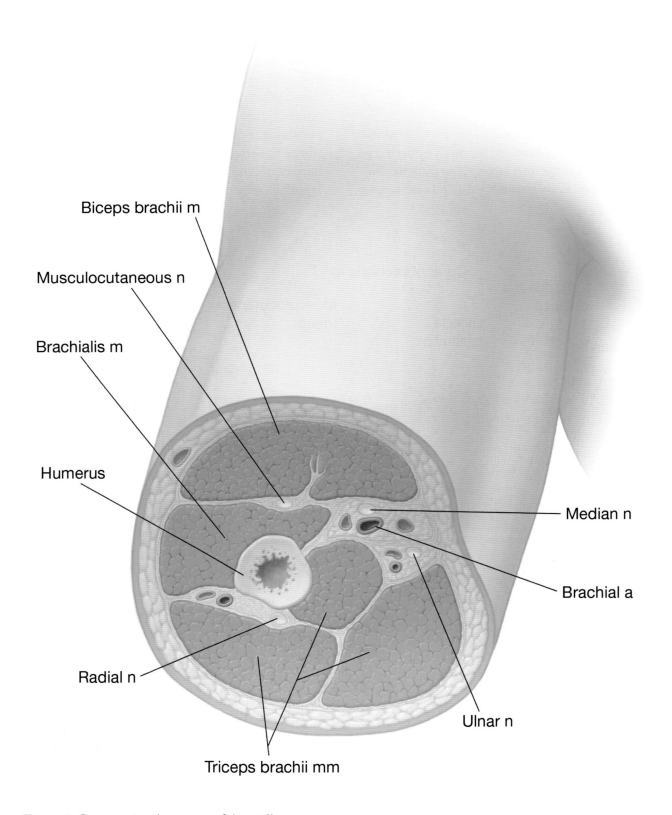

Biceps brachii m

Musculocutaneous n

Brachialis m

Humerus

Median n

Brachial a

Radial n

Ulnar n

Triceps brachii mm

Figure 3. Cross-sectional anatomy of the midhumerus.

descends in the groove between the biceps and brachialis muscles (Figure 3). The intercostobrachial nerve exits the humeral canal and resides within the subcutaneous tissue layer adjacent to the basilic vein.

Surface Anatomy

Despite its name, the midhumeral block is *not* performed at the level of the midhumerus. Rather, it is performed at the junction of the proximal and middle third of the arm where the brachial artery is most readily palpated. This location approximates the insertion of the deltoid muscle on the lateral aspect of the arm.

Patient Position

The patient is positioned supine with the head in a neutral position or rotated slightly away from the side to be blocked. The arm is abducted at the shoulder to approximately 80° to 90° and the forearm flexed at the elbow (Figure 4).

Technique

Neural Localization Techniques

The initial description by Dupré recommends anesthetizing the terminal nerves of the brachial plexus in the

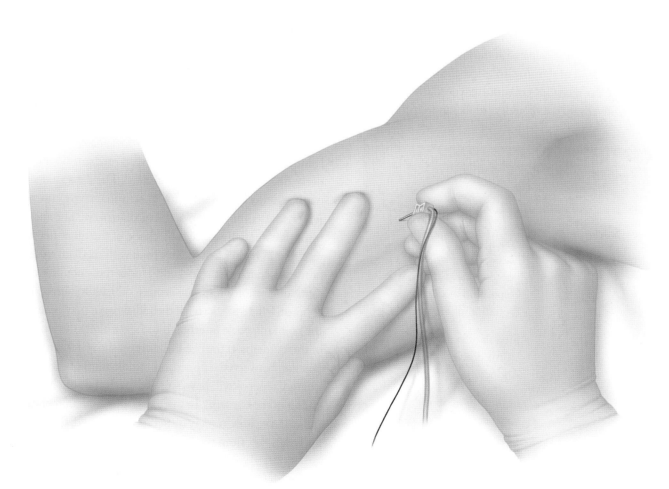

Figure 4. Patient position and needle insertion site for midhumeral blockade.

following order: median, ulnar, radial, and musculocutaneous. This sequence is thought to take advantage of the different onset times of the individual peripheral nerves. Traditionally, the technique has been performed using peripheral nerve stimulation (Table 1). However, ultrasound guidance may also be used for neural localization. Clinical experience, radiographic imaging, and anatomical dissections have shown the tremendous anatomical variation that occurs among peripheral nerves. Because of this, proponents of ultrasound-guided technology suggest that direct visualization of the neuroanatomy may facilitate neural localization, enhance block performance, and minimize complications such as inadvertent neural trauma or intraneural injection. However, additional studies are needed to fully support these claims within the literature.

Needle Insertion Site

The brachial artery is palpated at the junction of the upper and middle third of the arm. To locate the median nerve, a 22-gauge 1.5-inch (3.8-cm) insulated needle is advanced tangentially toward the shoulder, parallel and superficial to

the brachial artery until a median motor response is elicited at a current of 0.5 mA or less (Figure 5). Ulnar nerve blockade is performed by directing the needle through the same skin insertion site, medial to the artery and perpendicular to the operating table until an ulnar motor response is elicited at a current of 0.5 mA or less (Figure 6). The radial nerve is anesthetized by advancing the needle laterally through the same skin insertion site until contact is made with the humerus (Figure 4). At this point, the needle is "walked off" the humerus posteriorly until a radial motor response is elicited at a current of 0.5 mA or less (Figure 7). To locate the musculocutaneous nerve, the needle is again withdrawn to the subcutaneous tissue and redirected immediately posterior to the biceps muscle and toward the coracoid process until elbow flexion is elicited (Figure 8). Finally, the intercostobrachial nerve can be anesthetized with a subcutaneous injection of local anesthetic both anterior and posterior to the skin puncture site. In general, 5 to 8 mL of local anesthetic is injected onto each peripheral nerve to be blocked.

The most frequent stimulation failures include the ulnar and radial nerves. Failure to stimulate the ulnar nerve is believed to be due to the Martin-Gruber anastomosis—a common neural anastomosis between median and ulnar nerve fibers within the humeral canal. The consequence of this neural cross-linking is an ulnar-type motor response after stimulation of the median nerve. The anastomosis essentially mimics blockade of the ulnar nerve, resulting in higher failure rates than with median, radial, or musculocutaneous blockade. Under these conditions, a *true* ulnar motor response is often difficult to obtain. In contrast, failure to stimulate the radial nerve may occur if the point of needle insertion is too *distal* along the length of the humerus. If the needle insertion site is distal to the junction between the upper and middle third of the arm, the radial nerve will have spiraled around to the lateral border of the humerus. In this location, stimulation of the radial nerve is extremely difficult using a medial needle approach (i.e., from the humeral canal).

Alternative Techniques

A recent review by Guntz and colleagues used unintended nerve stimulation as a surrogate marker of potential

Table 1. Elicited Motor Responses of Terminal Nerves During Peripheral Nerve Stimulation	
Nerve	**Motor response**
Median	Flexion of wrist, second and third digits Opposition of thumb Pronation of forearm
Ulnar	Flexion of wrist, fourth and fifth digits Adduction of thumb
Radial	Extension of all digits Extension of wrist and forearm at the elbow Supination of forearm
Musculocutaneous	Flexion of forearm at the elbow

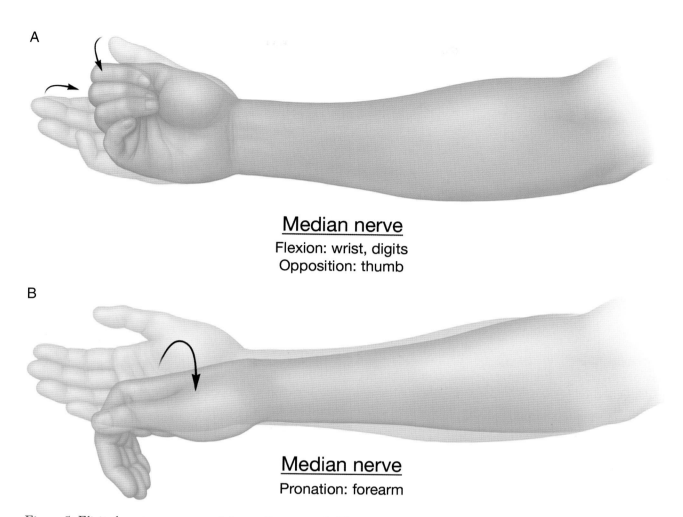

Median nerve
Flexion: wrist, digits
Opposition: thumb

Median nerve
Pronation: forearm

Figure 5. Elicited motor responses of the median nerve. A, Flexion of the wrist and digits. B, Pronation of the forearm.

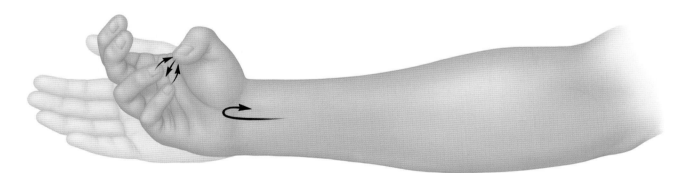

Ulnar nerve
Flexion: wrist, 4th and 5th digits
Adduction: thumb

Figure 6. Elicited motor responses of the ulnar nerve.

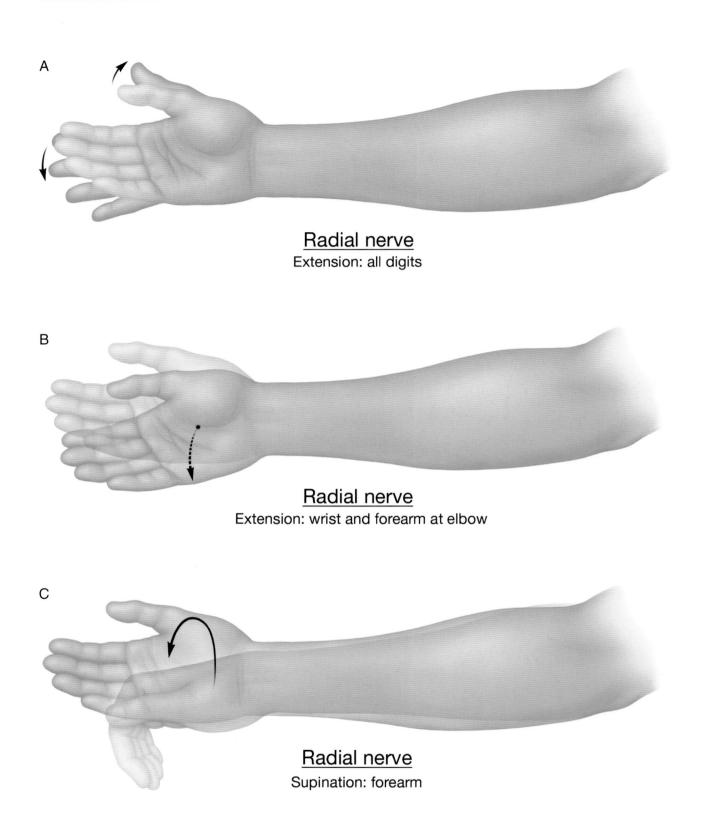

A

Radial nerve
Extension: all digits

B

Radial nerve
Extension: wrist and forearm at elbow

C

Radial nerve
Supination: forearm

Figure 7. Elicited motor responses of the radial nerve. A, Extension of all digits. B, Extension of the wrist and forearm at the elbow. C, Supination of the forearm.

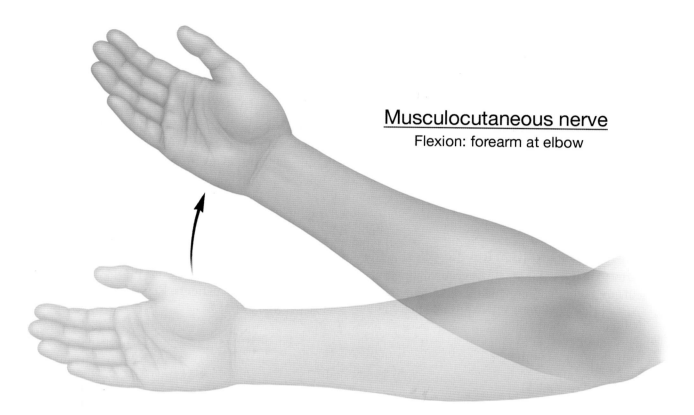

Musculocutaneous nerve
Flexion: forearm at elbow

Figure 8. Elicited motor response of the musculocutaneous nerve.

nerve injury. The authors reported that while searching for the radial nerve, an ulnar paresthesia was elicited in 50% of patients. However, when searching for the ulnar nerve, a radial response was elicited in only 10% of patients. Theoretically, if the more superficial ulnar nerve is anesthetized first, it could be injured during localization of the deeper radial nerve. Therefore, the following sequence of peripheral nerve blockade may be more appropriate during the midhumeral technique: median, radial, ulnar, and musculocutaneous nerves.

Side Effects and Complications
Side effects and complications during midhumeral blockade are similar to those with axillary approaches to the brachial plexus. Minor complications such as bruising and localized tenderness may be relatively common. However, true hematoma formation occurs significantly less often. The risk of local anesthetic toxicity appears to be minimized by the slow, incremental injection of small volumes of local anesthetic. Finally, because this technique may be used to supplement a failed proximal approach, there is always a theoretical risk of injury to partially anesthetized nerves.

Suggested Reading
Bouaziz H, Narchi P, Mercier FJ, Labaille T, Zerrouk N, Girod J, et al. Comparison between conventional axillary block and a new approach at the midhumeral level. Anesth Analg. 1997 May;84(5):1058-62.

Carles M, Pulcini A, Macchi P, Duflos P, Raucoules-Aime M, Grimaud D. An evaluation of the brachial plexus block at the humeral canal using a neurostimulator (1417 patients): the efficacy, safety, and predictive criteria of failure. Anesth Analg. 2001 Jan; 92(1):194-8.

Dupré LJ. [Brachial plexus block through humeral approach.] Cah Anesthesiol. 1994;42(6):767-9. French.

Frizelle HP. Technical note: the humeral canal approach to the brachial plexus. Yale J Biol Med. 1998 Nov-Dec;71(6):585-9.

Guntz E, Herman P, Delbos A, Sosnowski M. The radial nerve should be blocked before the ulnar nerve during a brachial plexus block at the humeral canal. Can J Anaesth. 2004 Apr;51(4):354-7.

Neal JM, Gerancher JC, Hebl JR, Ilfeld BM, McCartney CJ, Franco CD, et al. Upper extremity regional anesthesia: essentials of our current understanding, 2008. Reg Anesth Pain Med. 2009 Mar-Apr;34(2):134-70.

Selander D, Edshage S, Wolff T. Paresthesiae or no paresthesiae? Nerve lesions after axillary blocks. Acta Anaesthesiol Scand. 1979 Feb;23(1):27-33.

Sia S, Lepri A, Campolo MC, Fiaschi R. Four-injection brachial plexus block using peripheral nerve stimulator: a comparison between axillary and humeral approaches. Anesth Analg. 2002 Oct;95(4): 1075-9.

Stan TC, Krantz MA, Solomon DL, Poulos JG, Chaouki K. The incidence of neurovascular complications following axillary brachial plexus block using a transarterial approach: a prospective study of 1,000 consecutive patients. Reg Anesth. 1995 Nov-Dec;20(6):486-92.

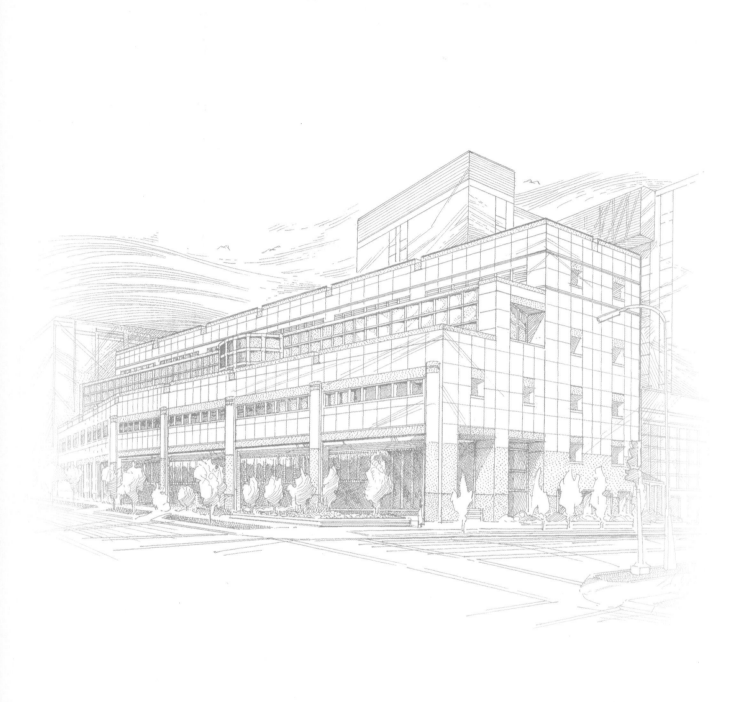

CHAPTER
17

Elbow Blockade

Steven R. Rettke, M.D.

Hugh M. Smith, M.D., Ph.D.

Clinical Applications

Nerve blocks at the elbow have limited but specific clinical applications. Although surgical procedures of the forearm, wrist, hand, or digits may be performed with peripheral blockade at the elbow, a significant limitation is the inability to use an upper arm tourniquet for prolonged periods. Although primarily intended for surgical anesthesia and postoperative analgesia, elbow blockade for minor hand trauma, local debridement, and foreign body removal in emergency departments and out-of-hospital settings has widespread utility. More commonly, elbow blocks are used to supplement inadequate anesthesia or analgesia after proximal approaches to the brachial plexus. This practice is controversial among providers concerned with unrecognized intraneural injection or neurologic injury in a partially anesthetized extremity.

Relevant Anatomy

Elbow blockade may involve one or more terminal branches of the brachial plexus (Figure 1). Although the terminal nerves are widely separated from one another at the level of the elbow, they are generally consistent in their anatomical location (Figures 2 and 3). The median nerve lies medial to the brachial artery and most commonly courses medial to the biceps tendon. Radial nerve anatomy is variable, but the nerve generally pierces the intramuscular septum and travels between the brachialis and brachioradialis muscles at a point approximately 6 cm proximal to the lateral humeral epicondyle. The ulnar nerve passes through the ulnar groove between the medial epicondyle of the humerus and the olecranon process (Figure 4). The musculocutaneous nerve travels within the fascia between the biceps and brachialis muscles. It emerges at the lateral border of the biceps tendon (Figure 2) immediately proximal to the elbow crease, where it becomes cutaneous within the forearm (Figures 2 and 5).

Surface Anatomy

Three of the four terminal nerves (radial, musculocutaneous, and median) are located in relation to the bicipital aponeurosis (i.e., biceps tendon) within the antecubital fossa. The radial nerve is found posterior (i.e., deep) to a point 1 to 2 cm lateral to the biceps tendon (Figure 2). The musculocutaneous nerve emerges at this same location lateral to the tendon, but in a more superficial tissue plane. The surface landmark for the median nerve is the brachial artery, which is located medial to the biceps tendon. Finally, the ulnar nerve is located proximal to the bony landmarks of the medial epicondyle of the humerus and the olecranon process.

Patient Position

The radial, musculocutaneous, and median nerves are blocked with the patient in the supine position with the arm partially abducted and the forearm extended (Figure 6). The ulnar nerve is blocked with the patient in the supine position with the elbow flexed (Figure 7).

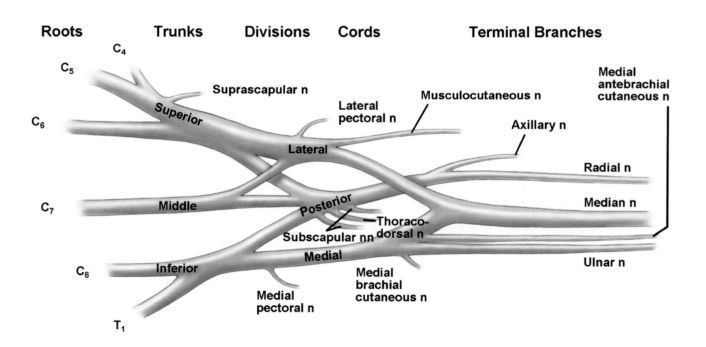

Figure 1. Brachial plexus anatomy.

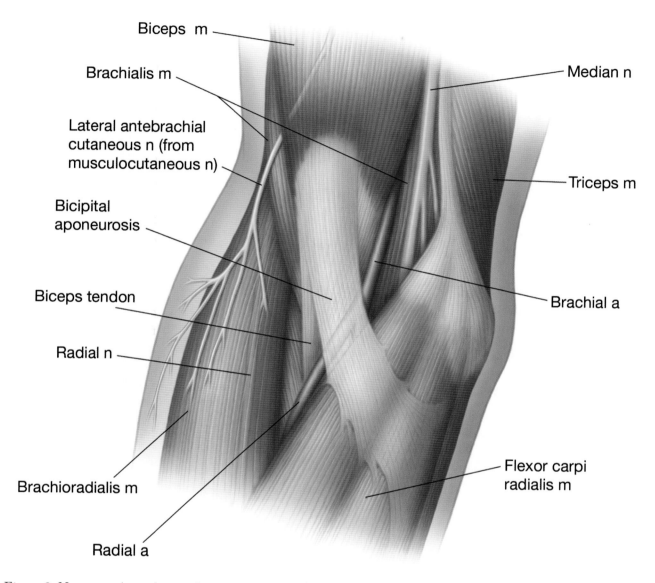

Biceps m

Brachialis m

Lateral antebrachial cutaneous n (from musculocutaneous n)

Bicipital aponeurosis

Biceps tendon

Radial n

Brachioradialis m

Radial a

Median n

Triceps m

Brachial a

Flexor carpi radialis m

Figure 2. Neurovascular and muscular anatomy of the antecubital fossa.

Alternatively, the ulnar groove may be identified by extending the elbow and internally rotating the arm.

Technique

Neural Localization Techniques

Nerve stimulation is most commonly used to identify the median and radial nerves at the elbow. In contrast, the musculocutaneous and ulnar nerves are typically blocked with either a field block or local infiltration at the level of the elbow. Paresthesia-seeking techniques have also been described for neural localization. More recently, ultrasonography provides both accurate neural localization and real-time imaging during neural blockade.

Needle Insertion Site

For median nerve blockade, a 22-gauge 2-inch (5-cm) insulated needle is inserted perpendicular to the skin or in a slightly cephalad direction 1 cm proximal to the elbow flexion crease and 1 cm medial to the brachial pulse. The needle is slowly advanced to obtain either a

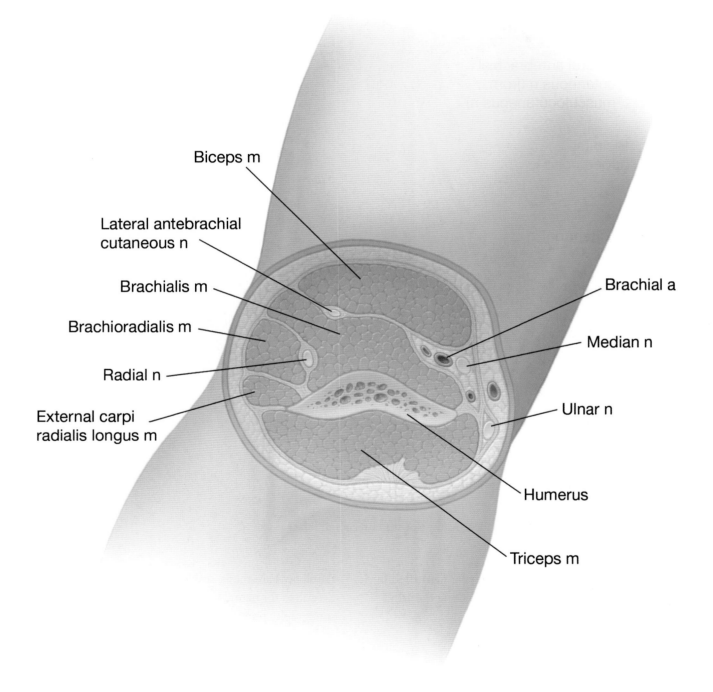

Figure 3. Cross-sectional anatomy of the antecubital fossa.

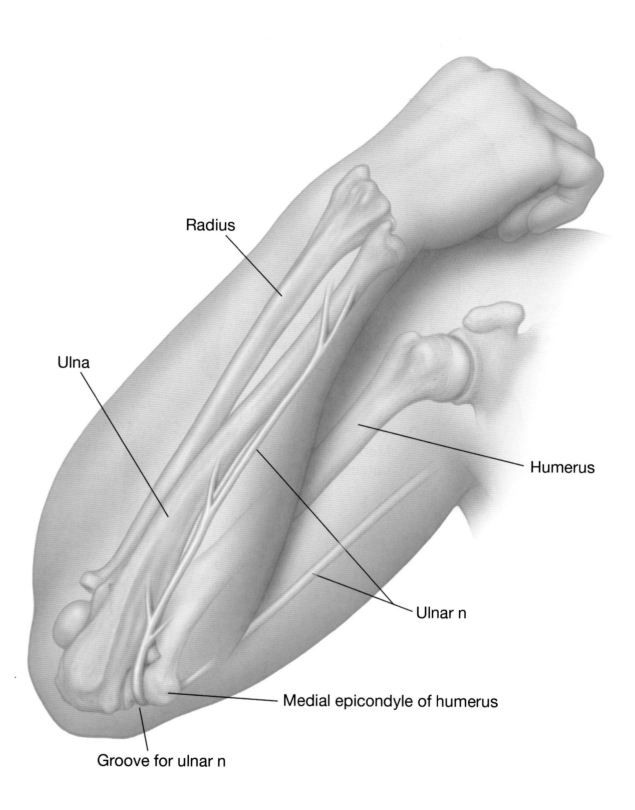

Radius

Ulna

Humerus

Ulnar n

Medial epicondyle of humerus

Groove for ulnar n

Figure 4. Ulnar nerve anatomy.

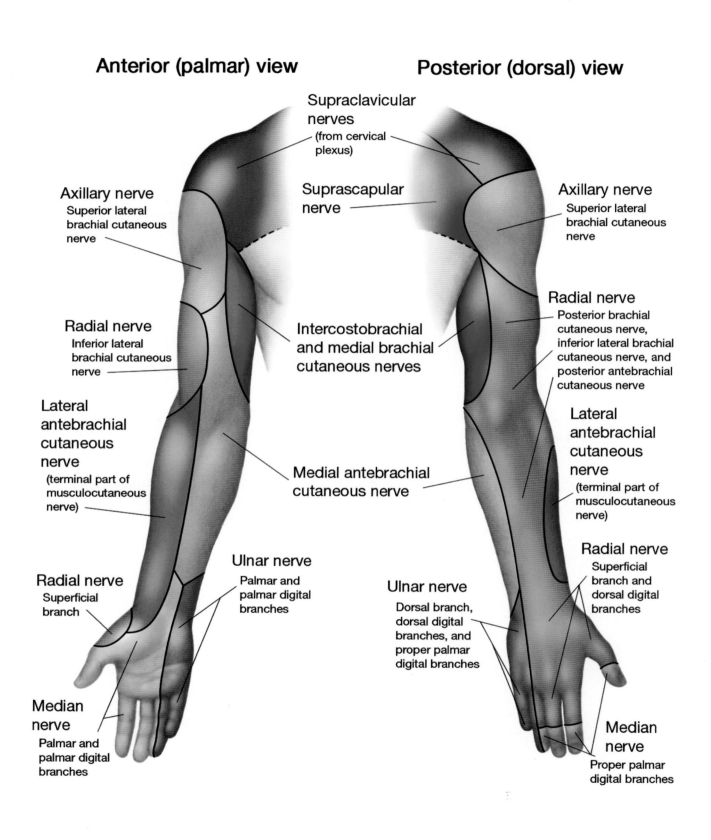

Figure 5. Cutaneous innervation of the upper extremity.

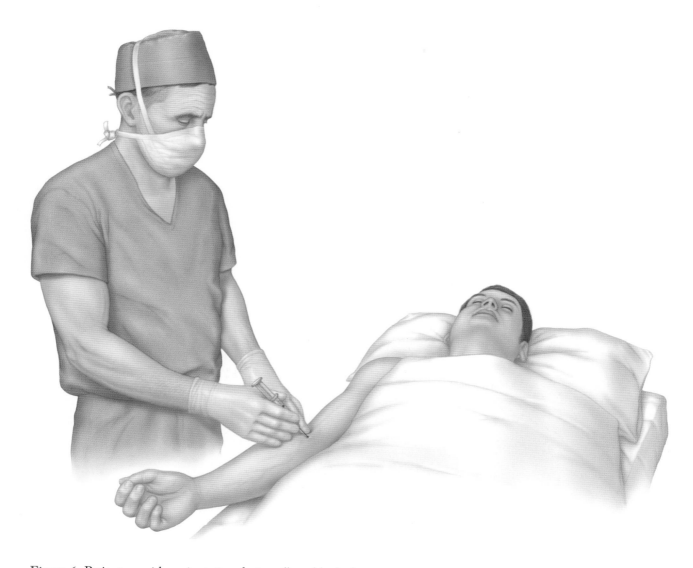

Figure 6. Patient-provider orientation during elbow blockade.

median motor response (Figure 8) or a paresthesia. After confirmation of negative aspiration, 5 to 8 mL of local anesthetic is injected. If necessary, initial needle redirection should be in a medial direction. Failure to elicit a motor response after medial repositioning should prompt needle lateralization, with care taken not to penetrate the brachial artery (Figure 2).

With use of a 22-gauge 2-inch (5-cm) insulated needle, the radial nerve is blocked lateral to the biceps tendon at a point 3 cm proximal to the elbow flexion crease. The needle is inserted perpendicular to the skin 1 to 2 cm

lateral to the tendon. The needle is advanced slowly until either a radial motor response (Figure 9) or paresthesia is elicited. Five to 8 mL of local anesthetic is injected. Initial redirection is in a lateral direction, followed by medial redirection if necessary.

Injection of local anesthetic directly over the ulnar groove may result in mechanical compression or ischemic injury of neural fibers. Therefore, the ulnar nerve should be blocked approximately 2 fingerbreadths (3-5 cm) *proximal* to the ulnar groove (Figure 7). An ulnar motor response (Figure 10) should be elicited

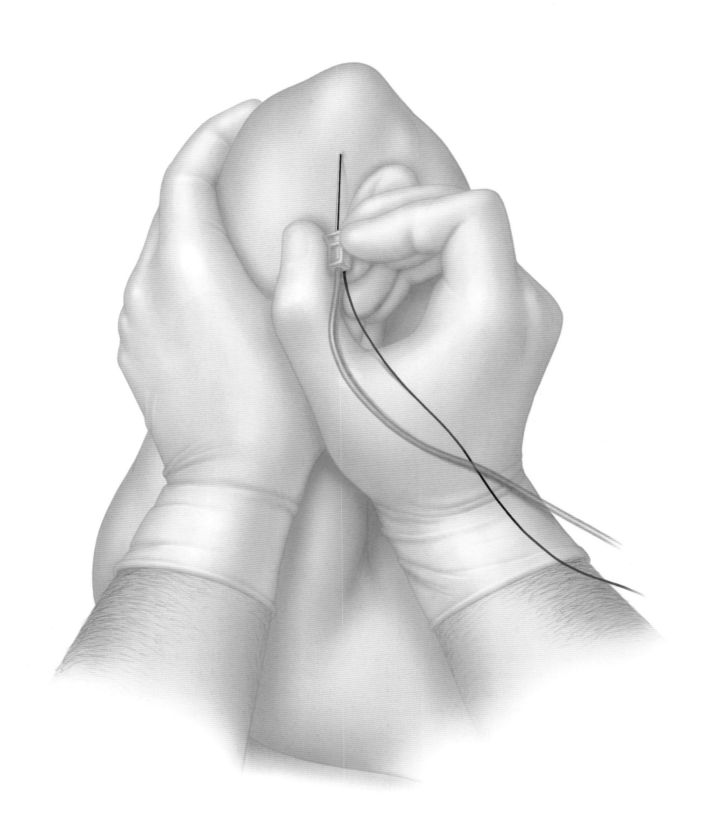

Figure 7. Ulnar nerve blockade at the elbow.

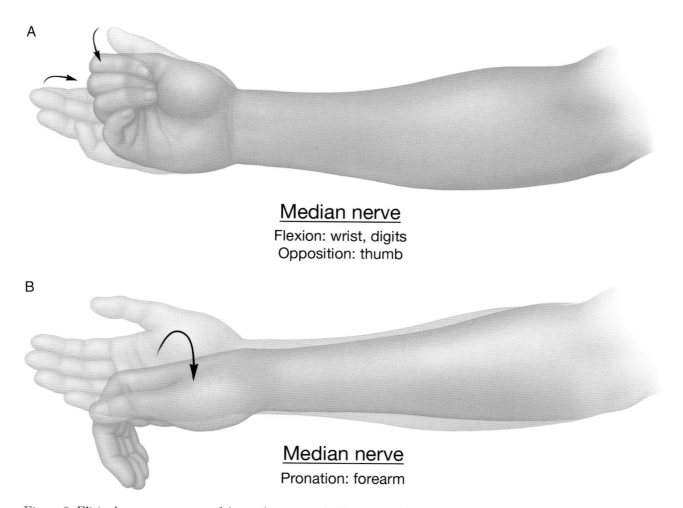

Figure 8. Elicited motor responses of the median nerve. A, Flexion of the wrist and digits. B, Pronation of the forearm.

at a fairly shallow depth. Slight medial or lateral needle redirection may be necessary if an appropriate motor response is not obtained. After confirmation of negative aspiration, 5 to 8 mL of local anesthetic is injected. Alternatively, local infiltration with 5 to 8 mL of local anesthetic may be performed 3 to 5 cm proximal to the ulnar groove in a fanlike distribution.

At the level of the elbow, the musculocutaneous nerve is a purely sensory nerve. Neural blockade is performed by inserting a 25-gauge 1.5-inch (3.8-cm) needle approximately 2.5 cm proximal to the elbow flexion crease. The needle is advanced subcutaneously along the lateral border of the biceps tendon and muscle to run parallel with the groove dividing the biceps and brachialis muscles.

Local anesthetic is injected where the lateral antebrachial cutaneous nerve emerges from the lateral border of the biceps muscle (Figure 2).

Ultrasound-Guided Peripheral Nerve Blockade at the Elbow

Anatomical variation, equipment imperfections, and operator limitations prevent anesthesia providers from achieving 100% success with *any* brachial plexus technique (e.g., supraclavicular, infraclavicular, axillary). Therefore, distal supplementation at the elbow may be necessary to provide a more complete or comprehensive block of the brachial plexus—particularly when incomplete anesthesia occurs within the surgical distribution.

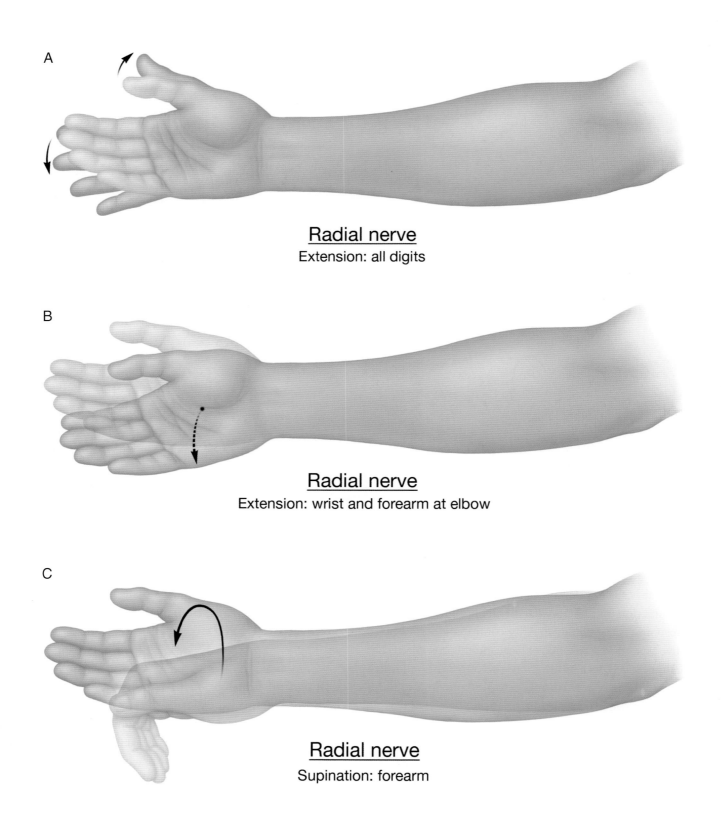

Figure 9. Elicited motor responses of the radial nerve. A, Extension of all digits. B, Extension of the wrist and forearm at the elbow. C, Supination of the forearm.

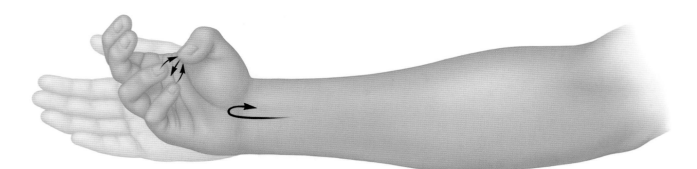

Ulnar nerve
Flexion: wrist, 4th and 5th digits
Adduction: thumb

Figure 10. Elicited motor responses of the ulnar nerve.

However, block supplementation in a partially anesthetized extremity may increase the risk of intraneural injection or neurologic injury. Although conclusive evidence of improved safety using ultrasound for supplementation is lacking, proponents believe that the ability to visualize both needle and neural target may prevent inadvertent nerve trauma and intraneuronal injection.

Scanning Technique

To scan peripheral nerves at the elbow, the ultrasound probe is oriented perpendicular to the axial direction of the limb so that each of the nerves is viewed in cross-section. The radial nerve is best seen proximal to the antecubital crease on the lateral aspect of the arm (Figure 11). The median nerve is most readily identified at a supracondylar location, with the probe on the biceps muscle and angled laterally (Figure 12). The ulnar nerve is best seen in the anterior aspect of the forearm, with the probe positioned slightly medial to the midline. Finally, the musculocutaneous nerve is difficult to visualize at the level of the elbow. However, the nerve can be easily identified and blocked in a more proximal location within the axilla.

Sonoanatomy

The sonographic appearance of the radial nerve just proximal to the elbow is typically elliptical, or even linear (Figure 13). By comparison, the median (Figure 14) and ulnar nerves are rounder. The radial nerve is viewed approximately 1 cm anterior to the humerus and should be traced both proximally and distally to confirm it as neural tissue. The median nerve is easily located by identifying the adjacent brachial artery. The brachial artery and vein and the median nerve form a distinct neurovascular bundle within the supracondylar region. The median nerve can be difficult to visualize at the level of the elbow because of shadowing caused by the bicipital aponeurosis. Therefore, it is recommended to block the nerve at a more proximal location within the supracondylar region (Figures 12 and 14).

The ulnar nerve may be viewed just proximal to the medial epicondyle of the humerus along the medial aspect of the arm (Figure 15). Alternatively, the ulnar nerve can be viewed in the midforearm, where the ulnar artery provides a clearly identifiable landmark. Pulsatility and color Doppler make identification of these vascular structures and adjacent nerves easy.

Ultrasound Approach

Supplementation of peripheral nerves proximal and distal to the elbow is performed using an *in-plane* (IP)

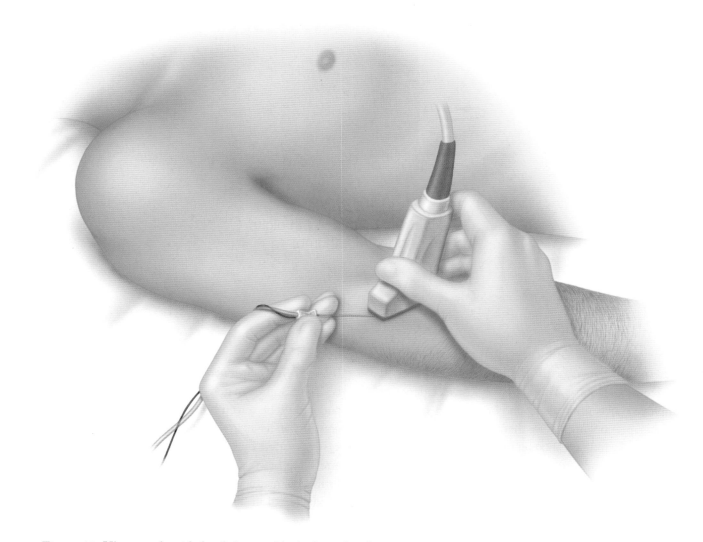

Figure 11. Ultrasound-guided radial nerve blockade at the elbow.

ultrasound approach. This is important for two reasons. First, the circumferential (i.e., rounded) configuration of the upper extremity and the superficial nature of the neural targets allow an almost perpendicular angle of incidence between the needle and the ultrasound beam. This favors optimal needle visualization. Second, the supplementation of partially anesthetized nerves should be performed with extreme caution. Clear identification of the needle tip in relation to the nerve is essential at all times and is best accomplished with an in-plane needle approach.

After identification and adequate visualization of the neural target, the needle is advanced in plane to a position directly above or below the nerve. Ideally, the needle should approach the nerve from the side opposite the vessels, so that vascular structures do not obstruct the needle path and increase the risk of intravascular injection. Nerve stimulation during needle placement is optional. Motor responses of proximally anesthetized nerves should remain intact. After needle placement and the elicitation of an appropriate motor response, the needle should be withdrawn several millimeters and 0.5 mL of local

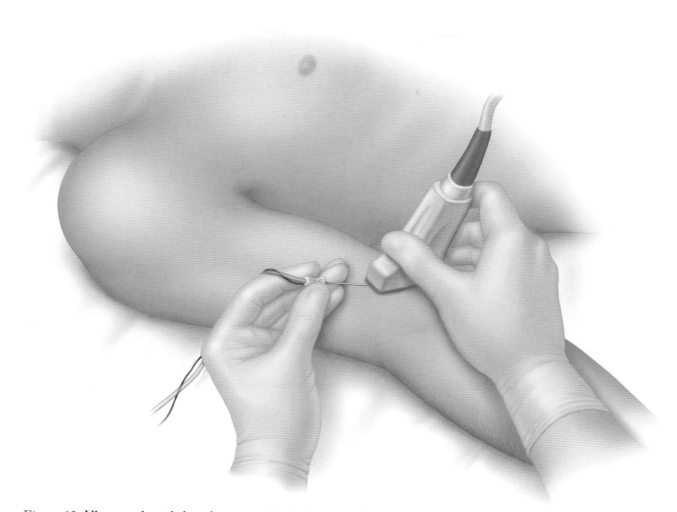

Figure 12. Ultrasound-guided median nerve blockade at the elbow.

anesthetic injected. This method of hydrodissection confirms the location of the needle tip and decreases the likelihood of inadvertent intraneural injection. The needle can then be safely advanced to distribute local anesthetic circumferentially around the nerve. Five to 7 mL of local anesthetic, depending on the volume used in the proximal approach, provides complete anesthetic blockade.

Side Effects and Complications
Although definitive data are lacking, there is a perception that *distal* peripheral nerve blocks may be associated with a slightly higher incidence of neural injury because of the proximity and anatomical relationship between neural structures and their bony and ligamentous surroundings. Furthermore, peripheral nerve blockade at the elbow—particularly in a partially anesthetized extremity—should be approached with extreme caution to avoid intraneural injection and subsequent neurologic injury. In particular, the risk of an unrecognized intraneural injection may be highest with traditional nerve stimulation techniques or generalized local infiltration. Finally, large volumes of local anesthetic should *not* be injected directly into the ulnar groove, because increased pressures within this tightly contained fascial and bony space may increase the risk of nerve injury.

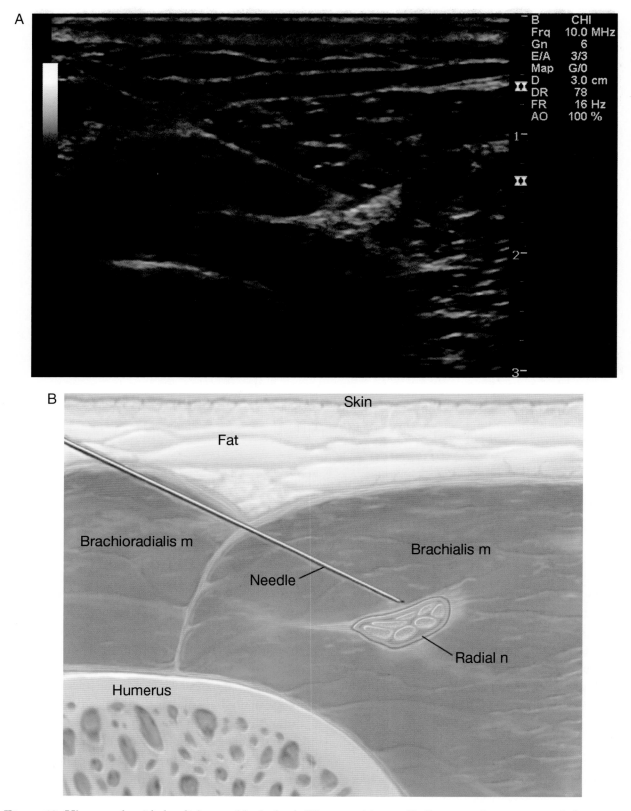

Figure 13. Ultrasound-guided radial nerve blockade. A, Ultrasound image. B, Corresponding anatomical illustration.

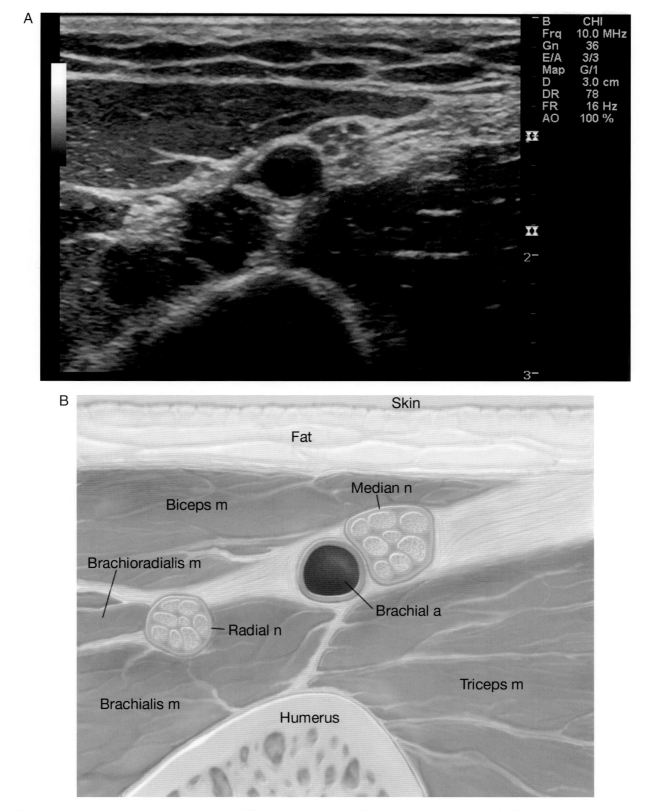

Figure 14. Median nerve at the elbow. A, Ultrasound image. B, Corresponding anatomical illustration.

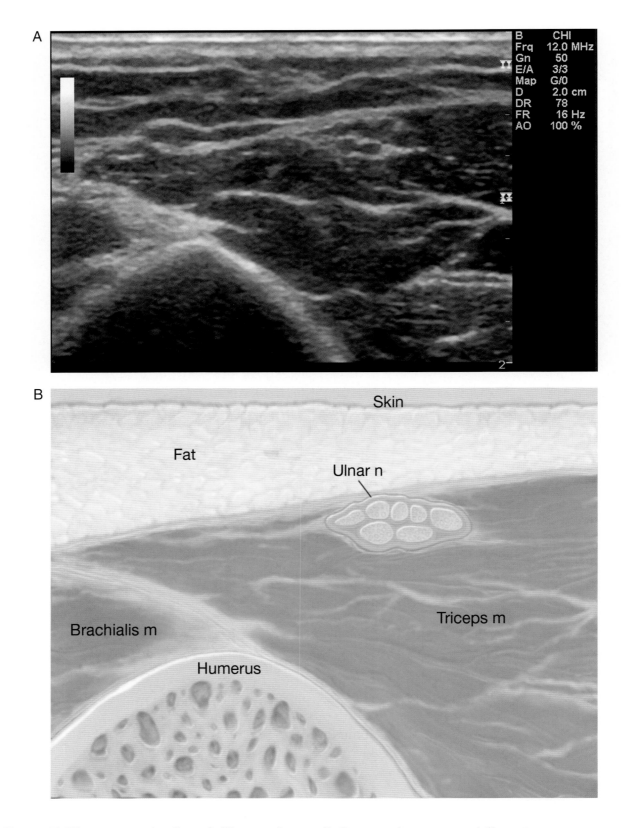

Figure 15. Ulnar nerve at the elbow. A, Ultrasound image. B, Corresponding anatomical illustration.

Suggested Reading

Brown AR. Anaesthesia for procedures of the hand and elbow. Best Pract Res Clin Anaesthesiol. 2002 Jun;16(2):227-46.

Brown DL. Atlas of regional anesthesia. 2nd ed. Philadelphia: W. B. Saunders Company; c1999. Chapter 7, Distal upper extremity blocks, p. 57-65.

Crews JC, Hilgenhurst G, Leavitt B, Denson DD, Bridenbaugh PO, Stuebing RC. Tourniquet pain: the response to the maintenance of tourniquet inflation on the upper extremity of volunteers. Reg Anesth. 1991 Nov-Dec;16(6):314-7.

deJong RH. Modified axillary block with block of the lateral antebrachial cutaneous (terminal musculocutaneous) nerve. Anesthesiology. 1965 Sep-Oct;26: 615-8.

Dilger JA, Wells RE Jr. The use of peripheral nerve blocks at the elbow for carpal tunnel release. J Clin Anesth. 2005 Dec;17(8):621-3.

Löfström JB. Ulnar nerve blockade for the evaluation of local anaesthetic agents. Br J Anaesth. 1975 Feb;47 Suppl:297-300.

Lopez S, Gros T, Deblock N, Capdevila X, Eledjam JJ. [Multitruncular block at the elbow for a major hand trauma for prehospital care.] Ann Fr Anesth Reanim. 2002 Dec;21(10):816-9. French.

McQuillan PM, Hahn MB. Does location matter in ulnar and common peroneal nerve block? Lancet. 1996 Aug 24;348(9026):490-1.

Melone CP Jr, Isani A. Anesthesia for hand injuries. Emerg Med Clin North Am. 1985 May;3(2):235-43.

Olson IA. The origin of the lateral cutaneous nerve of forearm and its anaesthesia for modified brachial plexus block. J Anat. 1969 Sep;105(Pt 2):381-2.

Warner MA, Warner ME, Martin JT. Ulnar neuropathy: incidence, outcome, and risk factors in sedated or anesthetized patients. Anesthesiology. 1994 Dec;81(6):1332-40.

CHAPTER

18

Wrist Blockade

David E. Byer, M.D.

Clinical Applications

Wrist blockade anesthetizes the median, ulnar, and radial nerves at the level of the wrist. The technique may be useful when clinical conditions such as infection or difficult anatomy limit more proximal approaches to the brachial plexus. Wrist blocks may also be used for bilateral surgery, when a limited surgical field is anticipated, or when an incomplete proximal block requires supplementation. In most patients, the entire hand may be anesthetized by separately blocking the median, ulnar, and radial nerves. Wrist blockade should be considered a suitable alternative to multiple digital blocks.

Relevant Anatomy

The three terminal branches of the brachial plexus (median, ulnar, and radial nerves) may be blocked at the level of the wrist. The median nerve passes through the carpal tunnel on the ventral aspect of the forearm in proximity to the flexor tendons (Figure 1). It provides sensation to the radial aspect of the palm, the palmar surface of the thumb and index and middle fingers, the radial half of the ring finger, and the dorsal nail beds of the same digits (Figure 2). The ulnar nerve travels along the ventromedial aspect of the forearm, medial to the ulnar artery and lateral to the flexor carpi ulnaris tendon (Figure 1). It provides sensation to the ulnar side of the hand, the fifth finger, and the ulnar half of the fourth finger. Finally, the radial nerve terminates as several small, subcutaneous branches across the lateral aspect of the wrist. It provides sensation to the dorsum of the hand and the proximal portion of the thumb and index, middle, and radial half of the fourth fingers on the dorsal surface (Figure 2).

Surface Anatomy

Several important surface landmarks should be identified before performing wrist blockade. The ulnar and radial styloid processes are palpated on the medial and lateral aspects of the wrist, respectively. Flexion of the wrist and fingers accentuates the flexor tendons within the ventral compartment of the forearm, particularly the palmaris longus and flexor carpi radialis tendons (Figure 1). Maximal thumb abduction defines the anatomical "snuffbox" on the dorsolateral aspect of the wrist between the tendons of the extensor pollicis longus, extensor pollicis brevis, and abductor pollicis longus. Finally, the ulnar artery—which lies immediately lateral to the ulnar nerve—is palpated on the ventromedial aspect of the wrist.

Patient Position

The patient is positioned supine with the forearm abducted and extended. A small towel roll is placed under the forearm during median and ulnar nerve blockade to facilitate hand supination and wrist dorsiflexion. During radial nerve blockade, the hand is placed on the procedural table in the pronated position.

Technique

Neural Localization Techniques

At the level of the wrist, the median, ulnar, and radial nerves are commonly anesthetized using a field block technique. However, median and ulnar nerve blockade may be performed using peripheral nerve stimulation, because these nerves contain both motor and sensory fibers in discrete, localized bundles. Alternatively, all three terminal branches of the brachial plexus can be localized using ultrasound guidance.

Needle Insertion Site

During median nerve blockade, a 25-gauge 1.5-inch (3.8-cm) needle is inserted 2 cm proximal to the wrist crease immediately adjacent to the radial edge of the palmaris longus tendon (Figures 1 and 3). If the palmaris longus tendon is absent, or cannot be palpated, the needle is introduced 1 cm medial to the ulnar edge of the flexor carpi radialis tendon. After negative aspiration is confirmed, 3 to 6 mL of local anesthetic solution is injected.

During ulnar nerve blockade, the ulnar artery is first identified on the ventromedial aspect of the wrist. The ulnar nerve is located medial and posterior (i.e., deep) to the artery (Figure 1). A 25-gauge 1.5-inch (3.8-cm) needle is inserted 2 cm proximal to the wrist crease at the radial edge of the flexor carpi ulnaris tendon and medial to the ulnar artery (Figure 4). After negative aspiration is confirmed, 3 to 6 mL of local anesthetic solution is injected.

At the level of the wrist, the radial nerve is unique in that it contains only sensory nerve fibers. These small subcutaneous fibers are anesthetized with local infiltration. A 25-gauge 1.5-inch (3.8-cm) needle is inserted in the center of the anatomical "snuffbox" at the level of the wrist crease (Figure 5). Five milliliters of local anesthetic is injected subcutaneously while the needle is advanced laterally to the dorsal surface of the wrist. An additional 5 mL of local anesthetic solution is injected subcutaneously in a medial direction from the anatomical "snuffbox."

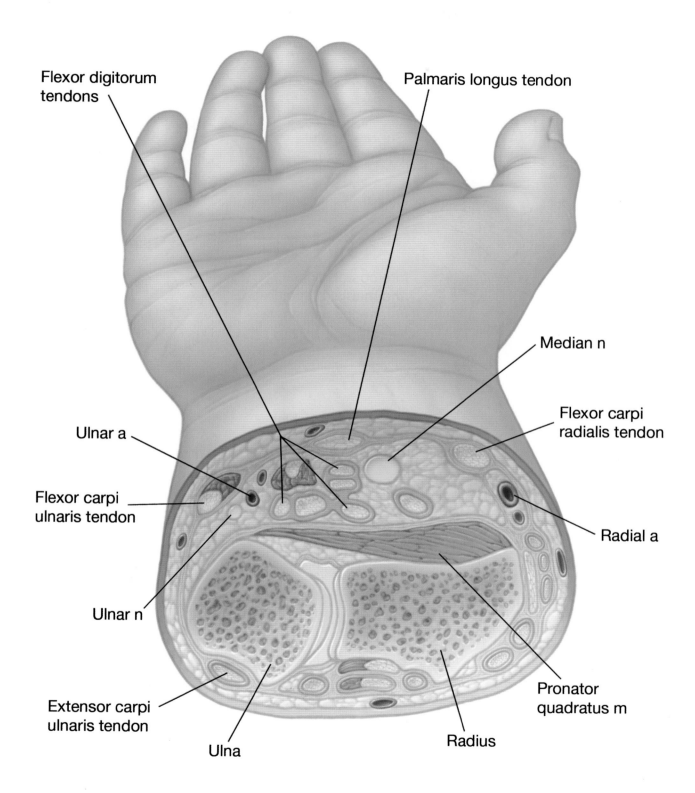

Flexor digitorum tendons

Palmaris longus tendon

Median n

Flexor carpi radialis tendon

Ulnar a

Flexor carpi ulnaris tendon

Radial a

Ulnar n

Extensor carpi ulnaris tendon

Pronator quadratus m

Ulna

Radius

Figure 1. Cross-sectional anatomy of the wrist.

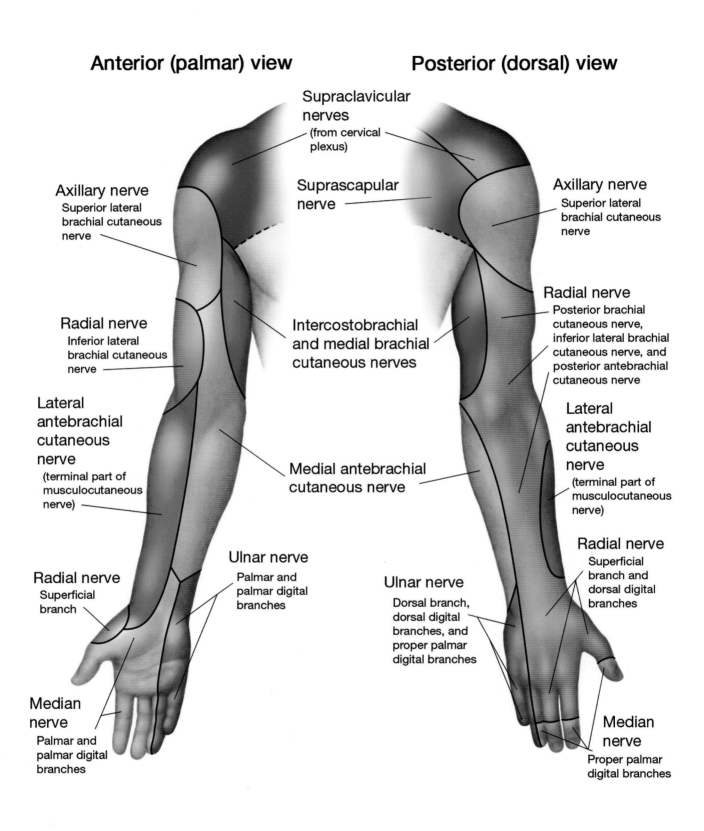

Anterior (palmar) view

Posterior (dorsal) view

Supraclavicular nerves (from cervical plexus)

Suprascapular nerve

Axillary nerve
Superior lateral brachial cutaneous nerve

Axillary nerve
Superior lateral brachial cutaneous nerve

Radial nerve
Inferior lateral brachial cutaneous nerve

Intercostobrachial and medial brachial cutaneous nerves

Radial nerve
Posterior brachial cutaneous nerve, inferior lateral brachial cutaneous nerve, and posterior antebrachial cutaneous nerve

Lateral antebrachial cutaneous nerve
(terminal part of musculocutaneous nerve)

Medial antebrachial cutaneous nerve

Lateral antebrachial cutaneous nerve
(terminal part of musculocutaneous nerve)

Radial nerve
Superficial branch and dorsal digital branches

Radial nerve
Superficial branch

Ulnar nerve
Palmar and palmar digital branches

Ulnar nerve
Dorsal branch, dorsal digital branches, and proper palmar digital branches

Median nerve
Palmar and palmar digital branches

Median nerve
Proper palmar digital branches

Figure 2. Cutaneous innervation of the upper extremity.

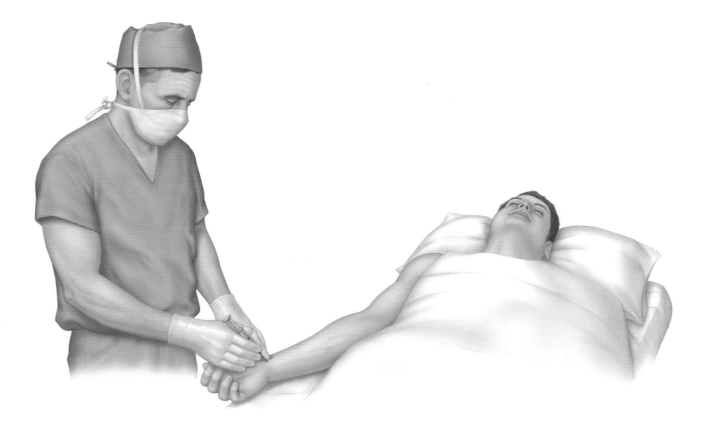

Figure 3. Median nerve blockade at the wrist.

Alternative Techniques

When anesthesia is inadequate, the failed block may be repeated and the tissue at the site of injection vigorously massaged. Alternative methods of median nerve blockade include the injection of local anesthetic as the needle is advanced in a stepwise manner from the palmaris longus tendon to the flexor carpi radialis tendon (i.e., in a medial to lateral direction) within the ventral compartment of the wrist. Ulnar nerve blockade may be modified by altering the point of needle insertion. The needle may be inserted on the ulnar side of the flexor carpi ulnaris tendon and directed radially for a distance of 1.5 cm. After negative aspiration is confirmed, 3 to 6 mL of local anesthetic solution is injected.

Side Effects and Complications

Although wrist blockade may provide adequate anesthesia for surgery on the hand or digits, the need for a proximal tourniquet significantly limits the clinical utility of this block technique. When clinically appropriate, surgical anesthesia may be achieved with minimal volumes of local anesthetic. Large volumes of injectate should be avoided to minimize the risk of nerve compression within the small, nonexpansive fascial compartments of the wrist. Other potential risks include intravascular injection or direct neural injury. However, both of these complications are exceedingly rare.

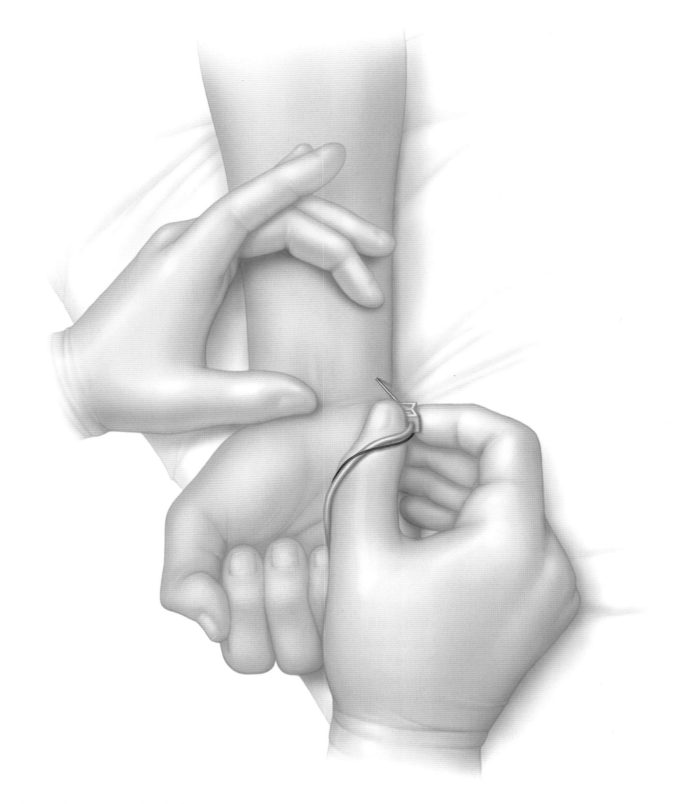

Figure 4. Ulnar nerve blockade at the wrist.

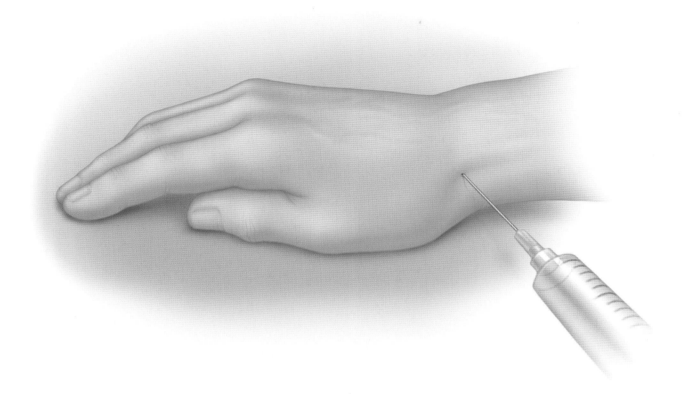

Figure 5. Radial nerve blockade at the wrist.

Suggested Reading

Bridenbaugh LD. The upper extremity: somatic blockade. In: Cousins MJ, Bridenbaugh PO, editors. Neuronal blockade in clinical anesthesia and management of pain. 2nd ed. Philadelphia: J. B. Lippincott Company; c1988. p. 387-416.

Brown DL. Atlas of regional anesthesia. 2nd ed. Philadelphia: W. B. Saunders Company; c1999. Chapter 7, Distal upper extremity blocks, p. 57-65.

Derkash RS, Weaver JK, Berkeley ME, Dawson D. Office carpal tunnel release with wrist block and wrist tourniquet. Orthopedics. 1996 Jul;19(7):589-90.

Sites BD, Spence BC. Ultrasound-guided rescue blocks: a description of a technique for the median and ulnar nerves. The Internet Journal of Anesthesiology. 2005;10(1).

CHAPTER

19

Digital Blockade

David E. Byer, M.D.

Clinical Applications

Digital nerve blocks are used to provide anesthesia of one or more fingers or toes. First described in 1889 for removal of an ingrown toenail, digital blocks have become commonplace in surgical suites, emergency departments, and other primary care settings. Various procedures can be performed under digital blockade, including laceration repair, nail removal, paronychia drainage, foreign body removal, and minor orthopedic interventions.

Relevant Anatomy

In the upper extremity, the common palmar digital nerves are terminal branches of the median and ulnar nerves. These nerves become the proper palmar digital branches that supply the medial, lateral, and palmar surfaces of the fingers, fingertips, and nail beds. The proper palmar digital nerves, together with the digital vessels, travel symmetrically within the ventrolateral and ventromedial aspects of the finger adjacent to the flexor tendon sheath (Figure 1).

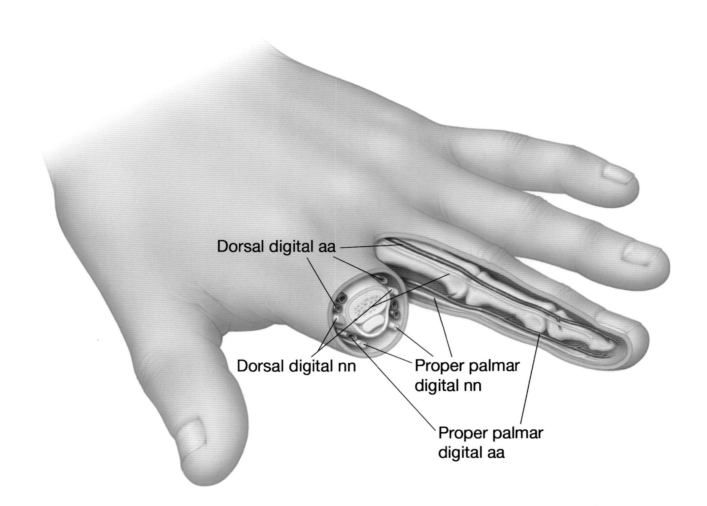

Dorsal digital aa

Dorsal digital nn

Proper palmar
digital nn

Proper palmar
digital aa

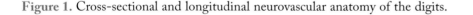

Figure 1. Cross-sectional and longitudinal neurovascular anatomy of the digits.

The smaller dorsal digital nerves, derived from the radial and ulnar nerves, travel on the dorsal aspect of each finger. The dorsal digital nerves supply sensation to the dorsal aspect of the finger to the level of the distal interphalangeal joint (Figure 1). Dorsal digital branches of the radial nerve and proper palmar digital branches of the median nerve innervate the thumb.

Surface Anatomy

The base of each digit and the adjacent web spaces may be readily palpated.

Patient Position

The patient should be resting supine with the operative hand pronated and resting on a flat surface.

Technique

Needle Insertion Site

The palmar and dorsal digital nerves may be blocked at the base of each digit. At the dorsolateral aspect of the finger base, a 25-gauge 1.5-inch (3.8-cm) needle is inserted and advanced anteriorly past the base of the phalanx until tenting of the palmar dermis is observed on the ventral surface of the web space. The proper palmar digital nerve is blocked by injecting 2 to 3 mL of local anesthetic solution. To block the dorsal digital nerve, the needle is withdrawn slightly and 1 mL of local anesthetic injected immediately anterior to the site of needle entry (Figure 2). This process is performed on both sides of the digit for both palmar and dorsal digital nerves.

Alternative Techniques

When inadequate anesthesia occurs, the block may be repeated and the tissue massaged at the site of injection to help facilitate the spread of local anesthetic and increase its absorption. Alternatively, the common volar digital nerves may be blocked at the site of their bifurcation between the metacarpal heads. During this technique, a 25-gauge 1.5-inch (3.8-cm) needle is inserted 2 to 3 mm into the web space in a cephalad direction, proximal to the junction of the web and the palmar skin. The needle is advanced proximally toward the hand in line with the extended fingers and 1 to 2 mL of local anesthetic is injected. The needle may also be redirected more posteriorly to block the dorsal segment of each nerve.

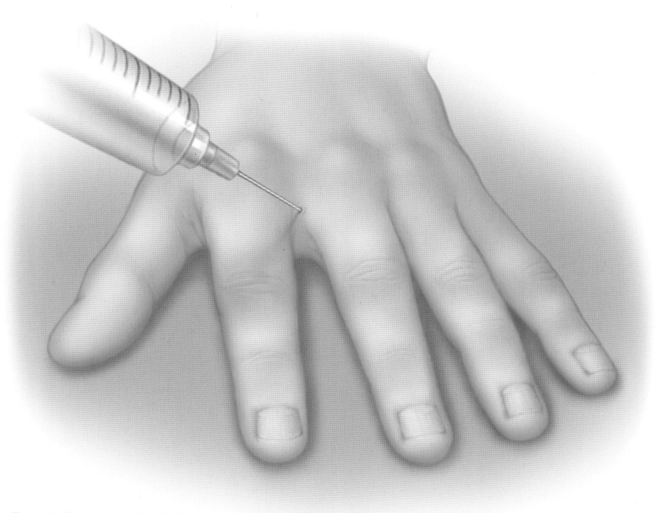

Figure 2. Digital nerve blockade.

Side Effects and Complications

In general, complications from digital blockade are rare. Because of concern about potential vascular insufficiency, digital ischemia, and necrosis, epinephrine-containing solutions and large injectate volumes are avoided. Direct vascular injury to the small vessels of the finger may also occur. Although the potential risk of nerve injury is small, patients should be cautioned that transient digital sensory loss can persist after the block, making the digit vulnerable to injury.

Suggested Reading

Bridenbaugh LD. The upper extremity: somatic blockade. In: Cousins MJ, Bridenbaugh PO, editors. Neural blockade in clinical anesthesia and management of pain. 2nd ed. Philadelphia: J. B. Lippincott Company; c1988. p. 387-416.

Flarity-Reed K. Methods of digital block. J Emerg Nurs. 2002 Aug;28(4):351-4.

Knoop K, Trott A, Syverud S. Comparison of digital versus metacarpal blocks for repair of finger injuries. Ann Emerg Med. 1994 Jun;23(6):1296-300.

O'Donnell J, Wilson K, Leonard PA. An avoidable complication of digital nerve block. Emerg Med J. 2001 Jul;18(4):316.

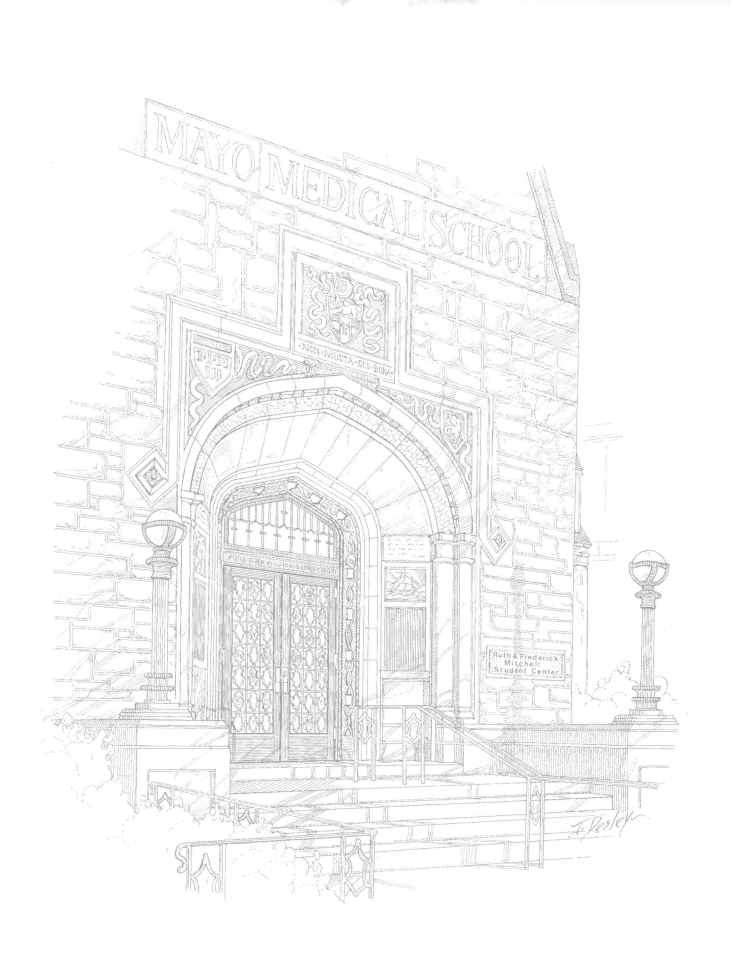

CHAPTER

20

Intravenous Regional Anesthesia

Edward D. Frie, M.D.

Clinical Applications

Intravenous regional anesthesia was first described by the German surgeon August Bier in 1908. The original Bier block technique involved intravenous injection of prilocaine into a previously exsanguinated limb to produce anesthesia for a short duration. In early descriptions of the block, the technique was used for surgical procedures involving the distal aspect of the arm or leg.

Soon after its introduction, Bier's technique lost popularity for an extended time because of associated complications and reports of death. However, in 1963 the technique was reintroduced by Holmes using lidocaine and has since become a popular method of upper extremity regional anesthesia.

In principle, the intravenous injection of local anesthetic into an exsanguinated limb provides anesthesia by diffusion of the drug to peripheral nerves supplied by small vessels. A proximal tourniquet that occludes both venous and arterial blood flow is used during the technique to prevent the mixing of local anesthetic with the systemic circulation. An important limitation of the technique is the inevitable pain from the proximal tourniquet. However, the use of a double-cuff tourniquet may help minimize patient discomfort and extend the duration of anesthesia. Regardless, surgical times should optimally be kept to less than 1 hour to ensure patient comfort and reduce the need to convert to a general anesthetic.

Intravenous regional anesthesia is most commonly used for surgical procedures on the hand, wrist, and digits. However, it may also be effective for minor surgery involving the foot and ankle. Emergency department and pain clinic physicians may use the Bier block technique outside the operating room for the closed reduction of extremity fractures and in the treatment of chronic pain syndromes (e.g., complex regional pain syndrome).

Patient Position

The patient is positioned supine with the operative extremity comfortably abducted.

Surface Anatomy

Temporary intravenous access is necessary in the operative extremity for the performance of the block. This is typically achieved in the dorsum of the hand in proximity to the surgical site. However, the block can be successfully accomplished using intravenous access anywhere distal to the tourniquet. Intravenous access is also established in the nonoperative extremity for use during the surgical procedure.

Technique

Intravenous regional anesthetic techniques essentially replace the intravascular blood volume of an exsanguinated extremity with local anesthetic. Intravenous access is established in the operative extremity in proximity to the proposed surgical site. The intravenous catheter and extension tubing are carefully secured to the skin to prevent dislodgment during extremity exsanguination. A double-cuff tourniquet (or two separate tourniquets) is placed as proximal on the extremity as possible. Standard blood pressure cuffs should *not* be used as tourniquets, because they do not reliably maintain constant pressure throughout the surgical procedure. Failure to maintain pressure may lead to a rapid and uncontrolled release of local anesthetic into the systemic circulation that causes local anesthetic toxicity.

After the tourniquet is in place, the extremity should be actively exsanguinated by elevating and wrapping the limb from distal to proximal using an Esmarch bandage (Figure 1). Historically, the quality of the block was believed to be related to the degree of limb exsanguination. However, recent evidence suggests that block density may not be influenced by limb exsanguination.

After extremity exsanguination, the *proximal* tourniquet (during a double-cuff technique) is inflated to 250 to 300 mm Hg. The Esmarch bandage may then be removed. If the tourniquet is functioning properly, the extremity will appear pale and mottled. A standard intravenous tourniquet can be placed proximal to the surgical site to increase venous hydrostatic pressure during injection of the local anesthetic to promote distal spread and thereby improve block density.

Several local anesthetics have been used for intravenous regional anesthetic techniques; lidocaine 0.5% at a dose of 1.5 to 3 mg/kg is the most common agent of choice. During injection (Figure 2), the patient may experience mild, local discomfort and the skin may become more mottled because of the peripheral displacement of venous blood by local anesthetic. The local anesthetic should be injected slowly and the patient monitored for signs and symptoms of systemic toxicity (e.g., tinnitus, lightheadedness, and perioral numbness).

Sensory changes may begin within 3 to 5 minutes of injection. However, reliable surgical anesthesia does not occur until approximately 10 minutes after the injection

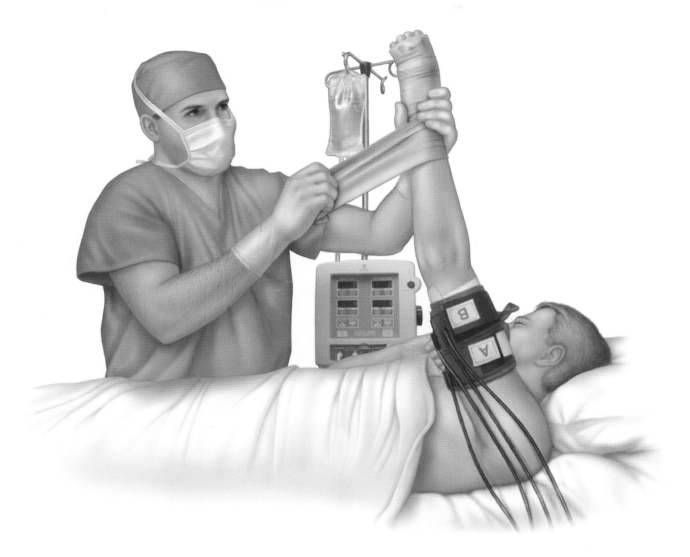

Figure 1. Exsanguination of the upper extremity using an Esmarch bandage.

of local anesthetic. Patients may begin to experience pain or discomfort from the tourniquet as soon as 10 to 15 minutes after tourniquet inflation. Inflation of the *distal* cuff (during a double-cuff technique) should alleviate this discomfort because the tissue underlying the cuff is anesthetized. When the cuffs are switched, the distal cuff should be inflated to the same pressure as the proximal cuff and its proper function confirmed *before* deflating the proximal cuff. The duration of the block is limited by pain from the tourniquet; patients seldom tolerate tourniquet times of more than 90 minutes.

Rapid resolution of the block occurs soon after tourniquet deflation. Therefore, distal tourniquet pressures should not be lowered until the surgical procedure is complete. To minimize the risk of rapidly introducing a large volume of local anesthetic into the systemic circulation, the tourniquet should remain inflated for a minimum of 45 minutes. After that time, the distal cuff should be deflated for approximately 5 seconds and then reinflated for 45 seconds. This deflation-reinflation sequence should be repeated 4 or 5 times before final cuff removal. Clinicians must remain cognizant that

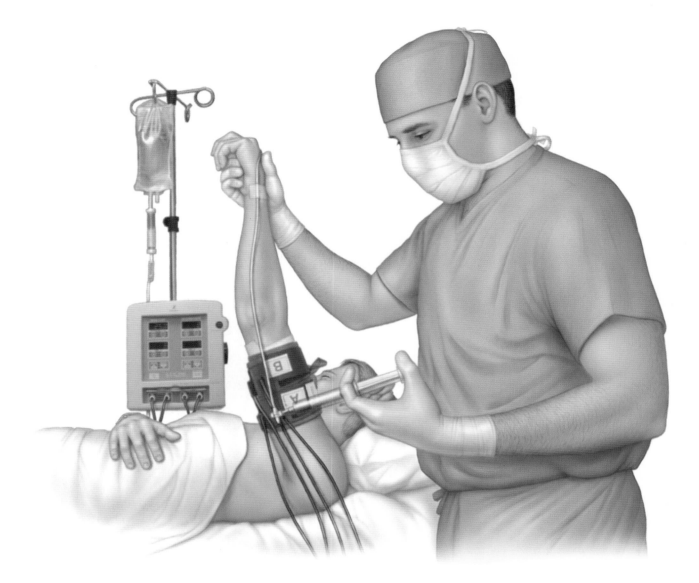

Figure 2. Intravenous regional anesthesia using a double-cuff tourniquet.

patients are at increased risk of systemic local anesthetic toxicity and should be monitored and closely observed.

Side Effects and Complications
Intravenous regional anesthesia is generally considered a safe technique. Although complications have been reported, their occurrence is extremely rare. The most common complication is local anesthetic toxicity due to cuff failure, technical error, or inadvertent cuff deflation. Interestingly, serum local anesthetic concentrations after intravenous regional anesthesia tend to be lower than after other commonly performed nerve blocks of the upper extremity (e.g., axillary blockade). Cases of compartment syndrome and tourniquet-related injuries (e.g., mechanical or ischemic myopathy or neuropathy) have also been reported.

Suggested Reading

Barnes CL, Blasier RD, Dodge BM. Intravenous regional anesthesia: a safe and cost-effective outpatient anesthetic for upper extremity fracture treatment in children. J Pediatr Orthop. 1991 Nov-Dec;11(6):717-20.

Blasier RD, White R. Intravenous regional anesthesia for management of children's extremity fractures in the emergency department. Pediatr Emerg Care. 1996 Dec;12(6):404-6.

Bolte RG, Stevens PM, Scott SM, Schunk JE. Mini-dose Bier block intravenous regional anesthesia in the emergency department treatment of pediatric upper-extremity injuries. J Pediatr Orthop. 1994 Jul-Aug;14(4):534-7.

Brown EM, McGriff JT, Malinowski RW. Intravenous regional anaesthesia (Bier block): review of 20 years' experience. Can J Anaesth. 1989 May;36(3 Pt 1):307-10.

Farrell RG, Swanson SL, Walter JR. Safe and effective IV regional anesthesia for use in the emergency department. Ann Emerg Med. 1985 Mar;14(3):239-43.

Hilgenhurst G. The Bier block after 80 years: a historical review. Reg Anesth. 1990 Jan-Feb;15(1):2-5.

Mabee J, Orlinsky M. Bier block exsanguination: a volumetric comparison and venous pressure study. Acad Emerg Med. 2000 Feb;7(2):105-13.

Rawlings ID, Staniforth P. Intravenous regional anaesthesia in upper limb trauma. Injury. 1979 Feb;10(3):231-4.

Roberts JR. Intravenous regional anesthesia: "Bier block." Am Fam Physician. 1978 Feb;17(2):123-6.

Rodolà F, Vagnoni S, Ingletti S. An update on intravenous regional anaesthesia of the arm. Eur Rev Med Pharmacol Sci. 2003 Sep-Oct;7(5):131-8.

Rosenberg PH, Kalso EA, Tuominen MK, Lindén HB. Acute bupivacaine toxicity as a result of venous leakage under the tourniquet cuff during a Bier block. Anesthesiology. 1983 Jan;58(1):95-8.

CHAPTER

21

Paravertebral Blockade

Sandra L. Kopp, M.D.

Hugh M. Smith, M.D., Ph.D.

Clinical Applications

Paravertebral blockade was first described by Hugo Sellheim in 1905. However, the technique was seldom used until its reassessment by Eason and Wyatt in 1979. Today, thoracic paravertebral blockade is commonly used for unilateral breast, axillary, or chest wall surgery and in the management of chronic pain syndromes. Cervical and lumbar paravertebral blockade have also been described. However, the usefulness of these techniques is limited by the improved efficacy and safety of alternative regional anesthetic techniques.

Thoracic paravertebral blockade is associated with fewer cardiovascular and respiratory alterations than neuraxial techniques. In addition, sensorimotor function *distal* to the anesthetized neural segments remains intact. Single-injection and continuous catheter techniques can be performed at various paravertebral levels to provide effective surgical anesthesia and postoperative analgesia (Table 1).

Relevant Anatomy

The anatomical borders of the wedge-shaped paravertebral space include the parietal pleura anteriorly; the vertebral body, intervertebral disk, and neural foramen medially; the posterior intercostal membrane laterally; and the superior costotransverse ligament posteriorly (Figure 1). Therefore, the thoracic paravertebral space is continuous with the epidural space medially, the intercostal space laterally, and the contralateral paravertebral space via the prevertebral fascia. Awareness of the spinous processes, transverse processes, ribs, and costotransverse ligaments is essential when performing the block. The neural structures within the paravertebral space include the ventral ramus (intercostal nerve), the dorsal ramus, the gray and white communications, and the sympathetic chain (Figure 1). The intercostal nerve itself is fragmented within the paravertebral space and easily anesthetized by local anesthetics.

Surface Anatomy

Correct needle placement is dependent on identification of the spinous processes at the targeted thoracic dermatomal levels. The prominent C7 spinous process and the inferior aspect of the scapula (T7) may help to correctly determine thoracic levels (Figure 2). Paramedian marks are made 2.5 cm lateral from the superior border of the spinous processes for each planned injection site (Figure 3). These marks correspond with the transverse process of the next *caudad* vertebrae.

Patient Position

The patient is placed in the sitting position with the neck flexed (Figure 4). This is the optimal position for paravertebral blockade because it offers easy access, accurate spinal alignment, and the best overall presentation of surface anatomy. Alternatively, the prone or lateral decubitus position may be used when patient comfort and safety are important considerations. However, both of these positions are suboptimal compared with an upright, sitting position.

Technique

Neural Localization Techniques

Conventionally, nerve roots within the paravertebral space are anesthetized using surface anatomical landmarks and tactile needle advancement. The safety of this procedure is highly dependent on limiting needle advancement to 1 cm beyond the transverse process. Deeper needle advancement may significantly increase the risk of inadvertent pneumothorax. Although a slight loss of resistance may be felt when the needle passes through the costotransverse ligament, this should be considered a nonspecific and unreliable clinical end point.

Peripheral nerve stimulation has been used to signify needle entry into the paravertebral space and guard against pleural puncture. The stimulating needle elicits a motor response of the intercostal muscles before entering the pleura. During a multilevel nerve stimulation technique, local anesthetic injected at one level may spread to contiguous levels and confound the intercostal motor response.

Ultrasound measurements of the depth from skin to the transverse process and from skin to the parietal pleura

Table 1. Recommended Levels of Paravertebral Blockade for Specific Surgical Procedures	
Type of surgery	**Level to be blocked**
Shoulder	C6
Mastectomy	C7 to T5
Breast biopsy	Level corresponding to the site of incision
Thoracotomy	T5 to T9
Inguinal herniorrhaphy	T10 to L2
Ventral hernia	T7 to T10

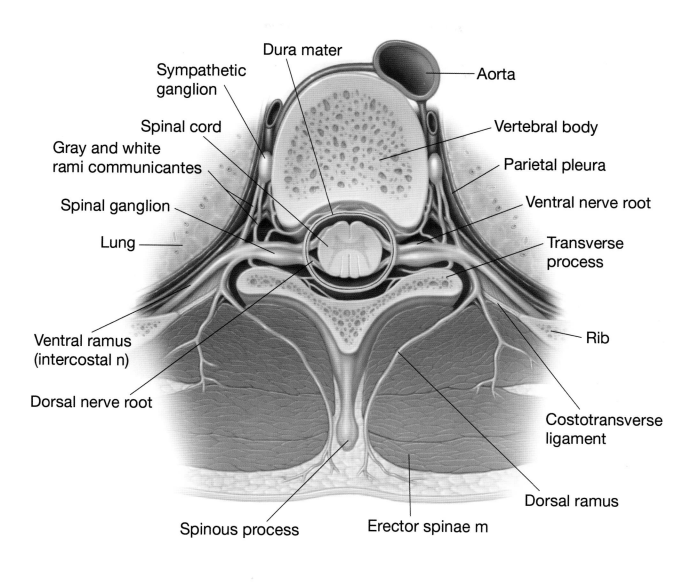

Figure 1. Cross-sectional paravertebral anatomy.

have been found to closely correlate with actual needle depth. Theoretically, knowing the maximum insertion depth should minimize the risk of pneumothorax.

Needle Insertion Site

After the spinous processes are identified, the points of needle insertion are marked 2.5 cm lateral to the superior border of each spinous process (Figure 3). Although many needle types may be used during the technique, the loss of resistance may be more pronounced with a 22-gauge (10-cm) Tuohy needle. The procedural needle should be inserted perpendicular to the skin (Figure 4) and advanced until the transverse process of the desired vertebra is contacted (2-4 cm in most adults). If the transverse process is not contacted, the needle should be redirected slightly cephalad and then caudad to identify the transverse process. To avoid inadvertent pleural puncture, it is imperative to identify the transverse process before advancing the needle beyond the expected depth.

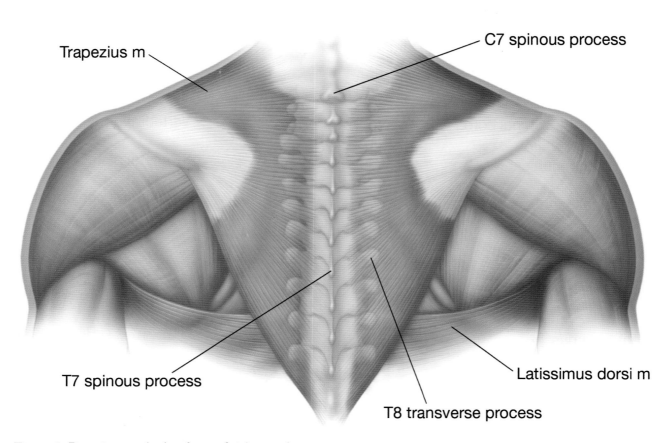

Figure 2. Posterior vertebral and superficial muscular anatomy.

After the transverse process is contacted, the needle is grasped at the point of skin entry and withdrawn to determine the distance from skin surface to transverse process. The needle is then reinserted to contact the transverse process, redirected to "walk off" the caudad aspect of the transverse process, and then advanced 1 cm past the predetermined skin-transverse process distance. If too much needle angulation is required to walk caudally off the transverse process, the cephalad portion of the transverse process has likely been contacted. At this point, the needle is returned to the skin and reinserted at a site 1 cm more caudad. If further attempts continue to result in an extreme needle angle, the needle is walked cephalad off the transverse process. However, this maneuver may result in the anesthetic blockade of a dermatome level higher than anticipated. After negative aspiration, approximately 5 mL

of local anesthetic is injected. This procedure is repeated at each targeted level.

If the planned surgery requires bilateral paravertebral blockade at multiple levels, reducing the amount of local anesthetic at each site to 3 mL is an acceptable alternative. Single injection techniques with up to 15 mL of local anesthetic have also been described. Under optimal conditions, this technique may provide adequate anesthesia for up to five dermatomal segments. However, there is considerable variation in the amount and direction of spread with single-injection techniques.

Needle Redirection Cues
The depth of each transverse process varies slightly based on the patient's body habitus and the spinal level of interest. The deepest levels are the high thoracic

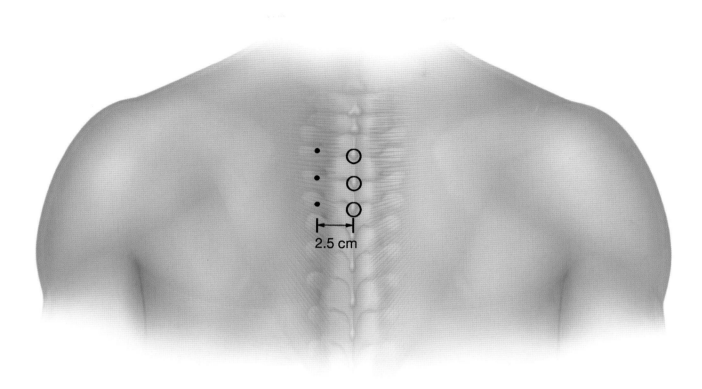

Figure 3. Surface anatomy and landmark identification for paravertebral blockade.

(T1-T2) and low lumbar (L4-L5) levels, where the transverse processes are an average of 6 to 8 cm below the skin surface in average-sized adults. The most superficial levels are in the midthoracic region (T5-T10), where the transverse processes are an average of 2 to 4 cm below the skin.

If resistance is encountered during injection of local anesthetic, the needle tip is likely adjacent to the superior costotransverse ligament. Under these circumstances, the needle is advanced slightly (2-3 mm) until injection pressures improve. Excessive needle advancement may increase the risk of pleural puncture. The needle should *never* be redirected medially toward the midline. Medial needle redirection may result in intraforaminal needle placement and subsequent spinal cord injury.

Alternative Techniques

The technique described above may also be used for lumbar paravertebral blockade. Because the transverse processes are much shorter and thinner than in the thoracic region, the point of needle insertion is only 2 cm lateral to the superior border of the transverse process. In addition, the needle is advanced only 0.5 cm beyond the transverse process before local anesthetic is injected. Insertion deeper than this may place the needle into the psoas muscle and subsequently decrease the effect of the block.

The cervical paravertebral approach was originally described by Kappis in 1919. However, the technique was recently modified by Boezaart and colleagues in 2003. The cervical approach consists of inserting a stimulating needle between the levator scapulae and

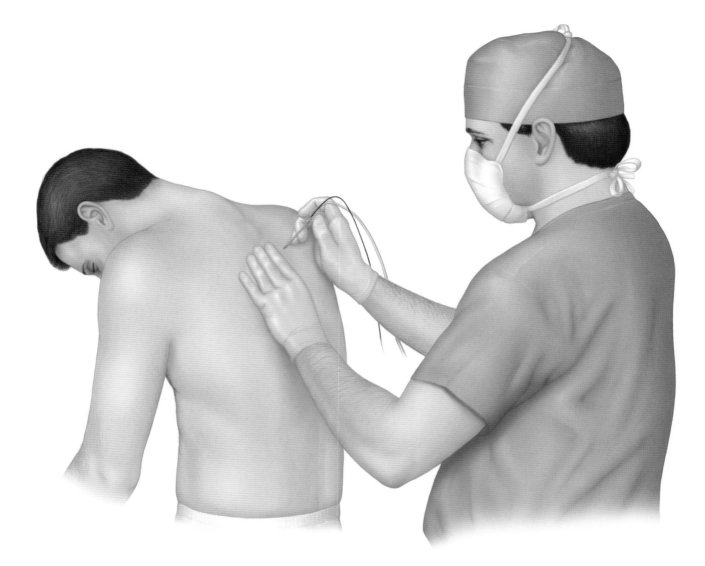

Figure 4. Patient position and provider orientation during paravertebral blockade.

trapezius muscles at the level of the C6 spinous process. The needle is advanced medially and approximately 30° caudad toward the suprasternal notch until the transverse process is encountered (approximately 4-6 cm from the skin). The needle is then walked off laterally until a distinct loss of resistance to air occurs along with the simultaneous motor response of the shoulder muscles. At this point (0.5-1.0 cm beyond bone), the paravertebral space is entered and local anesthetic injected or a catheter placed.

Side Effects and Complications

Potential complications associated with paravertebral blockade include pleural puncture and pneumothorax, epidural or intrathecal spread of local anesthetic, hypotension, hematoma or bleeding complications, neural injury, infection, and postdural puncture headache. Although intravascular injection may occur, systemic local anesthetic toxicity is rare. Failure rates during paravertebral blockade approach 6% to 10% and may be highly dependent on provider experience.

Suggested Reading

Boezaart AP, Koorn R, Rosenquist RW. Paravertebral approach to the brachial plexus: an anatomic improvement in technique. Reg Anesth Pain Med. 2003 May-Jun;28(3):241-4.

Buckenmaier CC III, Klein SM, Nielsen KC, Steele SM. Continuous paravertebral catheter and outpatient infusion for breast surgery. Anesth Analg. 2003 Sep;97(3):715-7. Erratum in: Anesth Analg. 2004 Jan;98(1):101.

Eason MJ, Wyatt R. Paravertebral thoracic block: a reappraisal. Anaesthesia. 1979 Jul-Aug;34(7):638-42.

Ganapathy S, Nielsen KC, Steele SM. Outcomes after paravertebral blocks. Int Anesthesiol Clin. 2005 Summer;43(3):185-93.

Karmakar MK. Thoracic paravertebral block. Anesthesiology. 2001 Sep;95(3):771-80.

Karmakar MK, Ho AM. Acute pain management of patients with multiple fractured ribs. J Trauma. 2003 Mar;54(3):615-25.

Klein SM, Bergh A, Steele SM, Georgiade GS, Greengrass RA. Thoracic paravertebral block for breast surgery. Anesth Analg. 2000 Jun;90(6):1402-5.

Lönnqvist PA, MacKenzie J, Soni AK, Conacher ID. Paravertebral blockade: failure rate and complications. Anaesthesia. 1995 Sep;50(9):813-5.

Naja Z, Lönnqvist PA. Somatic paravertebral nerve blockade: incidence of failed block and complications. Anaesthesia. 2001 Dec;56(12):1184-8.

Pusch F, Wildling E, Klimscha W, Weinstabl C. Sonographic measurement of needle insertion depth in paravertebral blocks in women. Br J Anaesth. 2000 Dec;85(6):841-3.

Richardson J, Lönnqvist PA. Thoracic paravertebral block. Br J Anaesth. 1998 Aug;81(2):230-8.

Terheggen MA, Wille F, Borel Rinkes IH, Ionescu TI, Knape JT. Paravertebral blockade for minor breast surgery. Anesth Analg. 2002 Feb;94(2):355-9.

SECTION

V

Lower Extremity Peripheral Nerve Block Techniques

CHAPTER

22

Posterior Lumbar Plexus (Psoas Compartment) Blockade

Sandra L. Kopp, M.D.

Clinical Applications

The posterior lumbar plexus block was first described by Winnie and colleagues in 1974 to provide comprehensive unilateral blockade of the lumbar plexus—including the lateral femoral cutaneous, femoral, and obturator nerves. The technique was later modified by Chayen and colleagues, who referred to the approach as the *psoas compartment block*. The posterior lumbar plexus block is primarily used to provide unilateral anesthesia and analgesia to the proximal aspect of the thigh and hip. However, it can be used for any procedure in which blockade of the lumbar plexus is required. Common indications include postoperative analgesia for total hip arthroplasty, pelvic surgery, femoral neck and shaft fractures, soft tissue procedures involving the thigh, and total knee arthroplasty. Because the posterior lumbar plexus block typically spares the sacral plexus, the technique must be combined with sciatic nerve blockade to provide complete anesthesia or analgesia of the lower extremity.

Both single-injection and continuous catheter techniques have been described for the block.

Relevant Anatomy

The lumbar plexus is derived from the anterior (ventral) primary rami of lumbar nerves one through four (L1-L4) with variable contributions from the 12th thoracic (T12) and 5th lumbar (L5) nerves (Figure 1). The ventral rami of these nerves converge to form the plexus anterior to the transverse processes of the lumbar vertebrae deep within the psoas major muscle or between the psoas major and quadratus lumborum muscles (Figure 2). The cephalad portion of the lumbar plexus (i.e., T12-L1) immediately divides into superior and inferior branches. The superior branch subsequently divides into the iliohypogastric and ilioinguinal nerves, and the inferior branch merges with a small branch from L2 to form the genitofemoral nerve (Figures 1 through 3).

The caudad portion of the lumbar plexus (L2-L4) forms three major nerves of the lower extremity—the lateral femoral cutaneous, femoral, and obturator nerves (Figure 1). These major nerves exit the pelvis anteriorly and provide the primary innervation to the ventral aspect of the lower extremity (Figure 3). The lateral femoral cutaneous nerve arises from the posterior divisions of the ventral rami of L2 and L3. It courses along the posterior abdominal wall until it crosses the iliac crest into the pelvis, where it descends posterior to the fascia iliaca and anterior to the iliacus muscle. The femoral nerve is the largest branch of the lumbar plexus and arises from the posterior division of the ventral rami of L2 to L4. It descends through the pelvis along the lateral border of the psoas major muscle within the groove between the psoas and iliacus muscles. The nerve passes under the inguinal ligament, deep to the fascia iliaca, and enters the femoral triangle where it lies lateral to the femoral artery and vein (Figure 4). The obturator nerve arises from the anterior division of the ventral rami of L2 to L4. It descends toward the pelvis along the posteromedial border of the psoas major muscle and passes under the fascia iliaca to reach the obturator foramen. The nerve accompanies the obturator artery and vein through the obturator canal and into the medial compartment of the thigh, where it branches into an anterior and posterior division (Figure 4).

Surface Anatomy

Important surface landmarks include the iliac crest, the posterior superior iliac spine, and the spinous processes of the lumbar vertebral column (Figure 5). The intercristal line connects one iliac crest to the other. The patient's midline is identified by a line connecting the spinous processes of the lumbar vertebral column. The posterior superior iliac spine, which may be difficult to identify in obese patients, is palpated along the posterior aspect of the ilium approximately 5 cm lateral to midline.

Patient Position

The patient is placed in the lateral decubitus position with the hips and knees flexed. The surgical extremity—or side to be blocked—is placed in the nondependent (i.e., upper) position (Figures 5 and 6).

Technique

Neural Localization Techniques

Initial descriptions of the psoas compartment block used a loss-of-resistance technique to identify the lumbar plexus. However, this technique of neural localization has since been replaced with peripheral nerve stimulation. Although any evoked motor response of the lumbar plexus may be acceptable, the preferred end point is stimulation of the quadriceps muscles. Ultrasound guidance may also be used to identify the lumbar plexus at this location. However, the depth of the lumbar plexus and associated poor imaging have prevented the widespread use of ultrasound with this block technique.

Needle Insertion Site

A vertical line is drawn to connect the iliac crests along the intercristal line. A second line is drawn along the midline connecting the spinous processes of the lumbar vertebrae. Finally, a third line is drawn parallel to the midline that originates at the posterior superior iliac spine

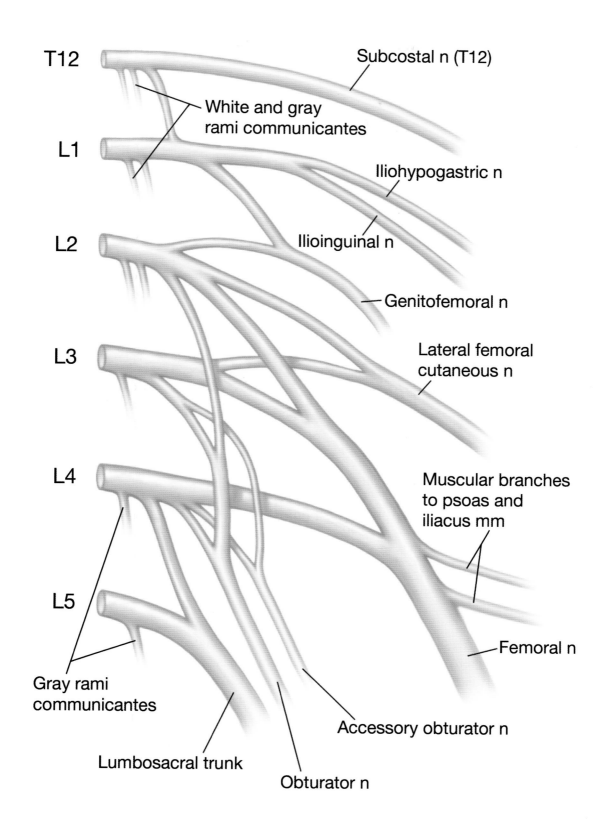

Figure 1. Lumbar plexus anatomy.

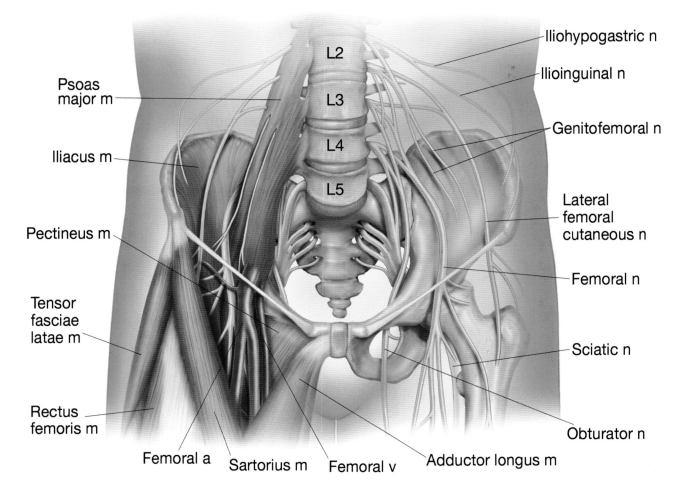

Figure 2. Anatomical location of the lumbar plexus in situ.

(Figure 7). The distance between the parallel lines is divided into thirds. The needle insertion site is 1 cm cephalad from the intercristal line at the junction of the middle and lateral thirds (Figure 7).

A 21-gauge 4-inch (10-cm) insulated needle is inserted perpendicular to the skin and advanced until contact is made with the transverse process of L4. The needle is then withdrawn slightly and redirected caudally to "walk off" the transverse process. Alternatively, the needle may be walked off the transverse process in a cephalad direction (Figure 8). The needle is advanced 1 to 2 cm beyond

the depth of the transverse process until a motor response of the lumbar plexus is elicited. Although the distance from the skin to lumbar plexus varies greatly with sex and body mass index, the distance from the L4 transverse process to the lumbar plexus is consistently 1.5 to 2 cm (Figure 9). If a motor response is not elicited after advancing the needle 1 to 2 cm beyond the depth of the transverse process, the needle should be slightly withdrawn and redirected medially in small incremental steps until a motor response is encountered. After an appropriate motor response (i.e., quadriceps muscle twitch) is elicited at a stimulating current of 0.7 mA or less, local

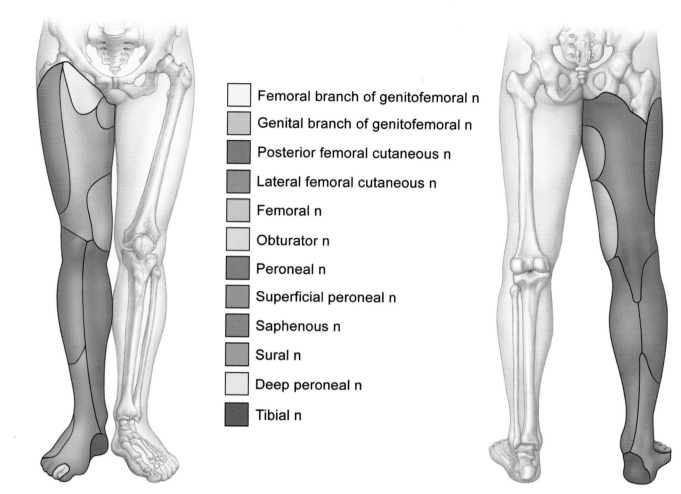

Femoral branch of genitofemoral n

Genital branch of genitofemoral n

Posterior femoral cutaneous n

Lateral femoral cutaneous n

Femoral n

Obturator n

Peroneal n

Superficial peroneal n

Saphenous n

Sural n

Deep peroneal n

Tibial n

Figure 3. Lower extremity cutaneous innervation.

anesthetic is slowly injected in 5-mL increments with intermittent aspiration to a total volume of 20 to 30 mL.

Needle Redirection Cues

If the L4 transverse process is not contacted during the first needle pass, the needle should be redirected slightly caudad until the transverse process is identified or an appropriate motor response is elicited. If the transverse process is not contacted or a desired motor response is not elicited despite caudal redirection, the needle should be redirected slightly cephalad. If the needle has been redirected both caudad and cephalad,

and the transverse process still has not been identified, the needle is redirected slightly medial and the above-described maneuvers are repeated. Extreme medial redirection of the needle should be avoided to minimize the risk of inadvertent dural puncture, neural trauma, or excessive neuraxial spread of local anesthetic.

Finally, if a motor response of the hamstring muscles is obtained, the needle has been inserted too caudally. The needle should be redirected in a more cephalad direction. Excessive needle depth may cause hip flexion due to direct stimulation of the psoas major muscle. In some

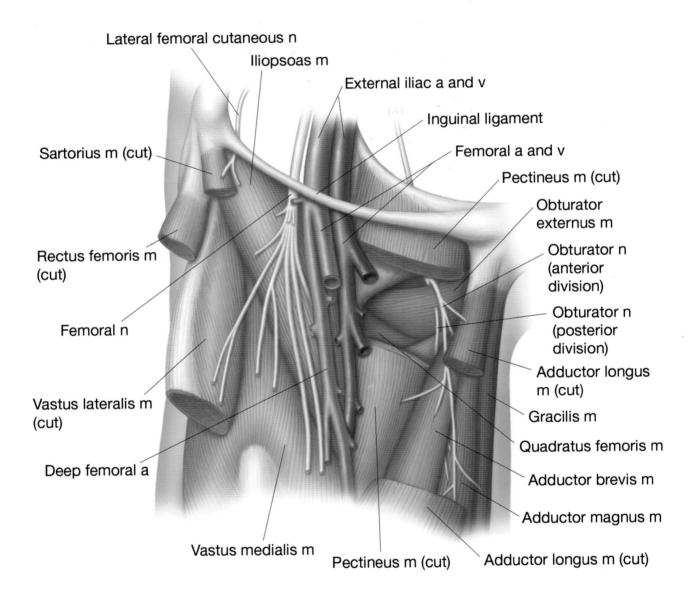

Lateral femoral cutaneous n

Iliopsoas m

External iliac a and v

Inguinal ligament

Sartorius m (cut)

Femoral a and v

Pectineus m (cut)

Obturator externus m

Rectus femoris m (cut)

Obturator n (anterior division)

Femoral n

Obturator n (posterior division)

Adductor longus m (cut)

Vastus lateralis m (cut)

Gracilis m

Quadratus femoris m

Deep femoral a

Adductor brevis m

Adductor magnus m

Vastus medialis m

Pectineus m (cut)

Adductor longus m (cut)

Figure 4. Neurovascular and muscular anatomy of the femoral region.

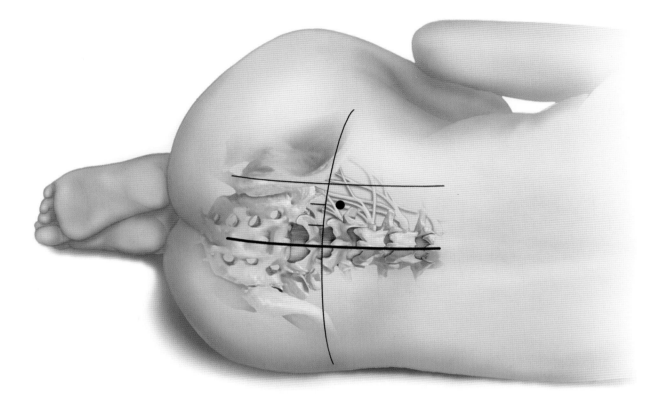

Figure 5. Surface landmarks for posterior lumbar plexus blockade.

patients, the inferior pole of the kidney may extend to the level of L3. Therefore, it is important to avoid extreme cephalad redirection when the needle is inserted at or above the level of L4 to minimize the risk of inadvertent renal trauma.

Continuous Peripheral Nerve Catheters

Continuous posterior lumbar plexus catheters are commonly used as an adjunct to intraoperative anesthesia and for postoperative pain management in patients undergoing lower extremity surgical procedures. The surface landmarks, patient position, neural localization technique, and needle insertion site for continuous catheter placement are the same as described above for single-injection techniques. An 18-gauge 4-inch (10-cm) insulated Tuohy needle is inserted perpendicular to the skin and advanced with the bevel

directed laterally. After an appropriate motor response (i.e., quadriceps muscle twitch) is elicited at a stimulating current of 0.7 mA or less, a 20-gauge multiorifice catheter is advanced 4 to 5 cm beyond the needle tip (Figure 10). Once the needle is removed, the catheter is secured to the patient's back with a sterile transparent adhesive dressing. The catheter should be aspirated for blood or cerebrospinal fluid before the injection of local anesthetic.

Side Effects and Complications

Many of the side effects and complications associated with posterior lumbar plexus blockade are similar to those occurring with other peripheral nerve blocks (e.g., localized discomfort, bruising, infectious complications). However, because of the proximity of the lumbar plexus to the central neuraxis, this block technique possesses

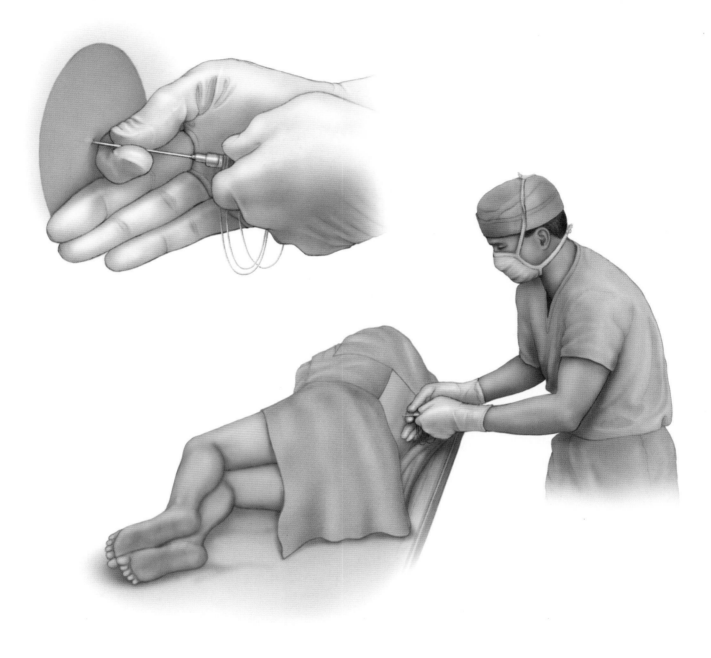

Figure 6. Patient-provider orientation during posterior lumbar plexus blockade.

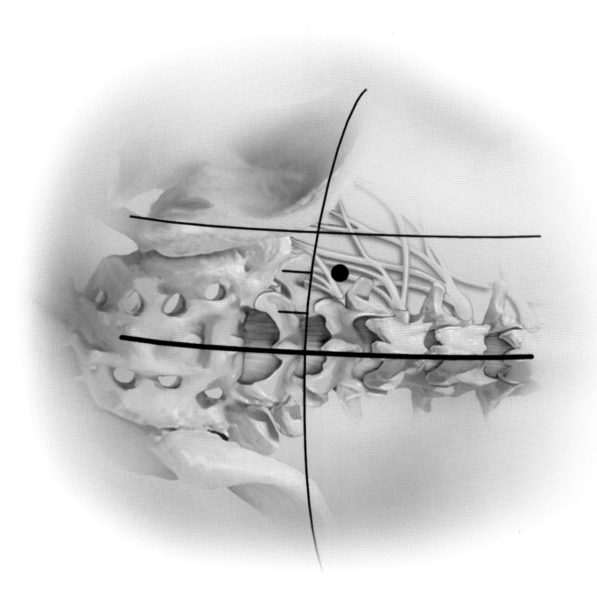

Figure 7. Surface landmarks and needle insertion site for posterior lumbar plexus blockade.

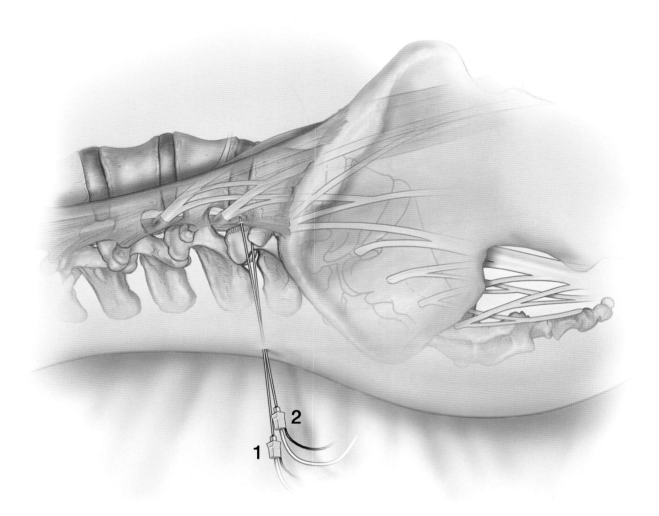

Figure 8. Needle redirection during posterior lumbar plexus blockade.

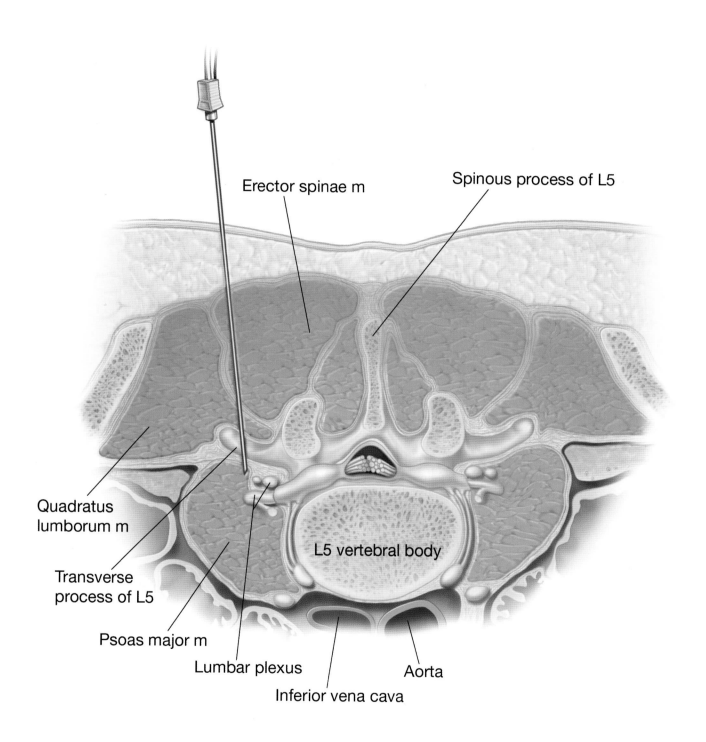

Figure 9. Cross-sectional anatomy of the lumbar region.

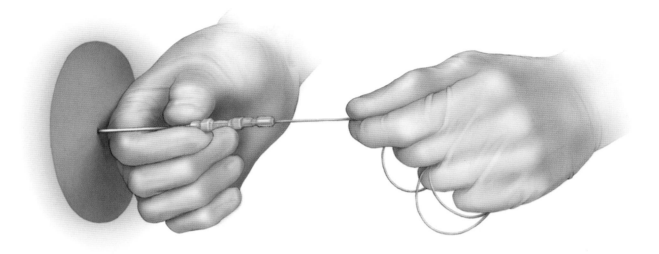

Figure 10. Peripheral nerve catheter insertion during posterior lumbar plexus blockade.

additional risks that warrant consideration. Intrathecal or epidural spread of local anesthetic may occur in 1.8% to 16% of patients. Factors that may contribute to the intrathecal or epidural spread of local anesthetic include a medially directed needle, large volumes of local anesthetic, and the proximity of a dural sleeve or spinal deformity (e.g., scoliosis). It has also been suggested that the incidence of epidural spread may be higher with more cephalad needle insertion sites (e.g., L3 versus L5). Ipsilateral sacral plexus blockade may also occur with extensive local anesthetic spread or a caudal needle insertion site.

The psoas major and quadratus lumborum muscles are richly vascularized anatomical structures. As a result, the injection of large volumes of local anesthetic during posterior lumbar plexus blockade may result in higher serum plasma levels of local anesthetic than with other peripheral nerve blocks. This potential risk requires vigilance and proper monitoring for signs and symptoms of systemic local anesthetic toxicity. Retroperitoneal and renal capsular hematomas have also been reported in patients who have undergone posterior lumbar plexus blockade. However, most of these reports have occurred in the setting of perioperative thromboprophylaxis.

Unlike the known risks of spinal hematoma arising from concomitant anticoagulation and neuraxial anesthesia, the risk of hemorrhagic complications after peripheral nerve blockade is not clearly defined, nor are there guidelines or recommendations available to guide clinical practice. A conservative approach may be to apply the recommendations from the American Society of Regional Anesthesia and Pain Medicine Consensus Conference on Neuraxial Anesthesia and Anticoagulation to *all* regional techniques—including peripheral nerve blocks. However, this may be an overly cautious approach. Rather, it may be prudent to take into consideration the compressibility of the needle insertion site, as well as the vascular structures at risk. From this, it may be recommended that the utilization of peripheral techniques in patients with coagulopathy be based on a careful risk-benefit analysis and that they be performed cautiously. This approach is particularly applicable if the block is to be performed in a region where an expanding hematoma could go unrecognized for several hours or days in a noncompressible site (e.g., posterior lumbar plexus) or compress the airway (e.g., interscalene). Regardless, communication between clinicians and subspecialists involved in the perioperative management of patients receiving anticoagulants is critical to providing optimal patient care and decreasing the risk of serious hemorrhagic complications.

Although uncommon, neural injury to the lumbar plexus has also been reported after continuous posterior lumbar plexus blockade. Nerve injury may be caused by direct mechanical trauma (i.e., from the needle or perineural catheter), local anesthetic toxicity (i.e., prolonged exposure with continuous infusions), or ischemia due to local anesthetic additives. Finally, posterior lumbar plexus blockade typically results in a unilateral sympathectomy. However, adverse sequelae from this—including hypotension—are quite rare.

Suggested Reading

Aida S, Takahashi H, Shimoji K. Renal subcapsular hematoma after lumbar plexus block. Anesthesiology. 1996 Feb;84(2):452-5.

Awad IT, Duggan EM. Posterior lumbar plexus block: anatomy, approaches, and techniques. Reg Anesth Pain Med. 2005 Mar-Apr;30(2):143-9.

Ben-David B, Joshi R, Chelly JE. Sciatic nerve palsy after total hip arthroplasty in a patient receiving continuous lumbar plexus block. Anesth Analg. 2003 Oct;97(4)1180-2.

Capdevila X, Macaire P, Dadure C, Choquet O, Biboulet P, Ryckwaert Y, et al. Continuous psoas compartment block for postoperative analgesia after total hip arthroplasty: new landmarks, technical guidelines, and clinical evaluation. Anesth Analg. 2002 Jun;94(6):1606-13.

Chayen D, Nathan H, Chayen M. The psoas compartment block. Anesthesiology. 1976 Jul;45(1):95-9.

Enneking FK, Chan V, Greger J, Hadzić A, Lang SA, Horlocker TT. Lower-extremity peripheral nerve blockade: essentials of our current understanding. Reg Anesth Pain Med. 2005 Jan-Feb;30(1):4-35.

Farny J, Drolet P, Girard M. Anatomy of the posterior approach to the lumbar plexus block. Can J Anaesth. 1994 Jun;41(6):480-5.

Horlocker TT, Wedel DJ, Benzon H, Brown DL, Enneking FK, Heit JA, et al. Regional anesthesia in the anticoagulated patient: defining the risks (the Second ASRA Consensus Conference on Neuraxial Anesthesia and Anticoagulation). Reg Anesth Pain Med. 2003 May-Jun;28(3):172-97.

Kirchmair L, Lirk P, Colvin J, Mitterschiffthaler G, Moriggl B. Lumbar plexus and psoas major muscle: not always as expected. Reg Anesth Pain Med. 2008 Mar-Apr;33(2):109-14.

Klein SM, D'Ercole F, Greengrass RA, Warner DS. Enoxaparin associated with psoas hematoma and lumbar plexopathy after lumbar plexus block. Anesthesiology. 1997 Dec;87(6):1576-9.

Parkinson SK, Mueller JB, Little WL, Bailey SL. Extent of blockade with various approaches to the lumbar plexus. Anesth Analg. 1989 Mar;68(3):243-8.

Pousman RM, Mansoor Z, Sciard D. Total spinal anesthetic after continuous posterior lumbar plexus block. Anesthesiology. 2003 May;98(5):1281-2.

Vaghadia H, Kapnoudhis P, Jenkins LC, Taylor D. Continuous lumbosacral block using a Tuohy needle and catheter technique. Can J Anaesth. 1992 Jan;39(1):75-8.

Weller RS, Gerancher JC, Crews JC, Wade KL. Extensive retroperitoneal hematoma without neurologic deficit in two patients who underwent lumbar plexus block and were later anticoagulated. Anesthesiology. 2003 Feb;98(2):581-5.

Winnie AP, Durrani Z, Radonjic R. Plexus blocks, for lower extremity surgery: new answers to old problems. Anaesthesiol Rev. 1974;1:11-6.

CHAPTER

23

Femoral Nerve Blockade

Kimberly P. Wynd, M.B., B.Ch.

Hugh M. Smith, M.D., Ph.D.

Clinical Applications

Femoral nerve blockade is one of the most common lower extremity regional anesthetic techniques performed by anesthesiologists. Blockade of the femoral nerve provides surgical anesthesia and postoperative analgesia to the anterior aspect of the thigh and knee. The technique is commonly used for soft tissue surgery of the thigh (e.g., muscle biopsy), knee arthroscopy, and anterior cruciate ligament repair. During more extensive lower extremity surgical procedures (e.g., total knee arthroplasty), femoral nerve blockade may be used in combination with sciatic, lateral femoral cutaneous, or obturator nerve blockade to achieve more dense and comprehensive analgesia. Although single injection techniques are common, continuous femoral nerve blockade has achieved widespread acceptance due to the simplicity of anatomical landmarks, ease of patient positioning during block placement (i.e., supine position), high success rates, and low incidence of complications.

Relevant Anatomy

The femoral nerve is the largest branch of the lumbar plexus and arises from the ventral rami of the second (L2) through fourth (L4) lumbar nerve roots (Figure 1), with variable contribution from the fifth lumbar (L5) nerve. The nerve emerges from the lateral border of the psoas muscle before descending in the groove between the psoas major and iliacus muscles. The nerve passes beneath the inguinal ligament and enters the proximal aspect of the thigh lateral to the femoral artery and deep to the fascia lata and fascia iliaca (Figure 2).

After passing below the inguinal ligament, the femoral nerve divides into several major and minor muscular and cutaneous branches that innervate the anterior compartment of the leg. The two major branches of the femoral nerve are the anterior (i.e., superficial) and posterior (i.e., deep) divisions. The anterior division provides motor innervation to the sartorius and pectineus muscles and cutaneous sensation to the anterior and medial aspects of the thigh (Figure 3). The posterior division provides motor innervation to the rectus femoris, vastus lateralis, vastus medialis, and vastus intermedius muscles (i.e., quadriceps muscles) and cutaneous innervation to the anterior, anteromedial, and anterolateral aspects of the knee. In addition, the posterior division of the femoral nerve provides sensory innervation to the articular surfaces of the knee joint, the patella, the anterolateral portion of the femur, and the anteromedial aspect of the tibial plateau.

Surface Anatomy

Important surface landmarks for femoral nerve blockade include the inguinal skin crease, the inguinal ligament, and the pulse of the femoral artery. The inguinal ligament is identified by drawing a line from the anterior superior iliac spine to the pubic tubercle. The pulse of the femoral artery is marked at the level of the inguinal skin crease (Figure 4).

Patient Position

The patient should be in a supine position with the surgical extremity neutral or slightly abducted. Internal or external rotation of the lower extremity should be avoided because it may alter the anatomical relationship of the neurovascular structures. The proceduralist generally stands on the side of the patient to be blocked (Figure 5). However, some providers elect to always stand on either the right (i.e., right-hand–dominant providers) or the left (i.e., left-hand–dominant providers) side of the patient—regardless of the side to be blocked—because of improved hand and body positioning.

Technique

Neural Localization Techniques

Peripheral nerve stimulation is one of the most common techniques used to identify the femoral nerve. Several motor responses may be elicited during femoral nerve blockade (Table 1). However, the ideal neuromotor response is contraction of the quadriceps muscles and patellar elevation. Elicitation of a quadriceps motor response indicates stimulation of the posterior division of the femoral nerve—an important indicator because articular branches to the knee joint are also derived from the posterior division. It is important to distinguish a quadriceps motor response from a sartorial muscle contraction, because a sartorial muscle contraction may indicate either direct muscle stimulation or stimulation of the anterior division of the femoral nerve. Incorrect identification of a quadriceps motor response may result in inadequate blockade. In addition to peripheral nerve stimulation, ultrasound guidance is also commonly used to identify the femoral nerve.

Needle Insertion Site

A line overlying the inguinal ligament is drawn by connecting the anterior superior iliac spine and the pubic tubercle. The femoral artery is palpated and marked along its course from the inguinal ligament to the inguinal skin crease. The site for needle insertion is commonly described as 1 cm lateral and 1 cm caudad to the intersection of the femoral artery with *either* the inguinal

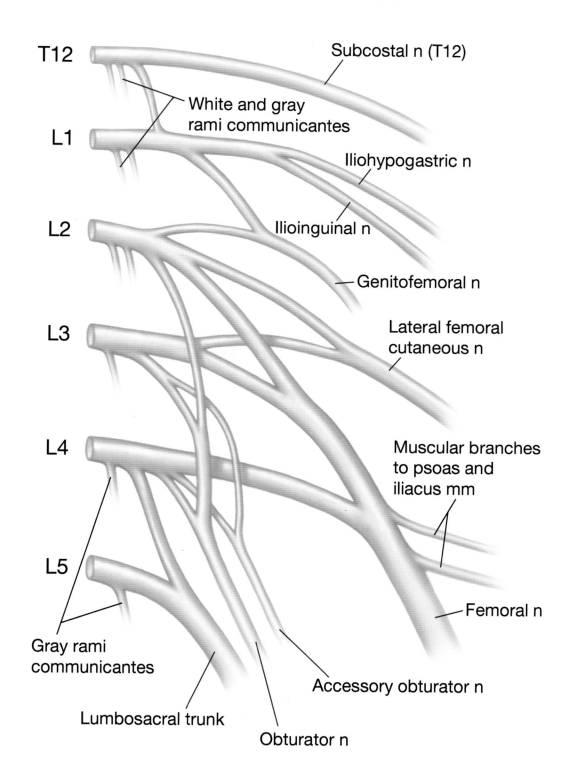

Figure 1. Lumbar plexus anatomy.

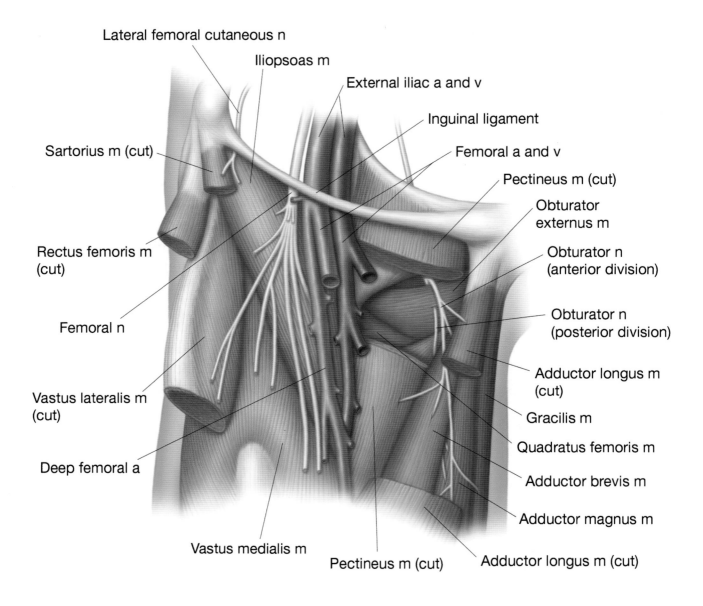

Figure 2. Neurovascular and muscular anatomy of the femoral region.

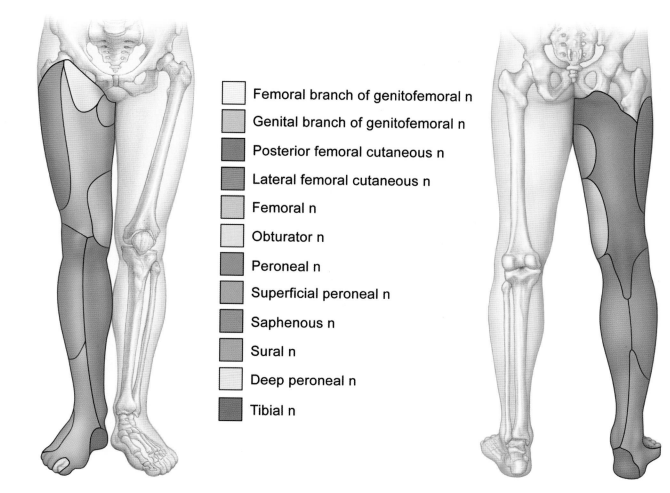

Figure 3. Lower extremity cutaneous innervation.

ligament or the inguinal skin crease (Figure 4). However, anatomical studies suggest that the femoral nerve may have a greater width and a more predictable location relative to the femoral artery at the level of the inguinal skin crease (Figure 6).

For a single injection technique, a 22-gauge 2-inch (5-cm) insulated needle is inserted at an angle 40° to 60° from the skin and advanced in a cephalad direction parallel to the femoral artery. The posterior division of the femoral nerve is generally encountered at a depth of 2 to 4 cm. However, the depth of neural structures may be highly dependent

on body habitus. Two distinct fascial "pops" are often felt as the needle passes through the fascia lata and fascia iliaca, respectively. After the desired motor response is elicited at a current of 0.5 mA or less, local anesthetic is slowly injected in 5-mL increments with intermittent aspiration to a total volume of 20 to 30 mL.

Needle Redirection Cues

The anterior division of the femoral nerve is often the first neural structure encountered during femoral nerve blockade—resulting in a sartorius motor response along the medial aspect of the thigh. Because the articular

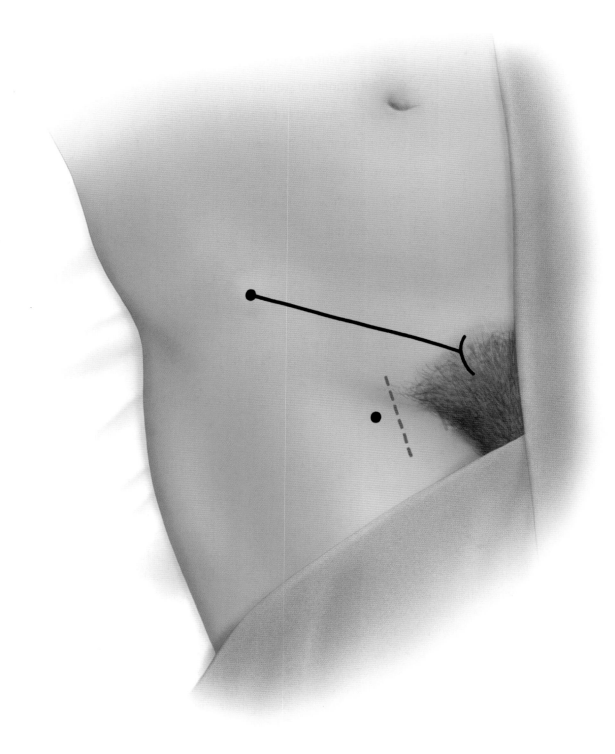

Figure 4. Surface landmarks for femoral nerve blockade.

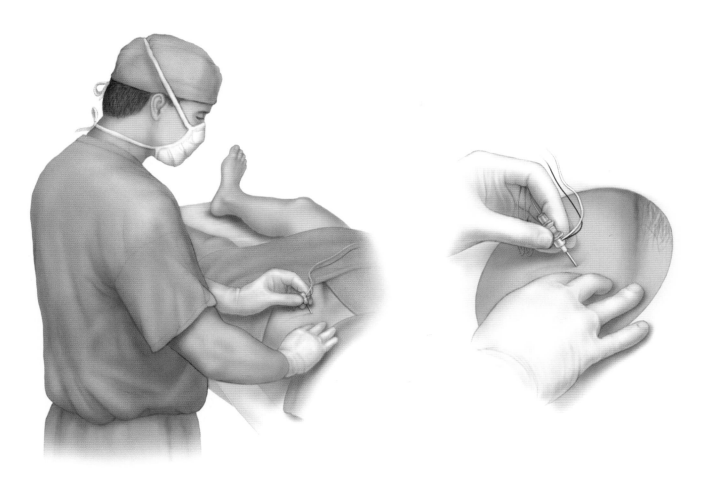

Figure 5. Patient-provider orientation during femoral nerve blockade.

branches to the knee are derived from the posterior division of the femoral nerve, a sartorius motor response (i.e., anterior division) is considered suboptimal for effective femoral nerve blockade. Therefore, if a sartorius motor response is elicited, the stimulating needle should be slowly advanced to a more posterior (i.e., deeper) location. If the desired motor response is not obtained (i.e., a quadriceps muscle contraction with associated patellar elevation), the needle should be redirected laterally in small incremental maneuvers. If a quadriceps twitch is still not identified, the needle should be redirected slightly medially in small increments. Providers need to be cautious not to puncture the femoral artery during medial redirection of the needle.

Ultrasound-Guided Femoral Nerve Blockade

Scanning Technique
The ultrasound probe is placed within the femoral region perpendicular to the long axis of the thigh (Figures 7 and 8). This orientation provides the best cross-sectional view of the femoral artery and relevant neurovascular anatomy. Ultrasound probes with mid- to high-range frequency (8-12 MHz) are most appropriate for imaging in this anatomical location.

Sonoanatomy
The ideal ultrasound image captures the femoral nerve in cross-section lateral to the femoral artery and deep to the

Table 1.   Elicited Motor Responses During Femoral Nerve Blockade

Elicited motor response	Clinical and anatomical correlation	Corrective maneuver
Quadriceps muscle contraction with patellar elevation that disappears with local anesthetic injection	Stimulating needle or catheter is in proximity to the posterior division of the femoral nerve—deep to the fascia iliaca	None—proper needle or catheter placement
Quadriceps muscle contraction with patellar elevation that persists with local anesthetic injection	Stimulating needle or catheter is in proximity to the posterior division of the femoral nerve—superficial to the fascia iliaca or within a vessel	Slightly advance the needle and repeat stimulation
Sartorius muscle contraction without associated patellar elevation	Stimulating needle or catheter is in proximity to the anterior division of the femoral nerve—superficial to the posterior division	Advance the needle more posterior (ie, deeper) and repeat stimulation. If no response, redirect the needle postero-laterally
Localized muscle contraction within the femoral region	Stimulating needle or catheter is directly stimulating the iliopsoas or pectineus muscle—posterior or cephalad to the femoral nerve	Withdraw the needle to the subcutaneous tissue and redirect the needle more caudad

fascia iliaca (Figure 9). The femoral artery is easily identified as a round, noncompressible, pulsatile, hypoechoic structure medial to the femoral nerve. In contrast, the compressible femoral vein is located medial to the femoral artery. Doppler may be used to confirm the vascular identity of both the artery and the vein. In general, the femoral nerve is identified 2 to 4 cm beneath the surface of the skin. However, this is highly dependent on the patient's body habitus. The sonographic appearance of the femoral nerve varies depending on the location of imaging. For example, at the level of the inguinal ligament, the nerve generally appears as a triangular or wedge-shaped hyperechoic structure (Figure 9), with central "honeycombing" that reflects the fascicular components of the peripheral nerve (Figure 10). However, at the level of the inguinal skin crease, the femoral nerve may appear more circular as the anterior and posterior divisions begin to form (Figure 11).

Ultrasound Approach

Ultrasound-guided femoral nerve blockade can be performed using either an in-plane or an out-of-plane needle approach. During an out-of-plane approach, the probe is positioned so that the femoral nerve is located near the center of the ultrasound image (Figure 12). A 22-gauge 2-inch (5-cm) stimulating needle is inserted 1 to 2 cm from the caudal edge of the transducer at an angle 45° to 60° from the skin (Figure 8). The needle is advanced to a position immediately lateral or medial to the femoral nerve. Fine needle movements, tissue displacement, and hydrodissection are useful indicators of needle position and direction. Peripheral nerve stimulation can be used to confirm neural localization—particularly if multiple neural structures are visible (Figure 11). After negative aspiration is confirmed, local anesthetic is slowly injected in 5-mL increments with intermittent aspiration to a total volume of 20 to 30 mL.

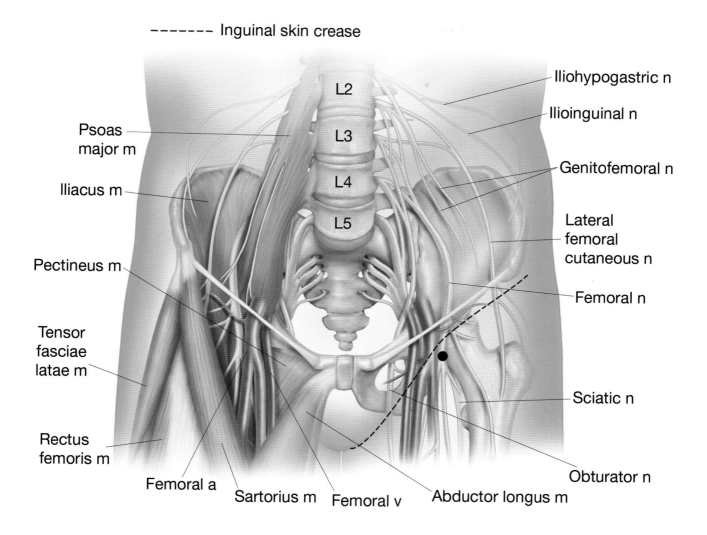

-------- Inguinal skin crease

Iliohypogastric n

Ilioinguinal n

Genitofemoral n

Lateral femoral cutaneous n

Femoral n

Sciatic n

Obturator n

L2

L3

L4

L5

Psoas major m

Iliacus m

Pectineus m

Tensor fasciae latae m

Rectus femoris m

Femoral a   Sartorius m   Femoral v   Abductor longus m

Figure 6. Anatomical landmarks and needle insertion site for femoral nerve blockade.

During an in-plane needle approach, the probe is positioned so that the femoral nerve is located on the medial third of the ultrasound image to enable continuous visualization of the entire needle. A 21-gauge 4-inch (10-cm) stimulating needle is inserted 1 to 2 cm from the lateral edge of the transducer at an angle 30° to 45° from the skin. Under direct visualization, the needle is slowly advanced in a medial direction to a location immediately posterior to the femoral nerve. Peripheral nerve stimulation can be used to confirm neural localization—particularly if multiple neural structures are visible. After negative aspiration is confirmed, local anesthetic is slowly injected in 5-mL increments with intermittent aspiration to a total volume of 20 to 30 mL.

Continuous Peripheral Nerve Catheters
Continuous peripheral nerve catheters are commonly used as an adjunct to intraoperative anesthesia and for extended postoperative pain management.

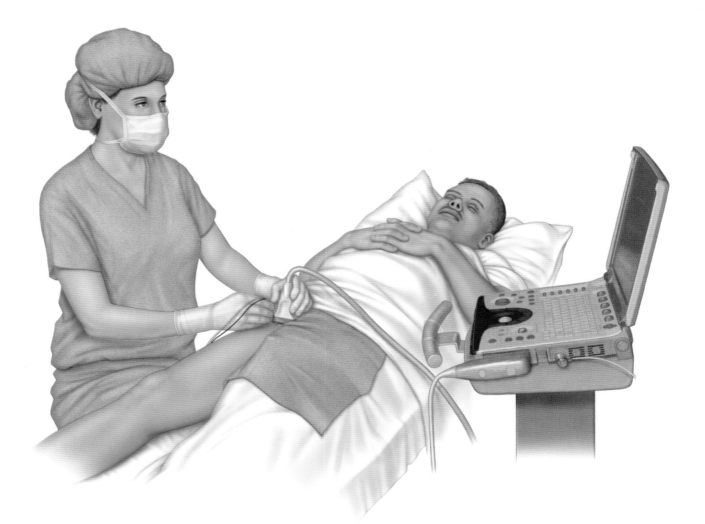

Figure 7. Patient-provider orientation during ultrasound-guided femoral nerve blockade.

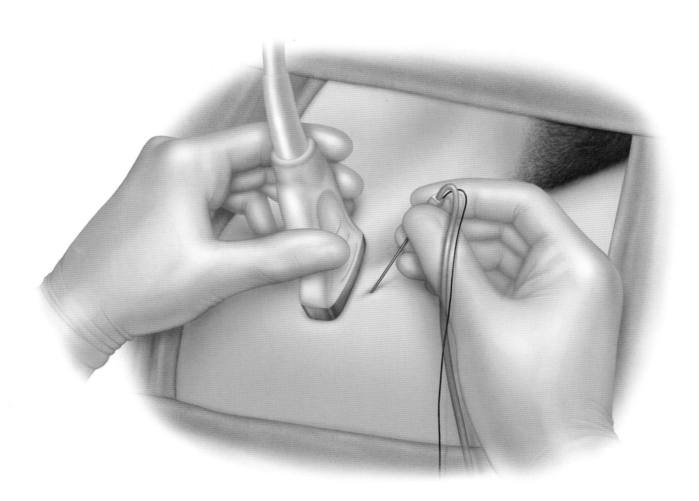

Figure 8. Probe and needle orientation during ultrasound-guided femoral nerve blockade.

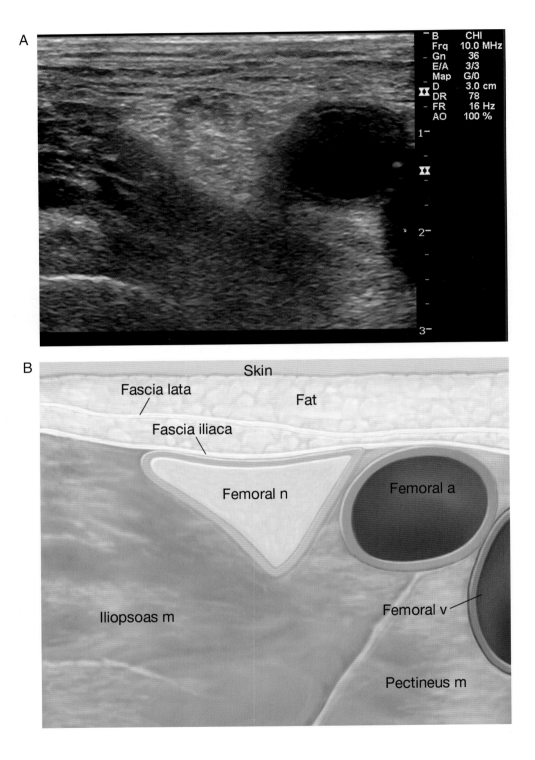

Figure 9. Femoral neurovascular anatomy in the proximal thigh. A, Ultrasound image. B, Corresponding anatomical illustration.

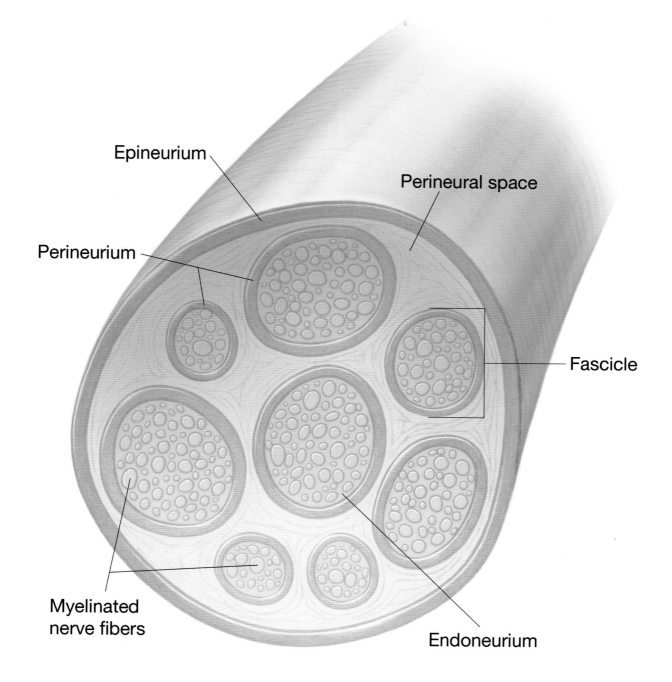

Figure 10. Peripheral nerve anatomy.

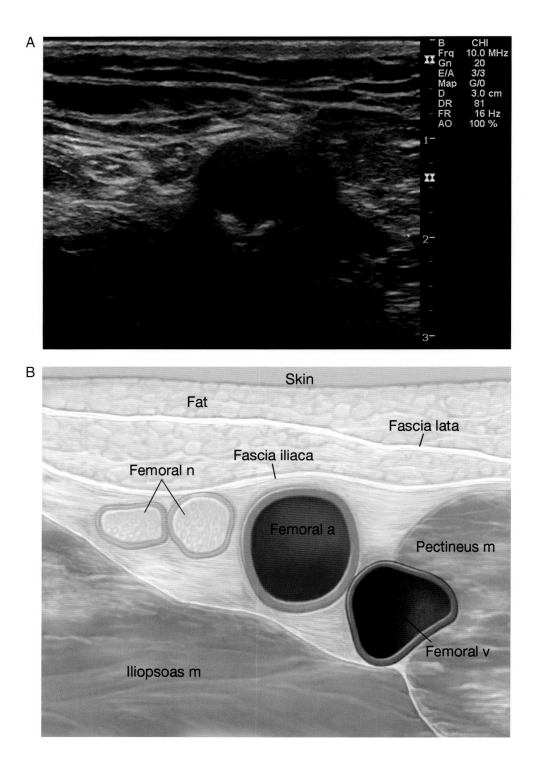

Figure 11. Femoral neurovascular anatomy in the proximal aspect of the thigh, showing anatomical variation. A, Ultrasound image. B, Corresponding anatomical illustration.

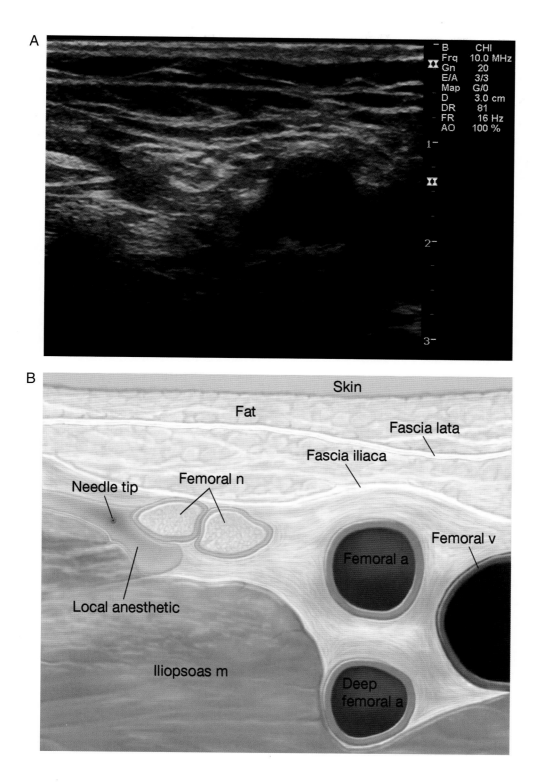

Figure 12. Ultrasound-guided femoral nerve blockade (out-of-plane approach). A, Ultrasound image. B, Corresponding anatomical illustration.

Both stimulating and nonstimulating femoral catheters have been used with success for patients undergoing inpatient and ambulatory lower extremity surgical procedures. Femoral nerve catheters have been shown to provide superior analgesia and improve postoperative rehabilitation after total knee arthroplasty compared with traditional intravenous opioids. Continuous perineural catheters also have several advantages over neuraxial techniques (e.g., epidural analgesia), including improved mobilization (i.e., unilateral blockade) and the avoidance of postdural puncture headache. In addition, concerns associated with the administration of low-molecular-weight heparin and thromboprophylaxis are generally avoided with the use of most peripheral nerve catheters. Although ultrasound technology can be used to accurately guide femoral nerve catheter placement, the evidence is currently insufficient to suggest that this technique is superior to more conventional methods of nerve stimulation.

Neural localization using peripheral nerve stimulation, including the site of needle insertion and needle redirection, is similar for both continuous and single-injection techniques. During femoral nerve catheter placement, an 18-gauge 2-inch (5-cm) insulated Tuohy needle is inserted and advanced until a quadriceps motor response with patellar elevation is elicited at a current of 0.5 mA or less. A 20-gauge catheter is then advanced 4 to 6 cm beyond the tip of the needle and secured with a sterile transparent dressing. Alternatively, the catheter may be tunneled subcutaneously to a location remote from the initial insertion site and covered with a protective dressing. The subcutaneous tunneling of catheters may decrease the risk of infectious complications or catheter dislodgement.

Ultrasound-guided femoral nerve catheter placement is similar to that described for out-of-plane single-injection ultrasound techniques. Under direct visualization, an 18-gauge 2-inch (5-cm) insulated Tuohy needle is inserted and advanced toward the femoral nerve with the bevel directed cephalad. Location of the needle tip can be confirmed by injecting either saline or a dextrose-containing solution. After optimal needle placement (i.e., immediately adjacent to the femoral nerve and deep to the fascia iliaca), a 20-gauge catheter is advanced 4 to 6 cm beyond the tip of the needle. The distribution of local anesthetic spread is confirmed using real-time ultrasound imaging. If circumferential spread of local anesthetic does not occur, catheter manipulation may be required with direct visualization. Once the catheter location has been optimized, the catheter is secured with a sterile transparent dressing.

Side Effects and Complications

Complications associated with femoral nerve blockade are extremely uncommon. Although localized bruising and tenderness may occur, true hematoma formation occurs much less often. Serious complications such as systemic local anesthetic toxicity or seizure-related events rarely occur when appropriate vigilance and cautious injection techniques are used during the block. Severe sensorimotor dysfunction and neurologic injury have been reported within the literature, but they are exceedingly rare. Inadvertent vascular puncture may also occur—particularly when using "blind" techniques. The performance of femoral nerve blockade in patients with a femoral artery graft should be carefully considered because mechanical puncture and infection of the prosthetic graft may be associated with significant comorbidities.

Suggested Reading

Allen HW, Liu SS, Ware PD, Nairn CS, Owens BD. Peripheral nerve blocks improve analgesia after total knee replacement surgery. Anesth Analg. 1998 Jul;87(1):93-7.

Berry FR. Analgesia in patients with fractured shaft of femur. Anaesthesia. 1977 Jun;32(6):576-7.

Capdevila X, Barthelet Y, Biboulet P, Ryckwaert Y, Rubenovitch J, D'Athis F. Effects of perioperative analgesic technique on the surgical outcome and duration of rehabilitation after major knee surgery. Anesthesiology. 1999 Jul;91(1):8-15.

Capdevila X, Coimbra C, Choquet O. Approaches to the lumbar plexus: success, risks, and outcome. Reg Anesth Pain Med. 2005 Mar-Apr;30(2):150-62.

Chelly JE, Greger J, Gebhard R, Coupe K, Clyburn TA, Buckle R, et al. Continuous femoral blocks improve recovery and outcome of patients undergoing total knee arthroplasty. J Arthroplasty. 2001 Jun;16(4):436-45.

Enneking FK, Chan V, Greger J, Hadzić A, Lang SA, Horlocker TT. Lower-extremity peripheral nerve blockade: essentials of our current understanding. Reg Anesth Pain Med. 2005 Jan-Feb;30(1):4-35.

Gjessing J, Harley N. Sciatic and femoral nerve block with mepivacaine for surgery on the lower limb. Anaesthesia. 1969 Apr;24(2):213-8.

Kaloul I, Guay J, Côté C, Fallaha M. The posterior lumbar plexus (psoas compartment) block and the three-in-one femoral nerve block provide similar postoperative analgesia after total knee replacement. Can J Anaesth. 2004 Jan;51(1):45-51. Erratum in: Can J Anaesth. 2005 Jan;52(1):119.

Marhofer P, Schrögendorfer K, Koinig H, Kapral S, Weinstabl C, Mayer N. Ultrasonographic guidance improves sensory block and onset time of three-in-one blocks. Anesth Analg. 1997 Oct;85(4):854-7.

Marhofer P, Schrögendorfer K, Wallner T, Koinig H, Mayer N, Kapral S. Ultrasonographic guidance reduces the amount of local anesthetic for 3-in-1 blocks. Reg Anesth Pain Med. 1998 Nov-Dec;23(6):584-8.

Oberndorfer U, Marhofer P, Bösenberg A, Willschke H, Felfernig M, Weintraud M, et al. Ultrasonographic guidance for sciatic and femoral nerve blocks in children. Br J Anaesth. 2007 Jun;98(6):797-801.

Patel NJ, Flashburg MH, Paskin S, Grossman R. A regional anesthetic technique compared to general anesthesia for outpatient knee arthroscopy. Anesth Analg. 1986 Feb;65(2):185-7.

Singelyn FJ, Deyaert M, Joris D, Pendeville E, Gouverneur JM. Effects of intravenous patient-controlled analgesia with morphine, continuous epidural analgesia, and continuous three-in-one block on postoperative pain and knee rehabilitation after unilateral total knee arthroplasty. Anesth Analg. 1998 Jul;87(1):88-92.

Vendittoli PA, Makinen P, Drolet P, Lavigne M, Fallaha M, Guertin MC, et al. A multimodal analgesia protocol for total knee arthroplasty: a randomized, controlled study. J Bone Joint Surg Am. 2006 Feb;88(2):282-9.

Vloka JD, Hadzić A, Drobnik L, Ernest A, Reiss W, Thys DM. Anatomical landmarks for femoral nerve block: a comparison of four needle insertion sites. Anesth Analg. 1999 Dec;89(6):1467-70.

CHAPTER
24

Fascia Iliaca Blockade

Thomas J. Jurrens, M.D.

James R. Hebl, M.D.

Clinical Applications

The fascia iliaca compartment block was first described by Dalens and colleagues in 1989. It was reported to be a safe and effective technique for anesthetizing the femoral, lateral femoral cutaneous, and obturator nerves in children undergoing lower extremity surgical procedures. At the time the fascia iliaca block was introduced into clinical practice, many clinicians, including Dalens, specifically compared the technique to Winnie's classic 3-in-1 approach. Although both techniques provided effective femoral nerve blockade, Dalens reported that the fascia iliaca approach provided lateral femoral cutaneous and obturator nerve blockade more consistently than the classic 3-in-1 technique. However, subsequent evidence has suggested that the fascia iliaca approach may also have its limitations—blocking the obturator nerve only one-third of the time. Currently, fascia iliaca blockade is used to provide postoperative analgesia in children and adults undergoing proximal lower extremity procedures. Common indications include postoperative analgesia for total hip arthroplasty, femoral neck and shaft fractures, soft tissue surgery of the anterior and lateral thigh, and total knee arthroplasty.

Relevant Anatomy

The iliac fascia (*fascia iliaca*) is formed from the aponeurosis of the psoas major, iliacus, and pectineus muscles. The fascial complex creates a potential triangular space within the proximal thigh called the fascia iliaca compartment. The anterior border (i.e., "roof") of the compartment is the iliac fascia, which attaches laterally to the iliac crest and medially with the pectineal fascia. The fascia iliaca also converges with the fascia covering the sartorius, psoas, and quadratus lumborum muscles. The remaining borders of the fascia iliaca compartment include the iliacus muscle posteriorly, the vertebral column and upper segment of the sacrum medially, and the inner border of the iliac crest laterally.

The caudad portion of the lumbar plexus (second lumbar nerve through the fourth lumbar nerve, L2-L4) forms three major nerves of the lower extremity—the lateral femoral cutaneous, femoral, and obturator nerves (Figure 1). These major nerves exit the pelvis anteriorly and are contained within the fascia iliaca compartment. The lateral femoral cutaneous nerve arises from the posterior divisions of the ventral rami of L2 and L3. It courses along the posterior abdominal wall until it crosses the iliac crest into the pelvis where it descends posterior to the fascia iliaca and anterior to the iliacus muscle. The nerve passes under the lateral segment of the inguinal ligament—medial to the anterior superior iliac spine—before dividing into two major sensory branches (Figure 2). The lateral femoral cutaneous nerve provides cutaneous innervation to the proximal two-thirds of the lateral aspect of the thigh and variable cutaneous innervation to the lateral aspect of the buttock distal to the greater trochanter (Figure 3).

The femoral nerve is the largest branch of the lumbar plexus and arises from the posterior division of the ventral rami of L2 to L4 (Figure 1). It descends through the pelvis along the lateral border of the psoas major muscle within the groove between the psoas and iliacus muscles. The nerve passes under the inguinal ligament—deep to the fascia iliaca—and enters the femoral triangle where it lies lateral to the femoral artery and vein (Figure 2). In contrast to the femoral nerve, the femoral artery and vein are commonly located *anterior* to the fascia iliaca within their own fascial compartment (Figure 4). Within the femoral triangle, the femoral nerve divides into anterior and posterior divisions, which provide motor innervation to the thigh extensor muscles and cutaneous innervation to the anterior thigh, femur, patella, and knee joint (Figure 3).

The obturator nerve arises from the anterior division of the ventral rami of L2 to L4 (Figure 1). It descends toward the pelvis along the posteromedial border of the psoas major muscle and passes under the fascia iliaca to reach the obturator foramen. The nerve accompanies the obturator artery and vein through the obturator canal and into the medial compartment of the thigh where it branches into anterior and posterior divisions (Figure 2). The anterior and posterior divisions of the obturator nerve provide motor innervation to the thigh adductor muscles and cutaneous innervation to the distal aspect of the medial thigh (Figure 3). However, cutaneous innervation of the obturator nerve has been shown to be extremely variable from one individual to another.

Surface Anatomy

Important surface structures to identify when performing the fascia iliaca compartment block include the anterior superior iliac spine, the pubic tubercle, and the femoral artery. A line drawn between the anterior superior iliac spine and the pubic tubercle demarcates the inguinal ligament. The pulse of the femoral artery should be identified at the midpoint and immediately caudad to the inguinal ligament.

Patient Position

The patient is positioned supine with the surgical extremity extended and slightly abducted. The proceduralist generally stands on the side of the patient to be blocked (Figure 5).

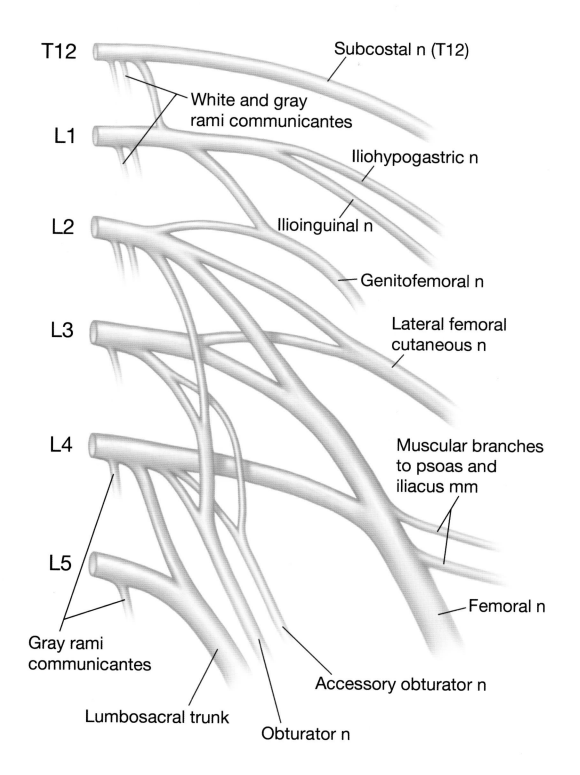

Figure 1. Lumbar plexus anatomy.

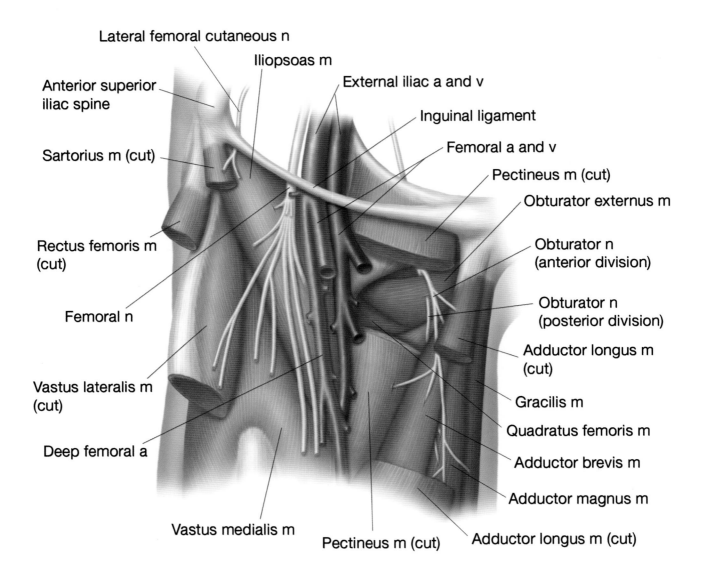

Figure 2. Neurovascular and muscular anatomy of the femoral region.

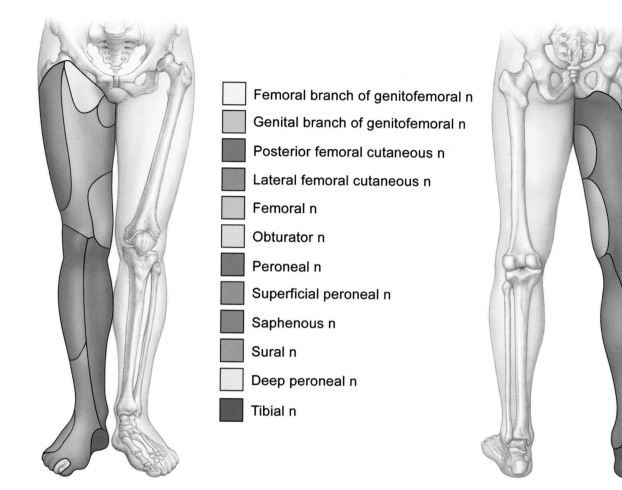

Femoral branch of genitofemoral n

Genital branch of genitofemoral n

Posterior femoral cutaneous n

Lateral femoral cutaneous n

Femoral n

Obturator n

Peroneal n

Superficial peroneal n

Saphenous n

Sural n

Deep peroneal n

Tibial n

Figure 3. Lower extremity cutaneous innervation.

Technique

Neural Localization Techniques

The location of the fascia iliaca compartment is identified using a loss-of-resistance technique. During needle advancement, two separate fascial "pops" occur, representing the fascia lata and fascia iliaca, respectively (Figure 4). Once the needle tip is determined to be within the fascia iliaca compartment, a relatively large volume of dilute local anesthetic is injected. The local anesthetic diffuses throughout the fascial compartment, anesthetizing the lateral femoral cutaneous, femoral, and obturator nerves.

Ultrasound guidance can also be used to directly visualize the needle entering the fascia iliaca compartment posterior (i.e., deep) to the iliac fascia.

Needle Insertion Site

A line is drawn from the anterior superior iliac spine to the ipsilateral pubic tubercle to demarcate the inguinal ligament. The line is divided into thirds and a point identified 1 cm caudal to the junction between the middle and lateral thirds (Figures 6 and 7). At this site, an 18-gauge Tuohy needle (22-gauge Tuohy needle for children under 25 kg) is inserted with the bevel facing cephalad

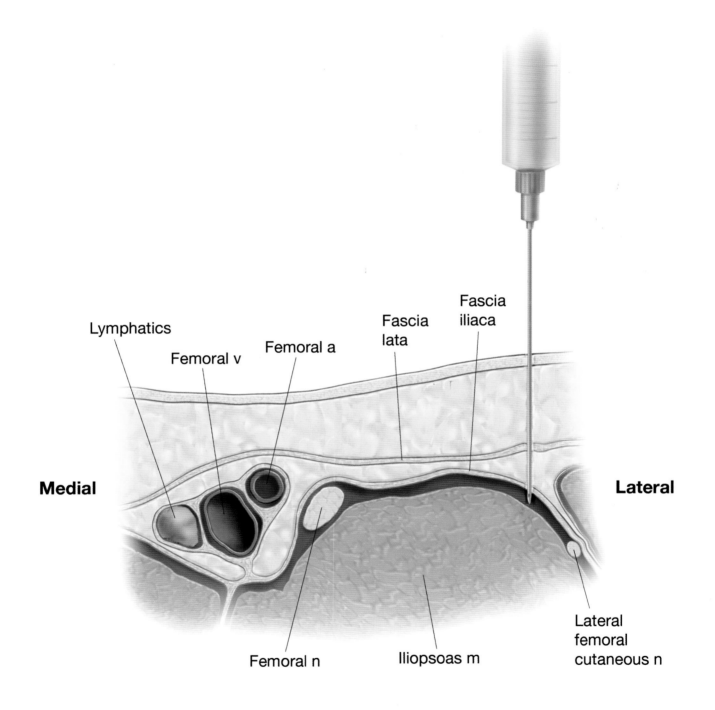

Figure 4. Cross-sectional anatomy of the fascia iliaca compartment.

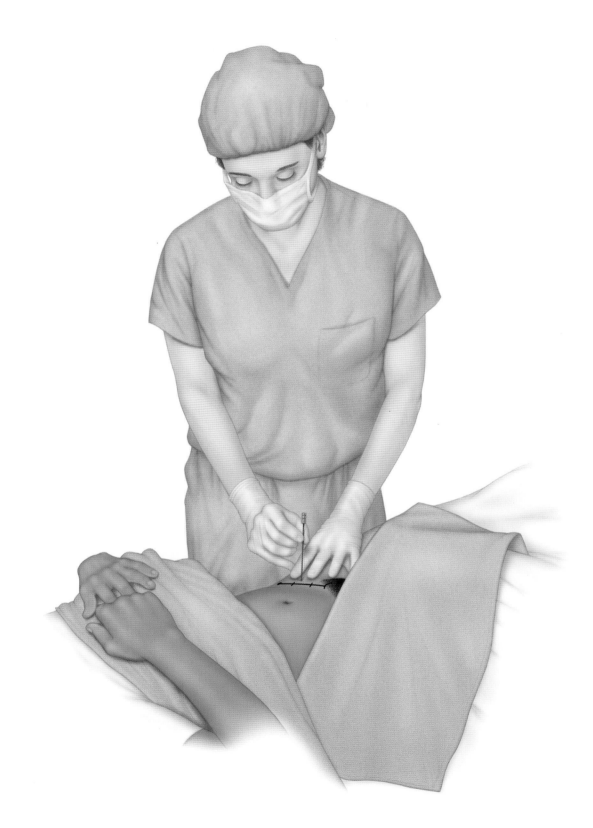

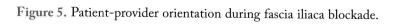

Figure 5. Patient-provider orientation during fascia iliaca blockade.

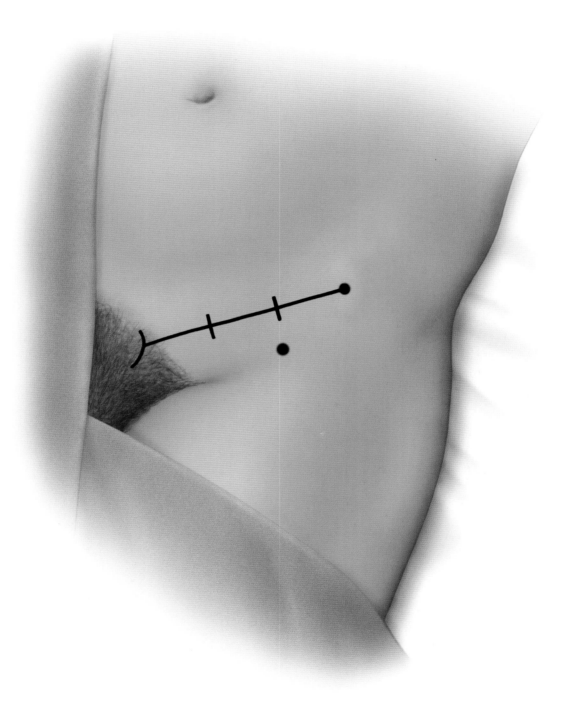

Figure 6. Surface landmarks for fascia iliaca blockade.

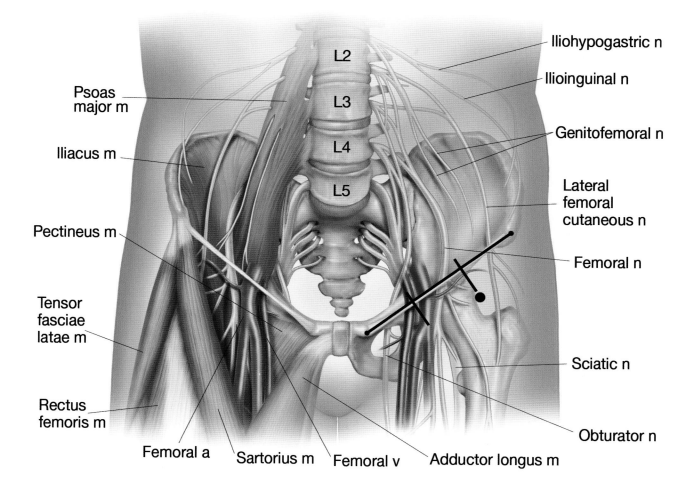

Psoas
major m

Iliacus m

Pectineus m

Tensor
fasciae
latae m

Rectus
femoris m

L2

L3

L4

L5

Femoral a

Sartorius m

Femoral v

Adductor longus m

Iliohypogastric n

Ilioinguinal n

Genitofemoral n

Lateral
femoral
cutaneous n

Femoral n

Sciatic n

Obturator n

Figure 7. Anatomical landmarks and needle insertion site for fascia iliaca blockade.

and advanced perpendicular to the skin (Figure 8). During slow needle advancement, an initial loss-of-resistance (i.e., "pop") is encountered as the needle passes through the fascia lata. As the needle is advanced further, a second loss of resistance is felt as the needle passes through the fascia iliaca and into the fascia iliaca compartment (Figure 4). At this point, 20 to 40 mL of local anesthetic is slowly injected in 5-mL increments with intermittent aspiration to minimize the risk of unrecognized intravascular injection. In general, large volumes of local anesthetic are required during fascia iliaca blockade to

provide adequate diffusion—and effective blockade—of local anesthetic throughout the fascial compartment. External compression caudad to the needle insertion site may also prevent the distal spread of local anesthetic away from the terminal branches of the lumbar plexus and improve block success.

Needle Redirection Cues

The most common miscue during fascia iliaca blockade is the absence of two distinct fascial "pops." Under these circumstances, the needle insertion site may be

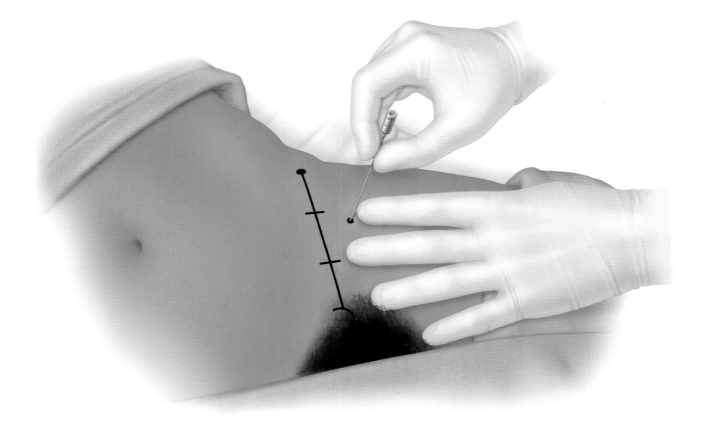

Figure 8. Needle insertion site for fascia iliaca blockade.

too medial, because the medial aspect of the fascia iliaca is relatively thin compared with the thick, lateral margin of the aponeurosis. Alternatively, surface landmarks may have been improperly identified or the needle advanced too rapidly through the fascial planes. As a result, reassessing surface landmarks, advancing the needle at a slower pace, or selecting a more lateral needle insertion site may be necessary to successfully identify the fascia iliaca compartment. The use of sharp cutting needles should also be avoided when performing the block, because these needles do not provide adequate tactile feedback when traversing fascial planes.

Ultrasound-Guided Fascia Iliaca Blockade

Scanning Technique
The ultrasound probe is placed over the femoral region at the level of the inguinal skin crease perpendicular to the long axis of the thigh (Figures 9 and 10). This orientation provides the best cross-sectional view of the femoral artery, relevant neurovascular anatomy, and fascial planes. The probe is directed laterally so that a cross-sectional view of the femoral artery is located along the medial edge of the ultrasound image. Although visualization of the femoral nerve and femoral

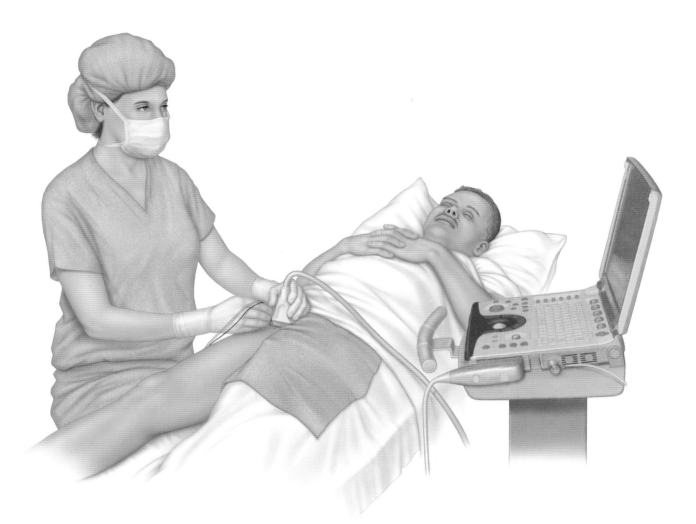

Figure 9. Patient-provider orientation during ultrasound-guided fascia iliaca blockade.

artery may be useful for orientation, the identification of two distinct fascial layers (fascia lata and fascia iliaca) overlying the iliopsoas muscle is most important (Figure 11). Ultrasound probes with mid- to high-range frequency (8-12 MHz) are most appropriate for imaging within this anatomical location.

Sonoanatomy

The ideal ultrasound image during fascia iliaca blockade captures the fascia lata and fascia iliaca as distinct hyperechoic lines overlying the heterogeneous, hypoechoic iliopsoas muscle with the femoral nerve, artery, and vein

positioned medially. The femoral artery is easily identified as a round, noncompressible, pulsatile, hypoechoic structure medial to the femoral nerve. In contrast, the compressible femoral vein is located medial to the femoral artery. Doppler may be used to confirm the vascular identity of both the artery and the vein. The sonographic appearance of the femoral nerve varies depending on the location of imaging. For example, at the level of the inguinal ligament, the nerve generally appears as a triangular or wedge-shaped hyperechoic structure (Figure 12), with central "honeycombing" that reflects the fascicular components of the peripheral nerve (Figure 13). However,

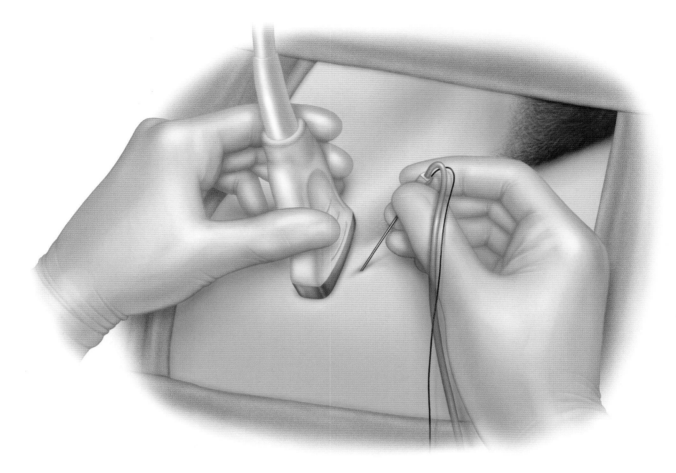

Figure 10. Probe and needle orientation during ultrasound-guided fascia iliaca blockade.

at the level of the inguinal skin crease, the femoral nerve may appear more circular as the anterior and posterior divisions begin to form (Figure 11).

Ultrasound Approach

Ultrasound-guided fascia iliaca blockade can be performed using either an in-plane or out-of-plane needle approach. During an out-of-plane approach, the ultrasound probe is placed immediately proximal to the needle insertion site described above for traditional single-injection techniques. A 21-gauge 4-inch (10-cm) insulated needle is inserted perpendicular to the skin and directed slightly

cephalad. Although the entire needle is not seen, tissue displacement of the fascial planes should be evident. Direct visualization of local anesthetic spread *below* the fascia iliaca confirms correct needle placement. After confirmation of negative aspiration, local anesthetic is slowly injected in 5-mL increments with intermittent aspiration to a total volume of 20 to 40 mL. During an in-plane needle approach, a 21-gauge 4-inch (10-cm) insulated needle is inserted 1 to 2 cm from the lateral edge of the transducer and advanced medially under direct visualization until the needle tip is located deep (i.e., posterior) to the fascia iliaca. After confirmation of

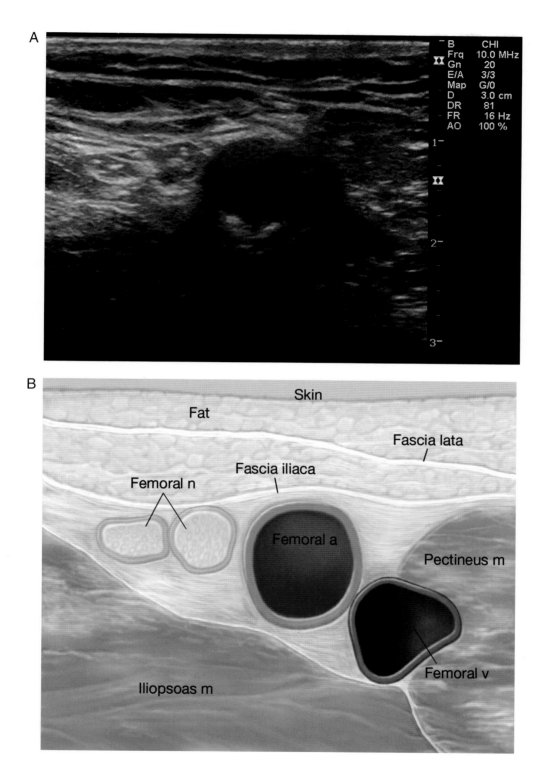

Figure 11. Femoral neurovascular anatomy in the proximal thigh. A, Ultrasound image. B, Corresponding anatomical illustration.

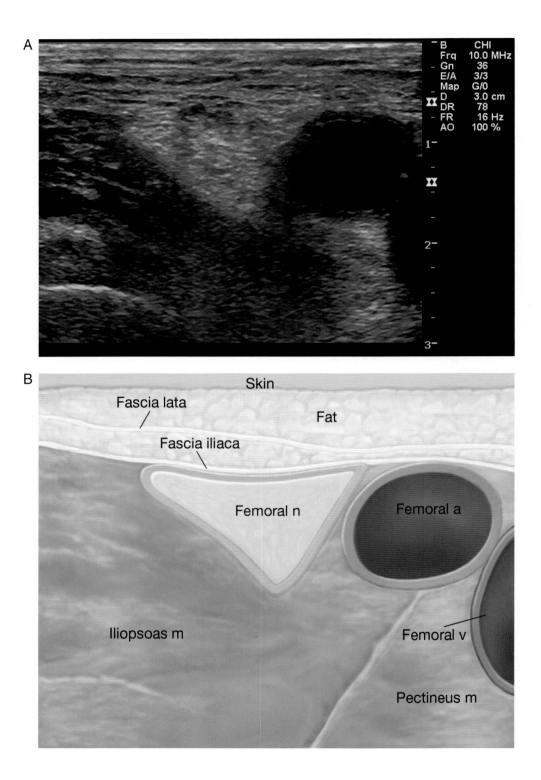

Figure 12. Femoral neurovascular anatomy in the proximal thigh, showing anatomical variation. A, Ultrasound image. B, Corresponding anatomical illustration.

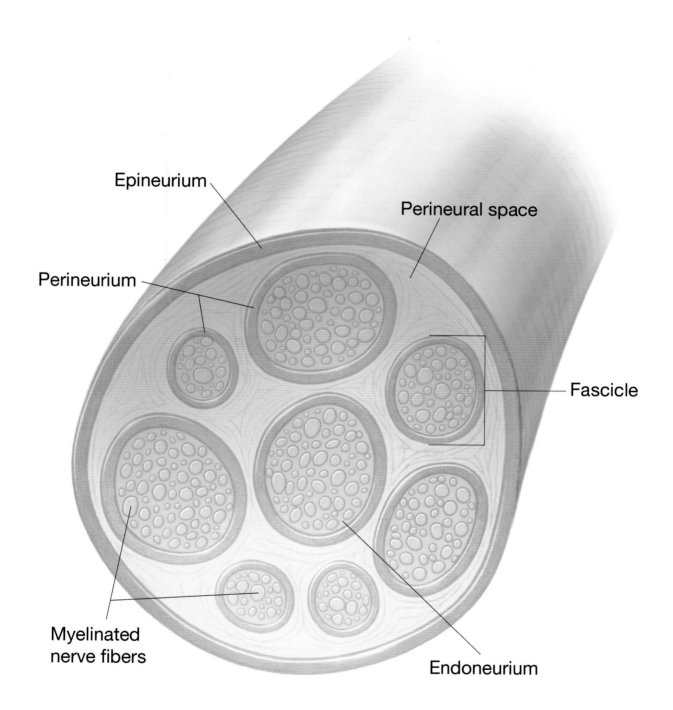

Figure 13. Peripheral nerve anatomy.

negative aspiration, local anesthetic is slowly injected in 5-mL increments with intermittent aspiration to a total volume of 20 to 40 mL.

Continuous Peripheral Nerve Catheters

Continuous fascia iliaca compartment blockade can be used as an adjunct to intraoperative anesthesia or to provide prolonged postoperative analgesia. The patient position, surface landmarks, needle insertion site, and block technique are similar for both single-injection and continuous techniques. An 18-gauge Tuohy needle is inserted as described above with the bevel directed cephalad. After a second distinct loss of resistance (i.e., "pop") is detected, the needle tip should be located posterior (i.e., deep) to the fascia iliaca. A 20-gauge multiorifice catheter is advanced 5 to 8 cm beyond the tip of the needle in a cephalad direction. Excessive needle advancement should be avoided to reduce the risk of inserting the perineural catheter into the hip joint capsule. The needle is removed and the catheter secured with a sterile transparent dressing. Alternatively, the catheter may be tunneled subcutaneously to a location remote from the initial insertion site and covered with a protective dressing. The subcutaneous tunneling of catheters may decrease the risk of infectious complications or catheter dislodgement.

Ultrasound-guided fascia iliaca catheter placement is similar to that described for out-of-plane single-injection ultrasound techniques. Under direct visualization, an 18-gauge 2-inch (5-cm) insulated Tuohy needle is inserted perpendicular to the skin and advanced toward the fascia iliaca (i.e., lateral to the femoral nerve) with the bevel directed cephalad. Location of the needle tip can be confirmed by injecting either saline or a dextrose-containing solution. After optimal needle placement (i.e., immediately posterior to the fascia iliaca and lateral to the femoral nerve), a 20-gauge catheter is advanced 5 to 8 cm beyond the tip of the needle. The distribution of local anesthetic spread is confirmed using real-time ultrasound imaging. If the spread of local anesthetic does not appear to be posterior to the fascia iliaca, the catheter may be manipulated (e.g., withdrawn) or replaced under direct visualization. Once the catheter location has been optimized, the catheter is secured with a sterile transparent dressing.

Side Effects and Complications

The fascia iliaca compartment block is a simple, efficacious, low-risk procedure. The needle insertion site is several centimeters lateral to major neurovascular structures, theoretically decreasing the risk of intravascular or intraneural injection. Despite this potential advantage, episodes of vascular puncture, intravascular injection, and transient postoperative neural injury have been reported after fascia iliaca blockade. Other potential complications include infection and local anesthetic toxicity. Local anesthetic toxicity may result from rapid vascular absorption from the large surface area within the fascial compartment or from intravascular injection into small circumflex veins located deep to the fascia iliaca.

Suggested Reading

Capdevila X, Biboulet P, Bouregba M, Barthelet Y, Rubenovitch J, d'Athis F. Comparison of the three-in-one and fascia iliaca compartment blocks in adults: clinical and radiographical analysis. Anesth Analg. 1998 May;86(5):1039-44.

Dalens B, Vanneuville G, Tanguy A. Comparison of fascia iliaca compartment block with the 3-in-1 block in children. Anesth Analg. 1989 Apr;69(6):705-13. Erratum in: Anesth Analg. 1990 Apr;70(4):474.

Foss NB, Kristensen BB, Bundgaard M, Bak M, Heiring C, Virkelyst C, et al. Fascia iliaca compartment blockade for acute pain control in hip fracture patients: a randomized, placebo-controlled trial. Anesthesiology. 2007 Apr;106(4):773-8.

Lopez S, Gros T, Bernard N, Plasse C, Capdevila X. Fascia iliaca compartment block for femoral bone fractures in prehospital care. Reg Anesth Pain Med. 2003 May-Jun;28(3):203-7.

Morau D, Lopez S, Biboulet P, Bernard N, Amar J, Capdevila X. Comparison of continuous 3-in-1 and fascia iliaca compartment blocks for postoperative analgesia: feasibility, catheter migration, distribution of sensory block, and analgesic efficacy. Reg Anesth Pain Med. 2003 Jul-Aug;28(4):309-14.

Tran D, Clemente A, Finlayson RJ. A review of approaches and techniques for lower extremity nerve blocks. Can J Anaesth. 2007 Nov;54(11):922-34.

Wambold D, Carter C, Rosenberg AD. The fascia iliaca block for postoperative pain relief after knee surgery. Pain Pract. 2001 Sep;1(3):274-7.

Wathen JE, Gao D, Merritt G, Georgopoulos G, Battan FK. A randomized controlled trial comparing a fascia iliaca compartment nerve block to a traditional systemic analgesic for femur fractures in a pediatric emergency department. Ann Emerg Med. 2007 Aug;50(2):162-71, 171.e1. Epub 2007 Jan 8.

CHAPTER

25

Lateral Femoral Cutaneous, Obturator, and Saphenous Nerve Blockade

Kimberly P. Wynd, M.B., B.Ch.

Hugh M. Smith, M.D., Ph.D.

Lateral Femoral Cutaneous Nerve Blockade

Clinical Applications

Lateral femoral cutaneous nerve blockade may be used in combination with other regional techniques to provide anesthesia and postoperative analgesia to the lower extremity—particularly after total knee arthroplasty. The block has also been used in conjunction with

femoral nerve blockade to provide surgical anesthesia during muscle biopsy for patients undergoing diagnostic evaluation for malignant hyperthermia. Other indications include skin graft harvesting on the lateral aspect of the thigh and the diagnosis and treatment of meralgia paresthetica. Local anesthetic administration during femoral nerve blockade frequently extends beneath the fascia iliaca to produce anesthesia of the lateral femoral cutaneous nerve. However, isolated lateral femoral cutaneous nerve blockade differs from traditional femoral nerve block techniques.

Relevant Anatomy

The lateral femoral cutaneous nerve arises from the posterior divisions of the ventral rami of the second and third lumbar nerves (L2 and L3) (Figure 1). It emerges from the lateral border of the psoas major muscle to cross the iliac crest and enter the pelvis where is descends anterior to the iliacus muscle (Figure 2). The nerve runs beneath the fascial layer of the iliacus muscle and passes through a fascial opening approximately 2 to 3 cm medial to the anterior superior iliac spine at the level of the inguinal ligament. After passing under the inguinal ligament, the nerve courses inferolaterally on the anterior surface of the sartorius muscle where it divides into anterior and posterior branches. The anatomical location at which the lateral femoral cutaneous nerve begins to ascend from the deep iliac fascia to the subcutaneous tissue is highly variable. However, ultrasound imaging has shown that the nerve is reliably located between the fascia lata and fascia iliaca at a location 2 cm medial and 8 cm caudal to the anterior superior iliac spine. The anterior branch of the lateral femoral cutaneous nerve subdivides further and runs subcutaneously to the anterolateral aspect of the thigh. Terminal fibers from the anterior branch form part of the patellar plexus—a collection of neural structures that need to be anesthetized for surgical procedures involving the knee. The posterior branch provides cutaneous innervation from the greater trochanter to the middle aspect of the lateral thigh (Figure 3).

Surface Anatomy

The anterior superior iliac spine is the primary surface landmark for lateral femoral cutaneous nerve blockade. A mark is made 2 cm caudad and 2 cm medial to the anterior superior iliac spine, just below the inguinal ligament (Figures 2 and 4).

Patient Position

The patient is positioned supine with the leg extended at the knee and the long axis of the foot at an angle of 90° to the table. Internal or external rotation of the lower extremity should be avoided because it may alter the anatomical relationship of neurovascular structures. The proceduralist generally stands on the side of the patient to be blocked.

Technique

Neural Localization Techniques

Lateral femoral cutaneous nerve blockade is commonly performed using a modified field block technique with attention to fascial "pops" as indications of needle depth and location. Although paresthesia-seeking techniques and peripheral nerve stimulation are generally not used for this block, ultrasound guidance may be used to identify anatomical landmarks and neural structures.

Needle Insertion Site

A 22-gauge 1.5-inch (3.8-cm) blunt-tipped needle is inserted perpendicular to the skin at a point 2 cm caudad and 2 cm medial to the anterior superior iliac spine. The needle is advanced in a perpendicular direction, passing through the fascia lata (i.e., felt as a distinct "pop"), and 10 to 15 mL of local anesthetic is administered in a fanlike pattern moving in a lateral to medial direction above and below the fascial layer (Figure 5).

Alternative Techniques

Lateral femoral cutaneous nerve blockade may also be performed by contacting the iliac bone between the anterior superior iliac spine and the anterior inferior iliac spine. The needle is inserted medial and inferior to the anterior superior iliac spine and directed slightly caudad toward the anterior inferior iliac spine, contacting the iliac bone. Approximately 10 to 15 mL of local anesthetic is injected in a fanlike pattern. Alternatively, ultrasound guidance may be used to identify the nerve between the fascia lata and the fascia iliaca medial to the insertion of the sartorius muscle.

Side Effects and Complications

The risk of side effects or complications associated with lateral femoral cutaneous nerve blockade is extremely low.

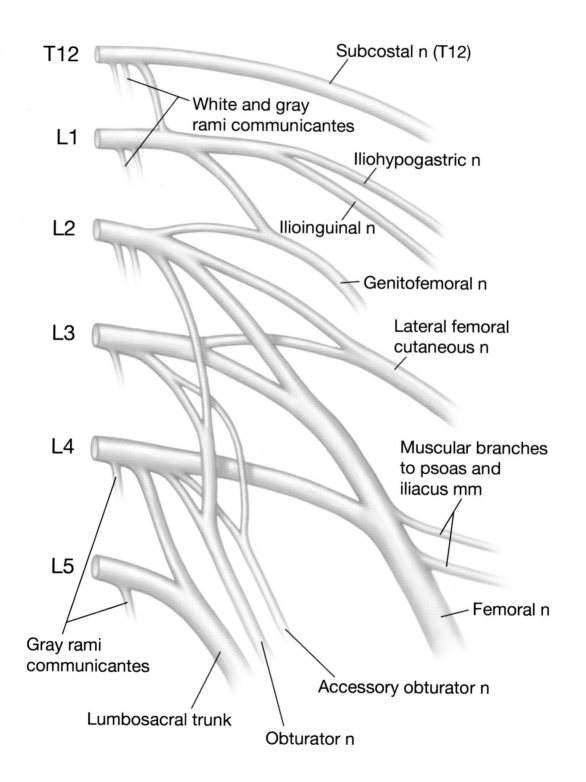

Figure 1. Lumbar plexus anatomy.

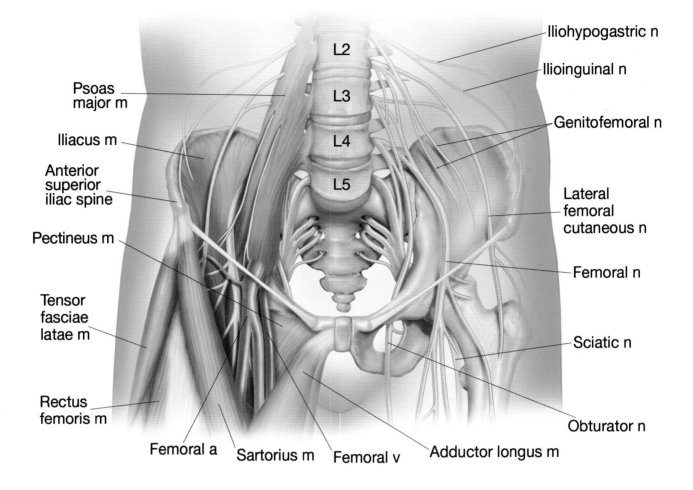

Figure 2. Anatomical location of the lateral femoral cutaneous and obturator nerves in situ.

Theoretical concerns include infection, bleeding, intravascular injection, local anesthetic toxicity, and neural injury. Incomplete blockade may occur as a result of anatomical variability and inadequate local anesthetic spread.

Obturator Nerve Blockade

Clinical Applications

Obturator nerve blockade has undergone significant modification since its first description by Gaston Labat in 1922.

In 1973, Winnie and colleagues described obturator nerve blockade as a component of the classic 3-in-1 technique, blocking the lateral femoral cutaneous, femoral, and obturator nerves with a single perivascular injection slightly distal to the inguinal ligament. However, subsequent studies demonstrated that the obturator nerve is inconsistently blocked with this technique. In 1993, the interadductor approach to the obturator nerve was described by Wassef, which was later modified by Pinnock and colleagues in 1997. Obturator nerve blockade is commonly used to supplement femoral and sciatic nerve blockade in patients undergoing lower

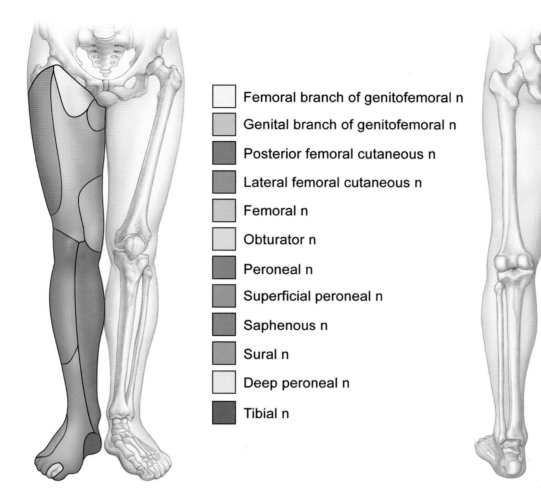

Femoral branch of genitofemoral n
Genital branch of genitofemoral n
Posterior femoral cutaneous n
Lateral femoral cutaneous n
Femoral n
Obturator n
Peroneal n
Superficial peroneal n
Saphenous n
Sural n
Deep peroneal n
Tibial n

Figure 3. Lower extremity cutaneous innervation.

extremity surgical procedures such as anterior cruciate ligament repair and total knee arthroplasty. Obturator blockade has also been used in the diagnosis and treatment of pain syndromes of the hip joint and adductor muscle spasm in patients with hemiplegia, paraplegia, and central neurologic disorders such as cerebral palsy and multiple sclerosis. Finally, selective obturator nerve block techniques may be used during urologic surgery to suppress the obturator reflex during transurethral resection of the lateral bladder wall. Relative contraindications to the block include inguinal lymphadenopathy, perineal infection, anticoagulation, and preexisting or degenerative neuropathies.

Relevant Anatomy

The obturator nerve arises from the anterior divisions of the ventral rami of the second lumbar nerve through the fourth lumbar nerve (L2-L4) (Figure 1). It descends toward the pelvis along the posteromedial border of the psoas major muscle, passes under the iliac vessels at the level of the fifth lumbar nerve (L5), and crosses inferior to the superior pubic ramus (Figure 2). The nerve accompanies the obturator artery and vein through the obturator canal and into the medial compartment of the thigh where it branches into anterior and posterior divisions. The anterior division of the obturator nerve courses deep to the

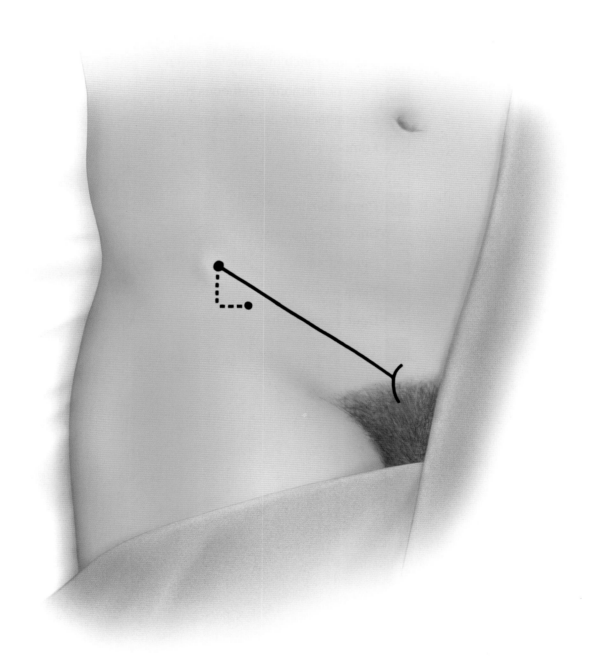

Figure 4. Surface landmarks for lateral femoral cutaneous nerve blockade.

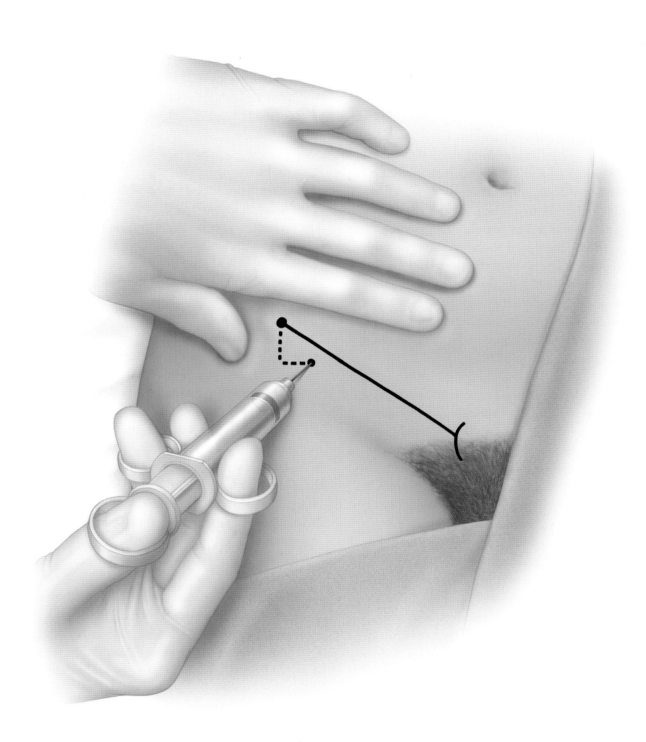

Figure 5. Needle insertion site for lateral femoral cutaneous nerve blockade.

pectineus and adductor longus muscles and anterior to the adductor brevis and obturator externus muscles before terminating within the gracilis muscle (Figure 6). The anterior division provides innervation to the superficial adductor muscles of the leg (i.e., adductor brevis, adductor longus, pectineus, and gracilis muscles), articular branches to the anteromedial hip capsule, and cutaneous branches to the skin overlying the posteromedial aspect of the thigh (Figure 3). However, cutaneous innervation has been shown to be extremely variable from one individual to another. The posterior division of the obturator nerve travels posterior to the adductor brevis muscle and anterior to the adductor magnus muscle (Figure 6). The posterior division provides innervation to the deep adductor muscles of the leg (i.e., obturator externus, adductor magnus, and adductor brevis muscles) and articular branches to the posterior knee joint. The posterior division of the obturator nerve has no cutaneous innervation.

The obturator nerve possesses numerous anatomical variants. For example, in approximately 75% of patients, the obturator nerve divides into its anterior and posterior divisions as is passes through the obturator canal. However, this division also may occur proximal (10% of patients) or distal (15% of patients) to the canal. In addition, up to 20% of patients may possess an accessory obturator nerve. The *accessory obturator nerve* is formed from variable contributions from the anterior divisions of the ventral rami of L2 to L4 (Figure 1). Unlike the obturator nerve, the accessory obturator nerve passes *anterior* to the superior pubic ramus to provide motor innervation to the pectineus muscle. The accessory obturator nerve also provides articular branches to the hip joint and commonly terminates by anastomosing with the obturator nerve within the proximal thigh.

Surface Anatomy

Important surface landmarks during obturator nerve blockade include the anterior superior iliac spine, the pubic tubercle, the femoral pulse, and the proximal insertion of the adductor longus muscle (Figure 6). A line overlying the inguinal ligament is drawn by connecting the anterior superior iliac spine with the pubic tubercle. At the level of the inguinal skin crease, the femoral artery and the medial border of the adductor longus muscle are palpated and marked (Figure 7).

Patient Position

The patient is positioned supine with the leg extended at the knee, abducted, and slightly rotated externally. The proceduralist generally stands on the side of the patient to be blocked.

Technique

Neural Localization Techniques

Although ultrasound-guided obturator nerve blockade has been described, peripheral nerve stimulation remains the most common technique of neural localization. In general, comprehensive blockade requires the elicitation of a motor response from both the anterior and the posterior divisions of the obturator nerve. Stimulation of the anterior division produces a motor response from the adductor longus and gracilis muscles (i.e., muscle twitch of the medial thigh). Stimulation of the posterior division produces a motor response from the adductor magnus muscle (i.e., hip adduction).

Needle Insertion Site

The paravascular inguinal approach to the obturator nerve is performed by identifying the femoral pulse and the medial border of the adductor longus muscle at the level of the inguinal skin crease (Figure 7). The tendon of the adductor longus muscle can be easily identified and marked with extreme leg abduction. A 22-gauge 3.25-inch (8-cm) insulated needle is inserted at the midpoint of a line drawn between the femoral artery and the medial border of the adductor longus muscle (Figure 8). The needle is advanced at a cephalad angle of 30° to the skin until a motor response is elicited from the anterior division of the obturator nerve (i.e., muscle

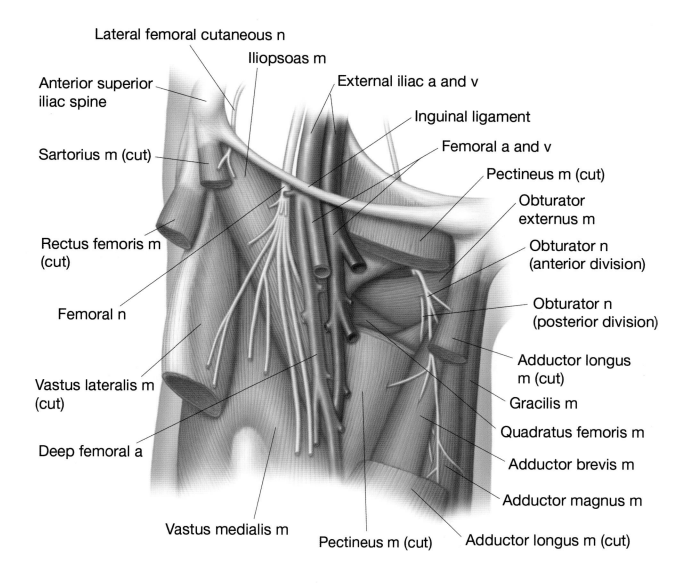

Figure 6. Neurovascular and muscular anatomy of the femoral region.

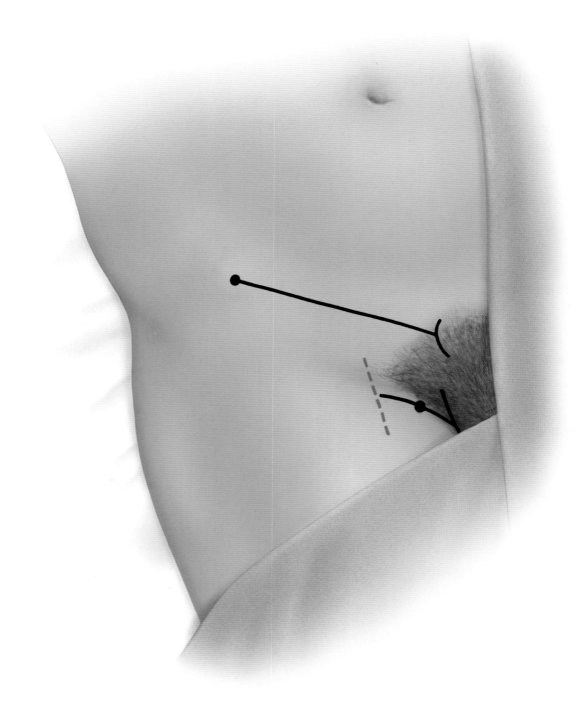

Figure 7. Surface landmarks for obturator nerve blockade.

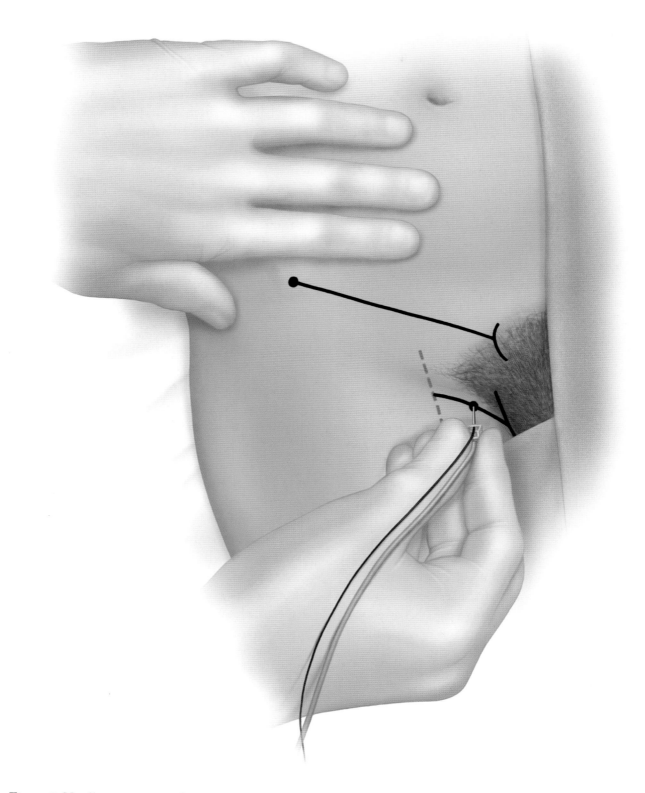

Figure 8. Needle insertion site for obturator nerve blockade.

twitch of the medial thigh) at a depth of approximately 1 to 2 cm. The needle is then advanced 0.5 to 1.5 cm deeper, and in a slightly lateral direction, until a motor response of the posterior division is elicited (i.e., hip adduction). After the desired motor response is acquired at a current of 0.5 mA or less, 5 to 7 mL of local anesthetic is slowly injected with intermittent aspiration. The needle is then slowly withdrawn until a motor response of the anterior division is once again elicited. After the desired motor response at a current of 0.5 mA or less is acquired, 5 to 7 mL of local anesthetic is slowly injected with intermittent aspiration. The administration of local anesthetic onto the deeper posterior division may minimize the risk of unrecognized needle trauma to an anesthetized anterior division. Because of the caudal location of local anesthetic injection, the paravascular inguinal approach to obturator nerve blockade may not adequately anesthetize the more proximal articular branches to the hip.

Needle Redirection Cues

If an appropriate motor response is not achieved during the first needle pass, the needle should be withdrawn and redirected in a more medial and cephalad direction using the same needle insertion site. If a motor response is not elicited with medial redirection, lateral redirection should be performed with small incremental maneuvers. However, clinicians must be mindful of the proximity of the femoral vein at this anatomical location.

Alternative Techniques

Several alternative techniques for obturator nerve blockade have been described. Labat's classic approach to the block was performed using a paresthesia-seeking technique. However, the approach is now commonly performed using peripheral nerve stimulation. With the patient lying supine, the limb to be blocked is abducted 30° from the midline. The site of needle insertion is a point 2 cm lateral and 2 cm caudad to the pubic tubercle. A 22-gauge 3.25-inch (8-cm) stimulating needle is inserted perpendicular to the skin and advanced 2 to 4 cm until it makes contact with the inferior border of the superior pubic ramus. The needle is then slightly withdrawn and redirected 45°

laterally and slightly caudad. The needle is advanced 2 to 3 cm beyond the pelvic ramus until an adductor motor response of the thigh is elicited. Once an appropriate motor response is achieved at a current of 0.5 mA or less, 10 to 15 mL of local anesthetic is slowly injected with intermittent aspiration. The classic Labat approach results in the injection of local anesthetic at a more proximal anatomical location (i.e., the obturator canal) than the previously described paravascular inguinal technique.

The interadductor approach to the obturator nerve is performed with the patient lying supine and the leg abducted 30° from the midline and externally rotated. A 22-gauge 3.25-inch (8-cm) stimulating needle is inserted at the posterior border of the most proximal (i.e., tendinous) segment of the adductor longus muscle. The needle is advanced 3 to 6 cm toward the obturator canal (i.e., 1 to 2 cm medial to the femoral pulse and immediately inferior to the inguinal ligament) until an appropriate paresthesia or motor response (i.e., thigh adduction) is elicited. After careful aspiration, 10 to 15 mL of local anesthetic is slowly injected with intermittent aspiration.

Side Effects and Complications

The risk of side effects or complications associated with the paravascular inguinal approach to obturator nerve blockade is extremely low. Theoretical concerns include infection, bleeding, intravascular injection, local anesthetic toxicity, and neural injury. Incomplete blockade may occur as a result of anatomical variability and inadequate local anesthetic spread. Because of the significant variability in cutaneous innervation of the obturator nerve, successful obturator nerve blockade should not be determined using sensory testing. Block evaluation using motor assessment (i.e., adductor muscle weakness) is a more reliable indicator of successful blockade. Intravascular injection, central nervous system toxicity, neural injury, hematoma formation, and organ penetration (e.g., bladder, rectum, vagina, spermatic cord) have been reported with Labat's classic approach to the block.

Saphenous Nerve Blockade

Clinical Applications

The saphenous nerve provides cutaneous innervation to the medial aspect of the lower extremity from the knee to the medial malleolus (Figure 3). It is commonly blocked in conjunction with the sciatic nerve to provide comprehensive anesthesia and analgesia of the distal extremity. Saphenous nerve blockade may also be performed to prevent pain and discomfort associated with the use of a lower extremity tourniquet or Esmarch bandage. Several approaches to the saphenous nerve have been described, including the paravenous, transsartorial, and field block techniques. Ultrasound-guided saphenous nerve blockade using a transsartorial approach (i.e., above the knee) and a paravenous approach (i.e., below the knee) have also been described. Saphenous nerve blockade at the level of the ankle is discussed in Chapter 28.

Relevant Anatomy

The saphenous nerve is the largest cutaneous sensory branch of the femoral nerve (Figures 1 and 6). It is derived from the posterior division of the femoral nerve and descends the leg within the adductor canal along the posterior surface of the sartorius muscle. At the level of the knee, the saphenous nerve emerges between the sartorius and gracilis muscles where it pierces the fascia lata and divides into infrapatellar and distal cutaneous branches (Figure 9). The saphenous nerve continues descending the leg along the medial border of the tibia within the subcutaneous tissue, immediately posterior to the great saphenous vein. At the level of the ankle, the saphenous nerve passes anterior to the medial malleolus where it subdivides into an extensive network of smaller subcutaneous nerve fibers (Figure 10). Saphenous sensory innervation to the foot is variable, but it may extend as far as the base of the great toe.

Surface Anatomy

At the level of the tibial tuberosity, the saphenous nerve is typically located 1 cm medial and 1 cm posterior to the great saphenous vein. With the patient in a sitting position, the saphenous vein may be identified by placing a tourniquet around the distal thigh and allowing the leg to hang in a dependent position. After several minutes, the vein can often be identified along the medial aspect of the leg, immediately distal to the knee, or overlying the proximal segment of the medial head of the gastrocnemius muscle.

Patient Position

The patient should be positioned supine with the leg extended at the knee, abducted, and slightly rotated externally. The proceduralist generally stands on the side of the patient to be blocked. Alternatively, the patient may be in a sitting position with the leg hanging in a dependent position.

Technique

The paravenous approach to saphenous nerve blockade is performed by infiltrating local anesthetic around the great saphenous vein at the level of the tibial tuberosity. Although variable, very high success rates have been reported with this approach.

Neural Localization Techniques

The saphenous nerve is a purely sensory neural target distal to the femoral triangle. Therefore, localized infiltration (i.e., field block technique) is one of the most common techniques used during saphenous nerve blockade. However, peripheral nerve stimulation, using a stimulating needle or a handheld cutaneous stimulator, may be used to elicit sensory pulsations (i.e., sensory paresthesias) and localize the nerve. Alternatively, ultrasound guidance may be used to identify anatomical landmarks and relevant neurovascular structures.

Needle Insertion Site

The needle insertion site is the anatomical location at which the great saphenous vein has been identified. A 25-gauge 2-inch (5-cm) needle is used to perform a perivascular injection immediately deep to the great saphenous vein. Local anesthetic (5-7 mL) is injected both medial and

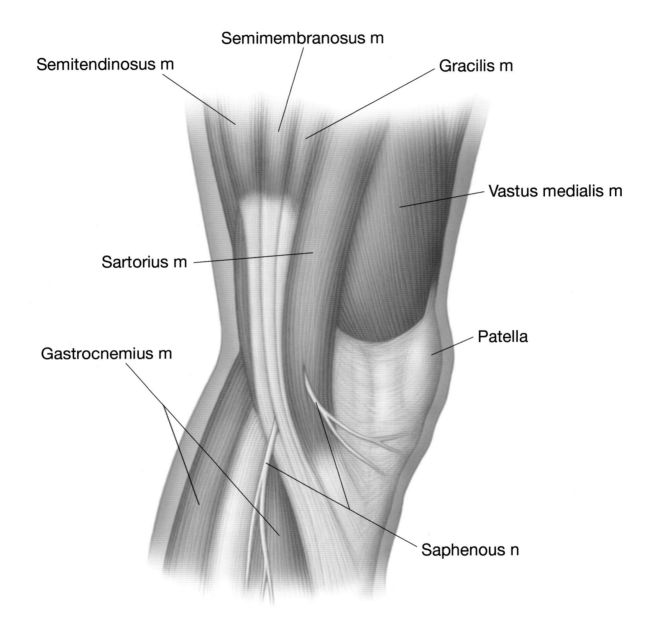

Figure 9. Saphenous nerve anatomy at the knee (medial view).

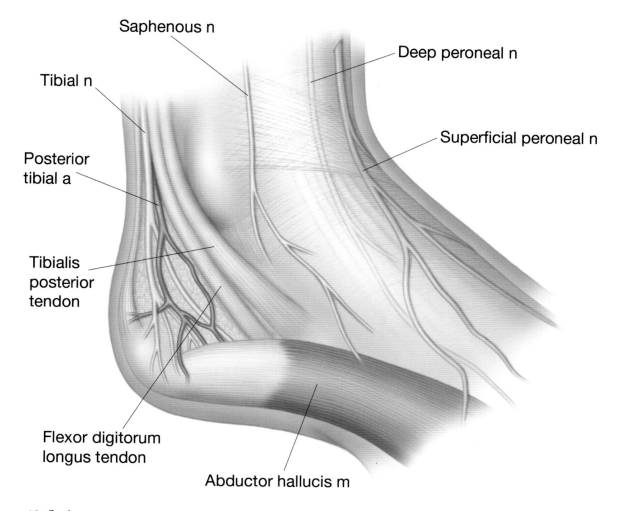

Saphenous n

Deep peroneal n

Tibial n

Superficial peroneal n

Posterior tibial a

Tibialis posterior tendon

Flexor digitorum longus tendon

Abductor hallucis m

Figure 10. Saphenous nerve anatomy at the ankle (medial view).

lateral to the vein. Clinicians should inform patients that localized bleeding and minor hematoma formation may commonly occur with this technique.

Alternative Techniques
Saphenous nerve blockade may also be performed using a localized field block technique. At the medial border of the knee, the saphenous nerve emerges between the sartorius and gracilis muscles where it pierces the fascia lata and divides into infrapatellar and distal cutaneous branches (Figure 9). With use of a 25-gauge 2-inch (5-cm) needle, 7 to 10 mL of local anesthetic is injected subcutaneously from the medial condyle of the tibia

anteriorly to the tibial tuberosity and posteriorly to the medial head of the gastrocnemius muscle (Figure 11). Extensive subcutaneous infiltration is required to adequately block both the infrapatellar and the distal cutaneous branches of the saphenous nerve. Success rates for the field block technique range from 33% to 65%.

The transsartorial approach to the saphenous nerve is commonly performed using a loss-of-resistance technique. The block technique anesthetizes the saphenous nerve as it descends the leg within the adductor canal along the posterior surface of the sartorius muscle. The site of needle insertion is located 3 to 4 cm cephalad and

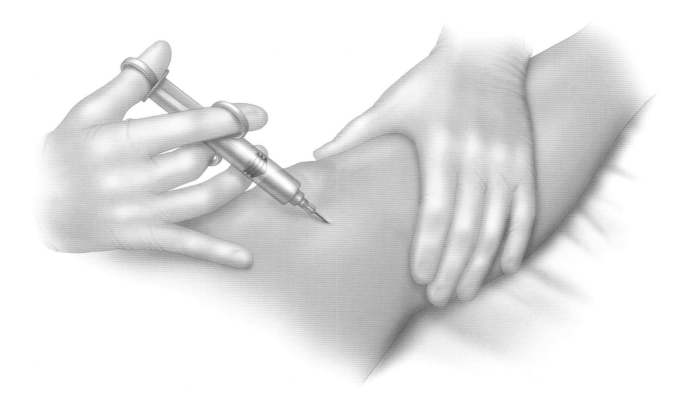

Figure 11. Needle insertion site during saphenous nerve blockade (medial view of the field block technique).

6 to 8 cm posterior to the superomedial border of the patella. The distal segment of the sartorius muscle can be identified with external rotation of the lower extremity and can often be palpated at the point of needle insertion. A 22-gauge 2-inch (5-cm) needle is inserted at a 45° angle from the coronal plane and advanced slightly caudad through the fascia lata and the muscle belly of the sartorius muscle until a fascial "pop," or "click," is noted. This loss-of-resistance typically occurs at a depth of 3 to 5 cm. Alternatively, a 22-gauge 2-inch (5-cm) stimulating needle may be used to elicit a sensory paresthesia that is referred to the medial malleolus. After acquiring a paresthesia at a current of 0.5 mA or less, 10 mL of local anesthetic is slowly injected with intermittent aspiration. Success rates for the transsartorial technique range from 70% to 80%.

Ultrasound-Guided Saphenous Nerve Blockade

Scanning Technique

Ultrasound-guided saphenous nerve blockade may be performed either above (i.e., transsartorial approach) or below (i.e., paravenous approach) the knee. During the paravenous approach, the patient is positioned supine with the leg extended at the knee, abducted, and slightly rotated externally. The proceduralist generally stands on the side of the patient to be blocked. Because of the superficial anatomical location of the saphenous nerve, a high-frequency ultrasound probe (10-12 MHz) is used to provide optimal images of the relevant neurovascular structures. The ultrasound probe is placed on the posteromedial aspect of the lower leg, perpendicular to the long axis of the extremity, and immediately caudad to the medial condyle of the tibia. The most important anatomical landmark to identify during ultrasound-guided paravenous saphenous nerve blockade is the great saphenous vein.

Sonoanatomy

The ideal ultrasound image captures the saphenous nerve in cross-section lying immediately posterior (i.e., deep) to the great saphenous vein (Figure 12). The great saphenous vein is a small, easily compressible, round or elliptical-shaped hypoechoic structure within the subcutaneous tissue of the posteromedial leg. Doppler imaging of the vessel reveals a continuous (i.e., nonpulsatile) color signature. The application of a distal thigh tourniquet and minimizing downward pressure on the ultrasound probe increase the likelihood of readily identifying the vein. The saphenous nerve is a small, circular, hyperechoic neural structure located posterior (i.e., deep) to the vein (Figure 12).

Ultrasound-guided saphenous nerve blockade may also be performed above the knee using the transsartorial approach. During ultrasound-guided transsartorial saphenous nerve blockade, the patient is placed in the supine position with the leg extended at the knee, abducted, and slightly rotated externally. A high-frequency ultrasound probe (10-12 MHz) is placed perpendicular to the limb on the medial aspect of the distal thigh. The saphenous nerve is identified as a round, hyperechoic structure within the fascia, medial to the vastus medialis muscle (Figure 13). It is beneficial to be familiar with both anatomical locations of the saphenous nerve (i.e., above and below the knee) because the sonographic image quality may differ significantly from patient to patient and from location to location (i.e., transsartorial versus paravenous approach).

Ultrasound Approach

Ultrasound-guided saphenous nerve blockade is commonly performed using an in-plane needle approach, which allows complete visualization of the needle and its advancement throughout the procedure. During the paravenous approach, the probe should be oriented so that the saphenous vein appears on the lateral third of the ultrasound image. A 22-gauge 2-inch (5-cm) stimulating needle is inserted and advanced in a medial to lateral direction. Continuous, real-time imaging is used to direct the needle toward a point inferior to the saphenous nerve. Once the needle tip is properly positioned, 5 to 8 mL of local anesthetic is slowly injected with incremental aspiration. The needle may need to be withdrawn and slightly redirected to ensure circumferential spread of the local anesthetic around the nerve (Figure 14). If the nerve cannot be visualized, 5 to 8 mL of local anesthetic should be injected inferior and medial to the saphenous vein.

Side Effects and Complications

Side effects and complications after saphenous nerve blockade are extremely rare. However, given the proximity of the saphenous nerve to the great saphenous vein, localized bleeding and painless hematoma formation may occur after the paravenous technique. Despite localized bleeding, intravascular injection and systemic local anesthetic toxicity are exceedingly rare. Infectious complications and neural injury due to mechanical trauma or intraneural injection are also theoretical concerns.

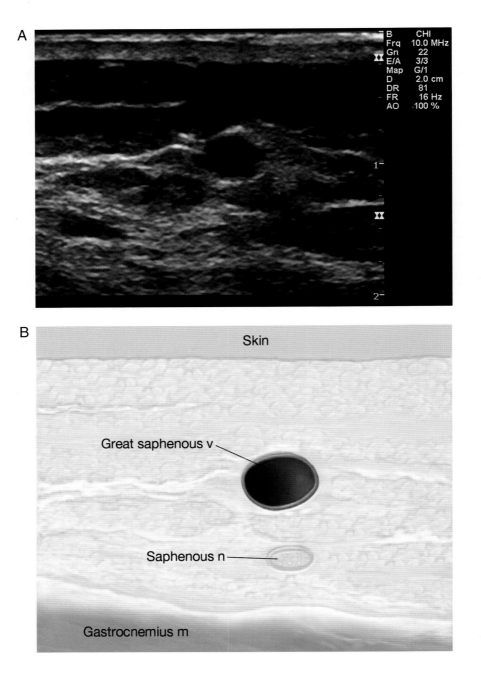

Figure 12. Paravenous view of the saphenous nerve. A, Ultrasound image. B, Corresponding anatomical illustration.

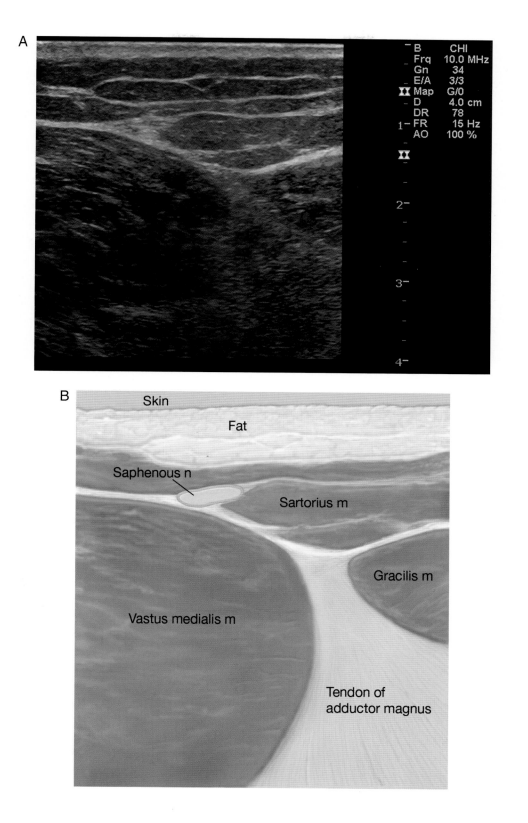

Figure 13. Transsartorial view of the saphenous nerve. A, Ultrasound image. B, Corresponding anatomical illustration.

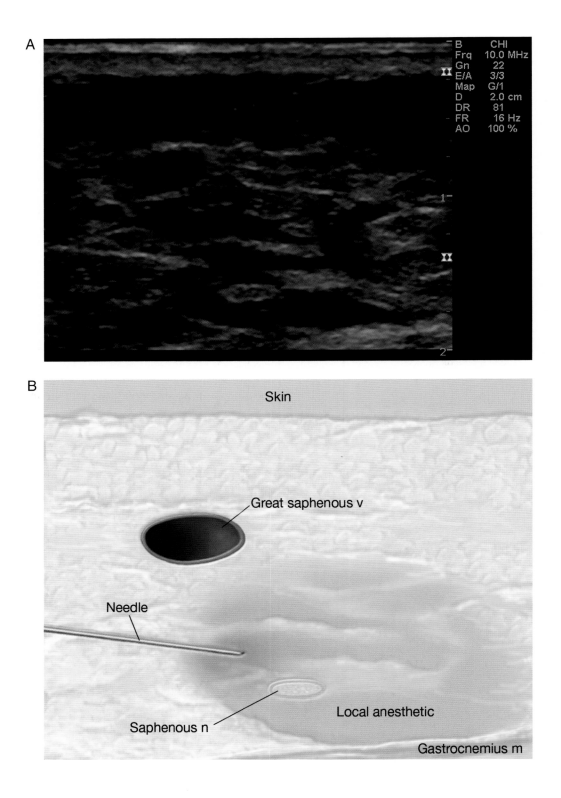

Figure 14. Ultrasound-guided paravenous saphenous nerve blockade. A, Ultrasound image. B, Corresponding anatomical illustration.

Suggested Reading

Benzon HT, Sharma S, Calimaran A. Comparison of the different approaches to saphenous nerve block. Anesthesiology. 2005 Mar;102(3):633-8.

Bouaziz H, Vial F, Jochum D, Macalou D, Heck M, Meuret P, et al. An evaluation of the cutaneous distribution after obturator nerve block. Anesth Analg. 2002 Feb;94(2):445-9.

Choquet O, Capdevila X, Bennourine K, Feugeas JL, Bringuier-Branchereau S, Manelli JC. A new inguinal approach for the obturator nerve block: anatomical and randomized clinical studies. Anesthesiology. 2005 Dec;103(6):1238-45.

Comfort VK, Lang SA, Yip RW. Saphenous nerve anaesthesia: a nerve stimulator technique. Can J Anaesth. 1996 Aug;43(8):852-7.

De Mey JC, Deruyck LJ, Cammu G, De Baerdemaeker LE, Mortier EP. A paravenous approach for the saphenous nerve block. Reg Anesth Pain Med. 2001 Nov-Dec;26(6):504-6.

Grothaus MC, Holt M, Mekhail AO, Ebraheim NA, Yeasting RA. Lateral femoral cutaneous nerve: an anatomic study. Clin Orthop Relat Res. 2005 Aug;437:164-8.

Hurdle MF, Weingarten TN, Crisostomo RA, Psimos C, Smith J. Ultrasound-guided blockade of the lateral femoral cutaneous nerve: technical description and review of 10 cases. Arch Phys Med Rehabil. 2007 Oct;88(10):1362-4.

Jochum D, Iohom G, Choquet O, Macalou D, Ouologuem S, Meuret P, et al. Adding a selective obturator nerve block to the parasacral sciatic nerve block: an evaluation. Anesth Analg. 2004 Nov;99(5):1544-9.

Kowbel MA, Comfort VK. Caudal epidural blood patch for the treatment of a paediatric subarachnoid-cutaneous fistula. Can J Anaesth. 1995 Jul;42(7):625-7.

Labat G. Regional anesthesia: its technic and clinical application. Philadelphia (PA): WB Saunders Company; 1922.

Macalou D, Trueck S, Meuret P, Heck M, Vial F, Ouologuem S, et al. Postoperative analgesia after total knee replacement: the effect of an obturator nerve block added to the femoral 3-in-1 nerve block. Anesth Analg. 2004 Jul;99(1):251-4.

Mansour NY. Sub-sartorial saphenous nerve block with the aid of nerve stimulator. Reg Anesth. 1993 Jul-Aug;18(4):266-8.

Ng I, Vaghadia H, Choi PT, Helmy N. Ultrasound imaging accurately identifies the lateral femoral cutaneous nerve. Anesth Analg. 2008 Sep;107(3):1070-4.

Pinnock CA, Fischer HBJ, Jones RP, Pinnock C, editors. Peripheral nerve blockade. Edinburgh: Churchill Livingstone, 1997.

Shannon J, Lang SA, Yip RW, Gerard M. Lateral femoral cutaneous nerve block revisited: a nerve stimulator technique. Reg Anesth. 1995 Mar-Apr;20(2):100-4.

van der Wal M, Lang SA, Yip RW. Transsartorial approach for saphenous nerve block. Can J Anaesth. 1993 Jun;40(6):542-6.

Wassef MR. Interadductor approach to obturator nerve blockade for spastic conditions of adductor thigh muscles. Reg Anesth. 1993 Jan-Feb;18(1):13-7.

Winnie AP, Ramamurthy S, Durrani Z. The inguinal para-vascular technic of lumbar plexus anesthesia: the "3-in-1 block." Anesth Analg. 1973 Nov-Dec;52(6):989-96.

CHAPTER

26

Sciatic Nerve Blockade

Adam K. Jacob, M.D.

Clinical Applications

The classic posterior approach to sciatic nerve blockade was first described in 1922 by Gaston Labat. However, Côté and colleagues subsequently discovered that the technique was likely pioneered by Labat's French mentor and surgical colleague, Victor Pauchet. Since its original description, several modifications and alternative approaches to sciatic nerve blockade have been described. In 1963, Beck described the anterior approach to the sciatic nerve. In 1975, Winnie and

Raj and colleagues described modifications of the Labat technique and the lithotomy approach, respectively. In 1993, Mansour described the parasacral approach to sciatic nerve blockade, which was later modified by di Benedetto and colleagues (i.e., subgluteal approach). Sciatic nerve blockade is performed to achieve anesthesia and analgesia of the distal lower extremity, including the anterior and posterolateral leg, ankle, and foot. Common indications include intraoperative anesthesia and postoperative analgesia for total knee arthroplasty, soft tissue surgery of the distal extremity, Achilles tendon reconstruction, and foot and ankle surgery. The sciatic nerve is commonly blocked in conjunction with the femoral nerve to achieve complete anesthesia and analgesia of the lower extremity. Because of its large diameter, the diffusion of local anesthetic to the inner core (i.e., axons) of the sciatic nerve is relatively slow, resulting in a prolonged onset of anesthesia.

Relevant Anatomy

The lumbosacral plexus is derived from the anterior (ventral) primary rami of the fourth lumbar nerve through the fourth sacral nerve (L4-S4) (Figure 1). It provides the primary sensory and motor innervation to the dorsal aspect of the upper leg and the majority of the sensorimotor innervation below the knee (Figure 2). The posterior femoral cutaneous nerve and the sciatic nerve are two of the most relevant neural structures for lower extremity peripheral nerve blockade.

The posterior femoral cutaneous nerve is derived from the anterior and posterior divisions of the ventral rami of S1 to S3 (Figure 1). The nerve courses inferolaterally and exits the pelvis with the sciatic nerve through the greater sciatic foramen (Figure 3). It enters the gluteal region inferior to the piriformis muscle and descends posterior to the superior gemellus, inferior gemellus, obturator internus, and quadratus femoris muscles. The posterior femoral cutaneous nerve provides sensory innervation to the posterior thigh from the inferior gluteal region to the popliteal fossa (Figure 2). Perineal branches of the posterior femoral cutaneous nerve emerge at the level of the ischial tuberosity and course posterior to the biceps femoris and semitendinosus muscles (Figure 3).

The sciatic nerve is the largest peripheral nerve in the body. It is formed from the convergence of two major nerve trunks—the tibial and common peroneal nerves (Figure 1). The tibial nerve arises from the anterior divisions of the ventral rami of L4 to S3. The common peroneal nerve is derived from the posterior divisions of the ventral rami of L4 to S2. The sciatic nerve courses inferolaterally and exits

the pelvis with the posterior femoral cutaneous nerve through the greater sciatic foramen (Figure 3). It enters the gluteal region inferior to the piriformis muscle and descends posterior to the superior gemellus, inferior gemellus, obturator internus, and quadratus femoris muscles lateral to the ischial tuberosity. The sciatic nerve passes between the ischial tuberosity and the greater trochanter before entering the posterior aspect of the thigh at the inferior border of the gluteus maximus muscle, posterior to the adductor magnus muscle and anterior to the long head of the biceps femoris muscle. It descends the leg toward the popliteal fossa within the groove between the semimembranosus and semi-tendinosus muscles medially and the long head of the biceps femoris muscle laterally (Figure 4). En route to the popliteal fossa, the tibial component of the sciatic nerve provides motor innervation to the adductor mag-nus, biceps femoris (long head), semitendinosus, and semimembranosus muscles.

Surface Anatomy

Important surface landmarks for the classic posterior approach to the sciatic nerve include the bony promi-nences of the posterior superior iliac spine, the greater trochanter, and the sacral hiatus (Figure 5). The sacral hiatus is palpated at the base of the vertebral column near the origin of the intergluteal cleft.

Patient Position

The classic posterior, subgluteal, and parasacral approaches to the sciatic nerve are performed with the patient in the modified Sims position (Figure 6). The nonoperative extremity (i.e., dependent leg) is fully extended, and the side to be blocked (i.e., nondepen-dent leg) is flexed at the hip and knee and positioned comfortably on the nonoperative extremity.

The anterior approach to the sciatic nerve is performed with the patient in the supine position with the surgical extremity neutral or slightly abducted. Internal or exter-nal rotation of the lower extremity should be avoided because it may alter the anatomical relationship of

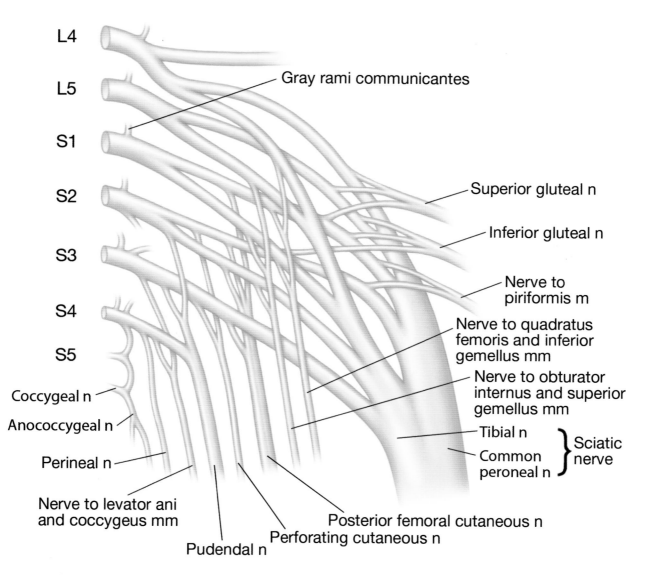

Figure 1. Lumbosacral plexus anatomy.

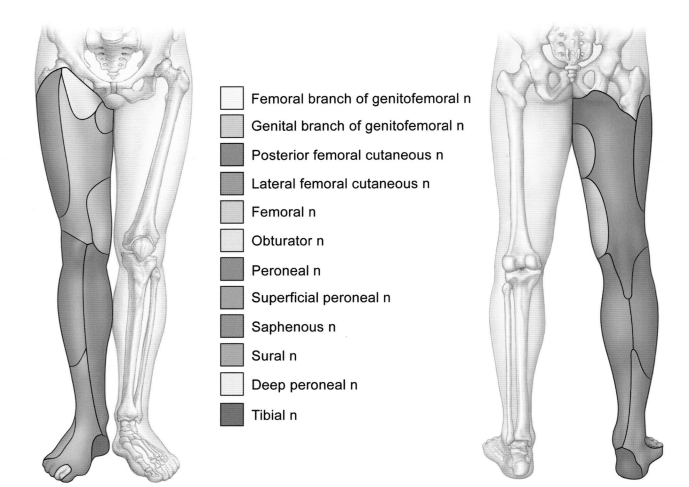

Femoral branch of genitofemoral n

Genital branch of genitofemoral n

Posterior femoral cutaneous n

Lateral femoral cutaneous n

Femoral n

Obturator n

Peroneal n

Superficial peroneal n

Saphenous n

Sural n

Deep peroneal n

Tibial n

Figure 2. Lower extremity cutaneous innervation.

neurovascular structures. The proceduralist generally stands on the side of the patient to be blocked (Figure 7).

Technique

Neural Localization Techniques
The most common method of neural localization during sciatic nerve blockade is peripheral nerve stimulation. An evoked motor response from the tibial component of the sciatic nerve produces plantar flexion at the ankle and foot inversion. Stimulation of the common peroneal

component evokes ankle dorsiflexion and foot eversion. Ultrasound guidance may also be used for neural localization during sciatic nerve blockade. Although the sciatic nerve is a deeper anatomical structure than most peripheral nerves, ultrasound guidance may be used to identify important anatomical landmarks (e.g., greater trochanter and ischial tuberosity) and neural structures.

Needle Insertion Site
Important anatomical landmarks for the classic posterior approach to sciatic nerve blockade include the posterior superior iliac spine, the greater trochanter, and the sacral

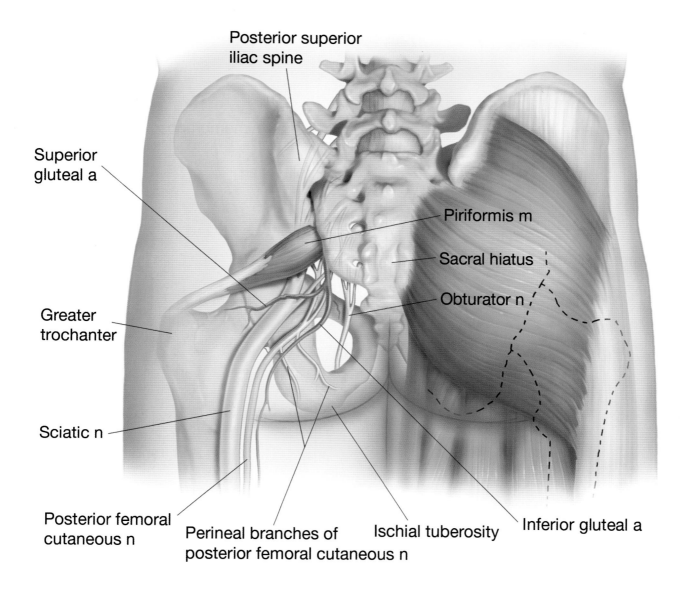

Posterior superior
iliac spine

Superior
gluteal a

Piriformis m

Sacral hiatus

Obturator n

Greater
trochanter

Sciatic n

Posterior femoral
cutaneous n

Perineal branches of
posterior femoral cutaneous n

Ischial tuberosity

Inferior gluteal a

Figure 3. Sciatic neuroanatomy.

hiatus. The needle insertion site is determined by first drawing a line connecting the posterior superior iliac spine and the posterior border of the greater trochanter. This line is then bisected and a second line drawn perpendicular to the first and extended 3 to 5 cm until it intersects with a line drawn from the greater trochanter to the sacral hiatus (Figure 5). The point of intersection between these two lines marks the site of needle insertion. A 21-gauge 4-inch (10-cm) insulated needle is inserted perpendicular to

the skin and advanced until a tibial or common peroneal motor response is elicited. After an appropriate motor response is elicited at a current of 0.5 mA, local anesthetic is slowly injected in 5-mL increments with intermittent aspiration to a total volume of 20 to 30 mL.

Needle Redirection Cues
If an appropriate motor response is not obtained during the first needle pass, the needle should be redirected

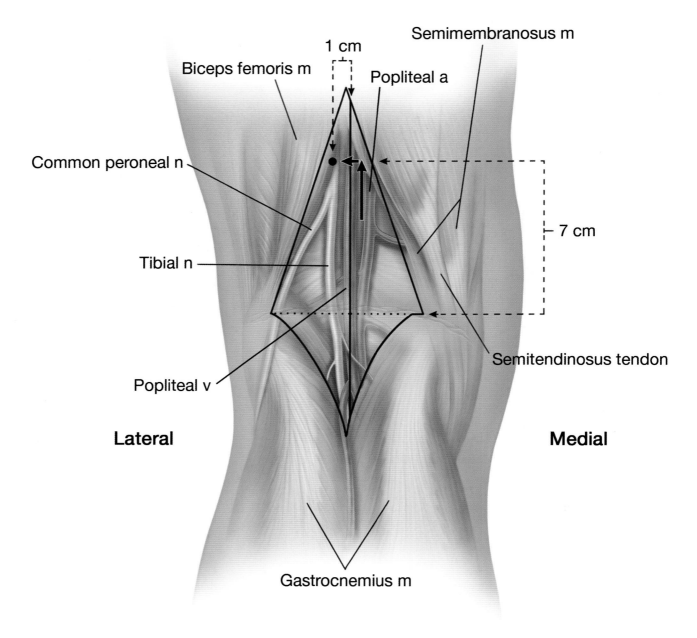

Figure 4. Neurovascular and muscular anatomy of the popliteal region.

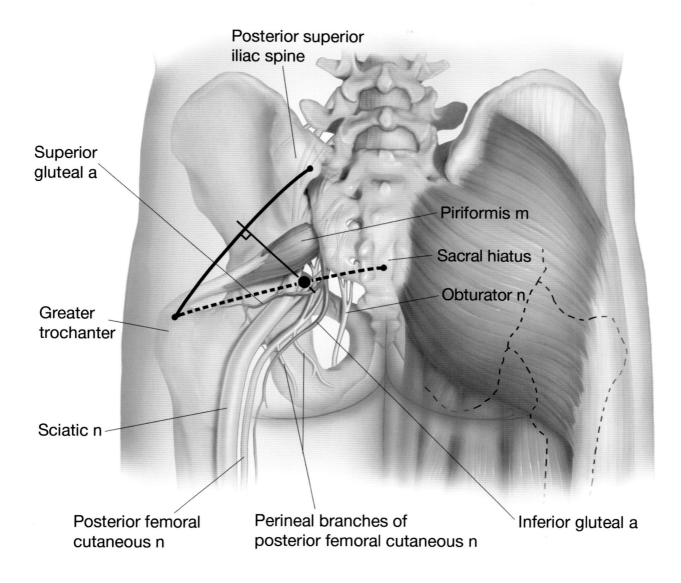

Figure 5. Anatomical landmarks and needle insertion site for sciatic nerve blockade (classic posterior approach).

slightly laterally in small incremental maneuvers along the line drawn between the sacral hiatus and the greater trochanter. If a motor response is not elicited despite lateral needle redirection, the needle should be redirected medially along the same line drawn between the sacral hiatus and the greater trochanter. If blood is aspirated during needle advancement, the needle may have penetrated the superior or inferior gluteal vessels—this situation requires lateral redirection of the needle.

If bone is contacted during needle advancement, the needle has likely contacted the ilium—this situation requires medial redirection of the needle.

Alternative Techniques
Several alternative techniques to sciatic nerve blockade have been described. The most common alternatives using a posterior approach include the subgluteal and parasacral techniques. Similar to the classic posterior

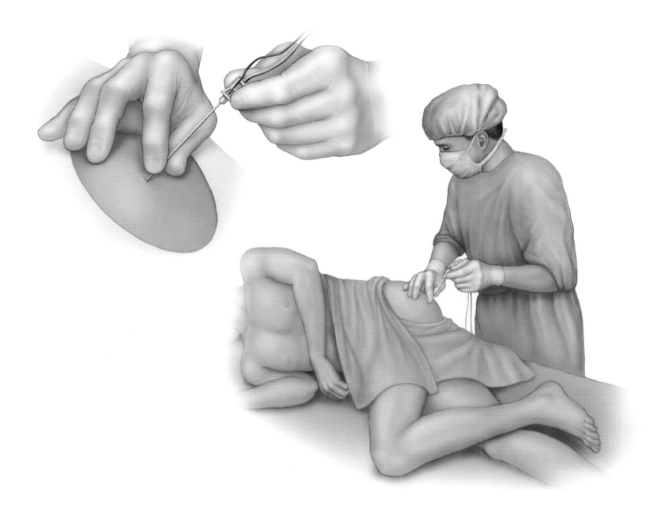

Figure 6. Patient-provider orientation during posterior sciatic nerve blockade.

approach, the patient is placed in the modified Sims position (Figure 6). For the subgluteal approach, a line is drawn between the ischial tuberosity and the greater trochanter—approximating the gluteal fold. This line is then bisected and a second line drawn perpendicular to the first, extending 4 cm in a caudal direction (Figure 8). The termination of this line marks the site of needle insertion. As confirmation, the point of needle insertion should approximate the palpable groove between the biceps femoris and vastus lateralis muscles.

A 21-gauge 4-inch (10-cm) insulated needle is inserted perpendicular to the skin and advanced until a tibial or common peroneal motor response is elicited. After an appropriate motor response is elicited at a current of 0.5 mA, local anesthetic is slowly injected in 5-mL increments with intermittent aspiration to a total volume of 20 to 30 mL. Because the subgluteal approach to the sciatic nerve is a more distal sciatic nerve block, the posterior femoral cutaneous nerve may be blocked with variable success.

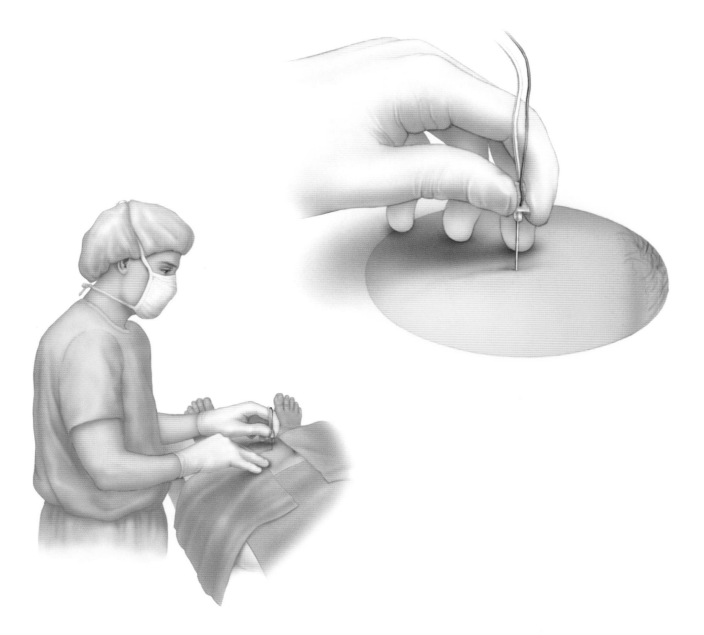

Figure 7. Patient-provider orientation during anterior sciatic nerve blockade.

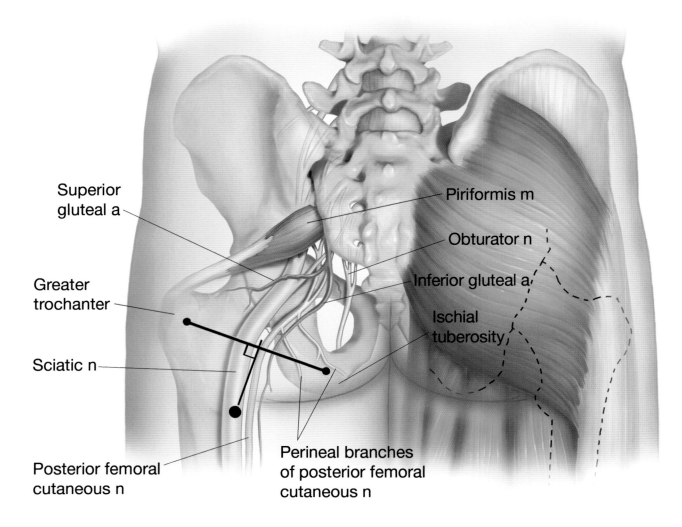

Figure 8. Anatomical landmarks and needle insertion site for sciatic nerve blockade (subgluteal approach).

The parasacral approach to sciatic nerve blockade is performed by placing the patient in the modified Sims position and drawing a line from the posterior superior iliac spine to the ischial tuberosity. The needle insertion site is identified and marked at a point 6 cm caudal from the posterior superior iliac spine (Figure 9). A 21-gauge 4-inch (10-cm) insulated needle is inserted perpendicular to the skin and advanced until a tibial or common peroneal motor response is elicited. After an appropriate motor response is elicited at a current of 0.5 mA, local anesthetic is slowly injected in 5-mL increments with intermittent aspiration to a total volume of 20 to 30 mL. The parasacral approach to the sciatic nerve may also block the pudendal (i.e., resulting in urinary retention) and obturator nerves because of its medial needle insertion site.

Finally, the anterior approach to sciatic nerve blockade is performed with the patient in the supine position (Figure 7). This approach may be advantageous when lateral positioning is difficult or painful for the patient. With the patient in the supine position and

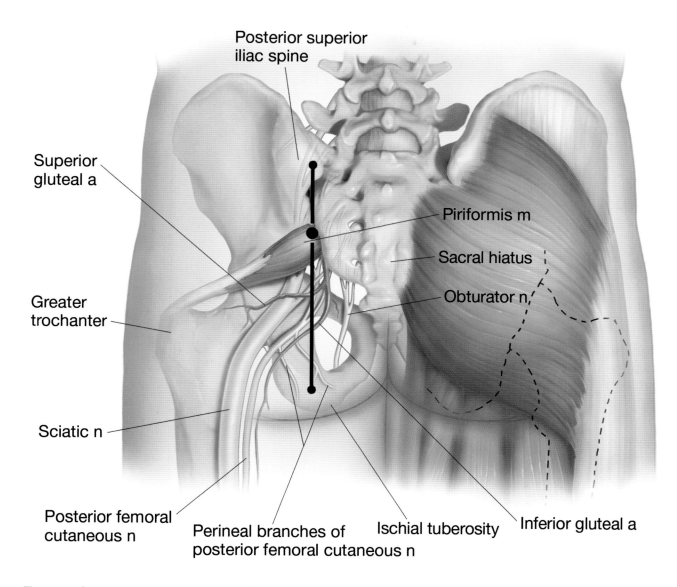

Figure 9. Anatomical landmarks and needle insertion site for sciatic nerve blockade (parasacral approach).

the surgical extremity neutral or slightly abducted, a line is drawn from the anterior superior iliac spine to the pubic tubercle and divided into thirds. At the junction of the middle and medial thirds, a second line is drawn perpendicular to the first and extended caudally to the proximal thigh (Figure 10). A third line is drawn from the greater trochanter across the anterior surface of the thigh, parallel to the inguinal ligament (i.e., the first line drawn). The point of intersection between the second line and the line extending from the greater trochanter marks the point of needle insertion (Beck approach). Alternatively, a line may be drawn between the inferior border of the anterior superior iliac spine and the superior angle of the pubic tubercle (Chelly approach). At the midpoint of this line, a second line is drawn perpendicular to the first and extended in a caudal direction. The site of needle insertion is identified and marked at a point 8 cm

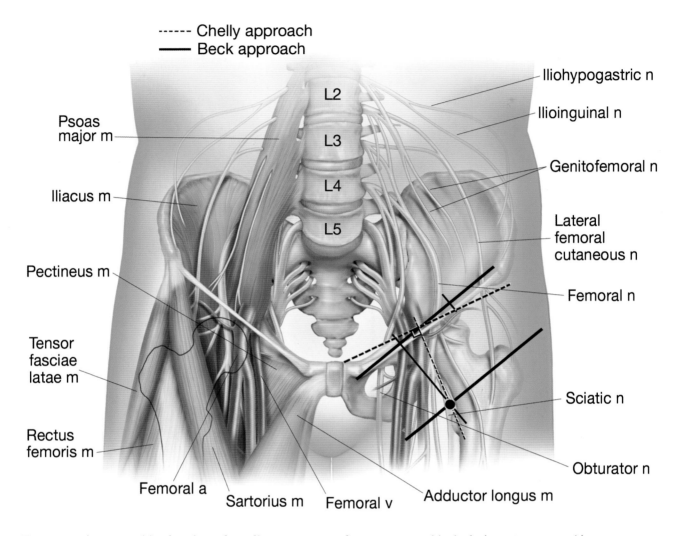

Figure 10. Anatomical landmarks and needle insertion site for sciatic nerve blockade (anterior approach).

caudad along this line (Figure 10). A 20-gauge 6-inch (15-cm) insulated needle is inserted perpendicular to the skin and advanced in a slightly lateral direction until bone (i.e., the lesser trochanter) is contacted or a motor response is elicited. If bone is contacted, the needle is redirected medially in small incremental maneuvers and advanced until a tibial or common peroneal motor response is elicited. After an appropriate motor response is elicited at a current of 0.5 mA, local anesthetic is slowly injected in 5-mL increments with intermittent aspiration to a total volume of 20 to 30 mL.

Ultrasound-Guided Sciatic Nerve Blockade

Scanning Technique

The ultrasound probe is placed in the subgluteal region, immediately caudad to the gluteal fold and perpendicular to the long axis of the thigh (Figures 11 and 12). Identification of the sciatic nerve within the subgluteal region is preferable to a more proximal site because of the anatomical location (i.e., shallower depth) of the nerve. Proper orientation of the probe in this position provides a cross-sectional view of the relevant anatomical structures (Figure 13). Optimal sonographic visualization may

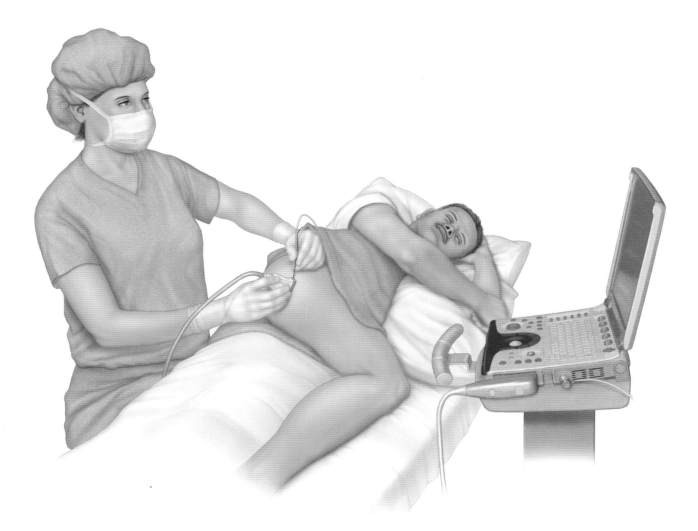

Figure 11. Patient-provider orientation during ultrasound-guided sciatic nerve blockade.

require minor adjustments in probe angulation to distinguish the sciatic nerve from adjacent muscular and fascial structures. Ultimately, the probe is oriented so that the sciatic nerve is positioned at the center of the ultrasound image. Because the sciatic nerve is quite deep at this location—even in thinner patients—a low-frequency (4-7 MHz) probe is generally required to obtain optimal images of important neurovascular structures.

Sonoanatomy

The ideal ultrasound image during subgluteal sciatic nerve blockade captures the sciatic nerve in cross-section between the hyperechoic ischial tuberosity and greater trochanter, deep to the gluteus maximus muscle (Figure 13). The sciatic nerve has a hyperechoic "honeycomb" appearance, representing the fascicular components of the peripheral nerve. The elliptical-shaped nerve is commonly surrounded by a dense hyperechoic border, representing the aponeurosis of the surrounding musculature.

Ultrasound Approach

Ultrasound-guided sciatic nerve blockade is commonly performed using an in-plane needle approach. The needle insertion site is generally located 1 to 2 cm from

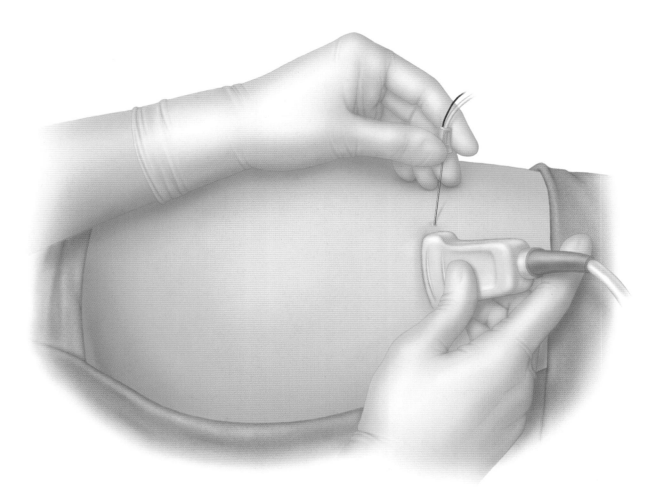

Figure 12. Probe and needle orientation during ultrasound-guided sciatic nerve blockade.

the lateral border of the transducer to improve the angle of incidence relative to the ultrasound beam (Figure 12). A 21-gauge 4-inch (10-cm) insulated needle is slowly advanced in a lateral to medial direction to a point immediately anterior or posterior to the nerve to minimize the risk of inadvertent needle trauma should the entire needle not be in view. If peripheral nerve stimulation is used for confirmation of neural identity, direct contact between the needle and the nerve may be necessary to elicit a motor response. Local anesthetic is then injected circumferentially around the nerve (Figure 14).

Side Effects and Complications

Side effects and complications associated with sciatic nerve blockade are relatively uncommon. Localized bruising and tenderness may be observed; however, true hematoma formation is quite rare. Although there is no major vasculature immediately adjacent to the sciatic nerve, the surrounding tissue is highly vascularized with an extensive vasonervorum. Serious complications resulting from systemic local anesthetic toxicity—including seizures and cardiovascular collapse—have been reported. However, the frequency of these events is extremely low.

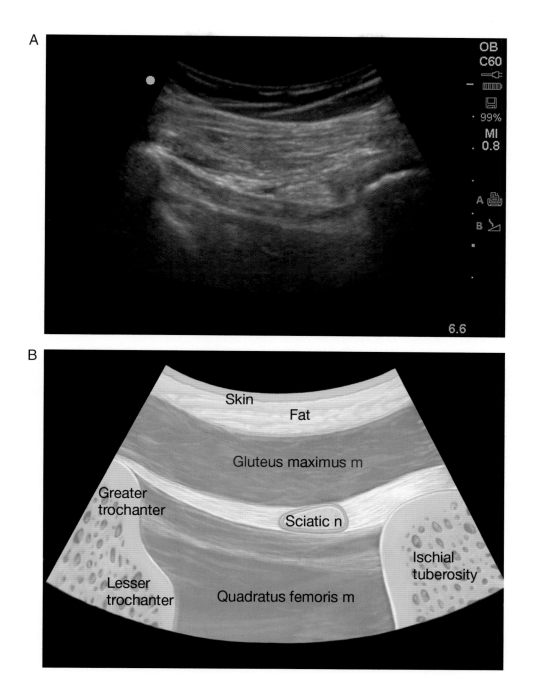

Figure 13. Subgluteal view of the sciatic nerve. A, Ultrasound image. B, Corresponding anatomical illustration.

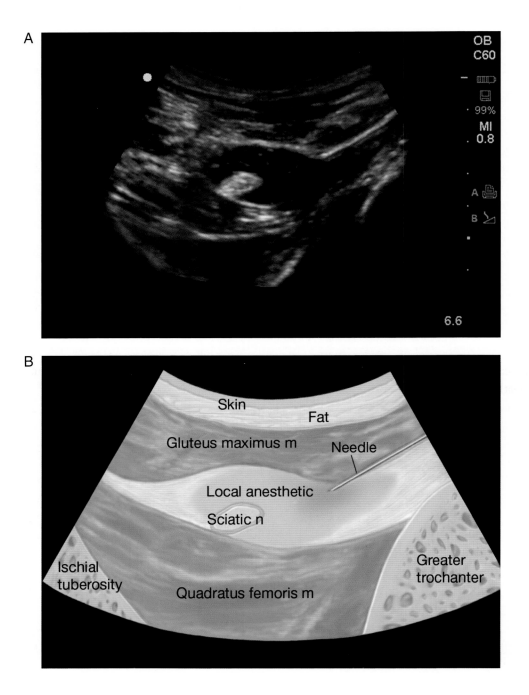

Figure 14. Ultrasound-guided sciatic nerve blockade. A, Ultrasound image. B, Corresponding anatomical illustration.

Postoperative sciatic nerve injury is one of the most feared complications of lower extremity regional blockade. The incidence of neural injury after sciatic nerve blockade is believed to be quite low. However, the precise role of neural blockade as a potential contributor to perioperative nerve injury remains undefined. Limited data suggest that the sciatic nerve may be more susceptible to mechanical, ischemic, or chemical injury than other peripheral nerves. Therefore, although definitive clinical evidence is lacking, it may be prudent to avoid sciatic nerve blockade in patients with multiple surgical or patient-related risk factors (e.g., prolonged tourniquet time, valgus knee deformity, new or progressive neurologic deficit) for peripheral nerve injury.

Suggested Reading

Auroy Y, Benhamou D, Bargues L, Ecoffey C, Falissard B, Mercier FJ, et al. Major complications of regional anesthesia in France: The SOS Regional Anesthesia Hotline Service. Anesthesiology. 2002 Nov;97(5):1274-80. Erratum in: Anesthesiology. 2003 Feb;98(2):595.

Beck GP. Anterior approach to sciatic nerve block. Anesthesiology. 1963 Mar-Apr;24:222-4.

Brown DL. Atlas of regional anesthesia. 2nd ed. Philadelphia: W. B. Saunders, c1999.

Chan VW, Nova H, Abbas S, McCartney CJ, Perlas A, Xu DQ. Ultrasound examination and localization of the sciatic nerve: a volunteer study. Anesthesiology. 2006 Feb;104(2):309-14.

Chelly JE, Delauney L. A new anterior approach to the sciatic nerve block. Anesthesiology. 1999 Dec;91(6):1655-60.

Côté AV, Vachon CA, Horlocker TT, Bacon DR. From Victor Pauchet to Gaston Labat: the transformation of regional anesthesia from a surgeon's practice to the physician anesthesiologist. Anesth Analg. 2003 Apr;96(4):1193-200.

di Benedetto P, Bertini L, Casati A, Borghi B, Albertin A, Fanelli G. A new posterior approach to the sciatic nerve block: a prospective, randomized comparison with the classic posterior approach. Anesth Analg. 2001 Oct;93(4):1040-4.

Enneking FK, Chan V, Greger J, Hadzić A, Lang SA, Horlocker TT. Lower-extremity peripheral nerve blockade: essentials of our current understanding. Reg Anesth Pain Med. 2005 Jan-Feb;30(1):4-35.

Hebl JR. Peripheral nerve injury. In: Neal JM, Rathmell JP, editors. Complications in regional anesthesia and pain medicine. Philadelphia: W.B. Saunders; c2007. p.125-40.

Karmakar MK, Kwok WH, Ho AM, Tsang K, Chui PT, Gin T. Ultrasound-guided sciatic nerve block: description of a new approach at the subgluteal space. Br J Anaesth. 2007 Mar;98(3):390-5.

Labat G. Regional anesthesia: its technic and clinical application. Philadelphia: W. B. Saunders; c1922.

Mansour NY. Reevaluating the sciatic nerve block: another landmark for consideration. Reg Anesth. 1993 Sep-Oct;18(5):322-3.

Mansour NY, Bennetts FE. An observational study of combined continuous lumbar plexus and single-shot sciatic nerve blocks for post-knee surgery analgesia. Reg Anesth. 1996 Jul-Aug;21(4):287-91.

Raj PP, Parks RI, Watson TD, Jenkins MT. A new single-position supine approach to sciatic-femoral nerve block. Anesth Analg. 1975 Jul-Aug;54(4):489-93.

Winnie AP. Regional anesthesia. Surg Clin North Am. 1975 Aug;55(4):861-92.

CHAPTER

27

Popliteal Blockade

James R. Hebl, M.D.

Adam K. Jacob, M.D.

Clinical Applications

Popliteal sciatic nerve blockade was first described by Gaston Labat in 1922. However, widespread use of the technique was initially limited because of concerns that blocking the sciatic nerve at this location may be associated with a higher incidence of complications or residual paresthesias. In 1980, Rorie and colleagues reassessed the block technique and demonstrated that popliteal blockade could be successfully performed without a higher incidence of serious complications or neurologic deficits. Since that time, popliteal blockade has become one of the most commonly used and widely accepted peripheral nerve block techniques for lower extremity surgery. Common indications include foot and ankle reconstructive surgery, soft tissue debridement, below-the-knee amputations, Achilles tendon repair, ankle arthrodesis, and saphenous vein stripping.

Popliteal sciatic nerve blockade does *not* provide comprehensive anesthesia or analgesia of the entire distal extremity. Cutaneous innervation of the medial leg and ankle is provided by the saphenous nerve (Chapter 25). Therefore, a supplemental saphenous nerve block is often necessary to achieve comprehensive blockade below the knee. In contrast to more proximal sciatic nerve block techniques, popliteal blockade preserves motor function of the hamstring muscles—allowing patients to maintain knee flexion and the ability to crutch-walk with assistance.

Relevant Anatomy

The sciatic nerve is formed from the convergence of two major nerve trunks—the tibial and common peroneal nerves. The tibial nerve is derived from the anterior divisions of the ventral rami of the fourth lumbar nerve through the third sacral nerve (L4-S3) and the common peroneal nerve arises from the posterior divisions of the ventral rami of L4 to S2 (Figure 1). The tibial and common peroneal nerves and their derivatives provide most of the sensory and motor innervation to the distal lower extremity (Figures 2 and 3).

The sciatic nerve descends the leg to the popliteal fossa within the groove between the semimembranosus and semitendinosus muscles medially and the long head of the biceps femoris muscle laterally (Figure 4). En route to the popliteal fossa, the tibial and peroneal components of the sciatic nerve diverge into the tibial and common peroneal nerves. The popliteal artery and vein are located medial and deep to both the tibial and the common peroneal nerves (Figure 5).

The tibial nerve exits the popliteal fossa and courses deep (i.e., anterior) to the soleus muscle where it descends within the posterior compartment of the leg with the posterior tibial artery. The nerve and artery travel within the groove between the tibialis posterior and flexor digitorum longus muscles before passing posterior to the medial malleolus. At the level of the medial malleolus, the tibial nerve separates into the medial plantar, lateral plantar, and medial calcaneal nerves, which provide sensorimotor innervation to the plantar aspect of the foot (Figure 3). The medial sural cutaneous nerve is a proximal branch of the tibial nerve that provides cutaneous innervation to the posterolateral aspect of the leg. It branches from the tibial nerve within the popliteal fossa and descends through the superficial compartment of the leg between the two heads of the gastrocnemius muscle. The medial sural cutaneous nerve becomes the sural nerve at the level of the mid-calf after receiving crossover innervation from the lateral sural cutaneous nerve. The sural nerve descends the leg along the lateral border of the Achilles tendon and passes posterior to the lateral malleolus. At the level of the lateral malleolus, the sural nerve branches into the lateral calcaneal and lateral dorsal cutaneous nerves, which provide sensory innervation to the lateral aspect of the foot and ankle (Figure 3).

The common peroneal nerve courses inferolaterally along the border of the biceps femoris muscle and its tendon insertion onto the head of the fibula. At the inferior neck of the fibula, the common peroneal nerve divides into its deep and superficial components. The deep peroneal nerve travels within the anterior compartment of the leg with the anterior tibial artery between the tibialis anterior and extensor digitorum longus muscles. It crosses the ankle immediately lateral to the extensor hallucis longus tendon and medial to the extensor digitorum longus tendon. The deep peroneal nerve provides motor innervation to the tibialis anterior, extensor digitorum longus and brevis, and extensor hallucis longus and brevis muscles. It provides sensory innervation to the deep dorsal structures of the foot and the web space between the first and second toes (Figure 3). The superficial peroneal nerve travels within the lateral compartment of the leg between the peroneus longus and extensor digitorum longus muscles and terminates in the foot anterior (i.e., superficial) and medial to the lateral malleolus. It provides motor innervation to the peroneus longus and brevis muscles and sensory innervation to the dorsal aspect of the foot (Figure 3).

Surface Anatomy

Important surface landmarks for the posterior approach to popliteal sciatic nerve blockade include the popliteal skin crease, the medial border of the biceps femoris muscle, and

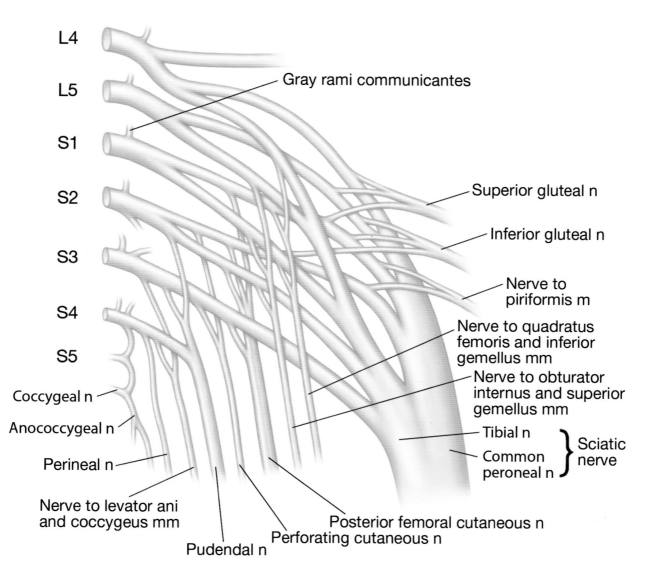

Figure 1. Lumbosacral plexus anatomy.

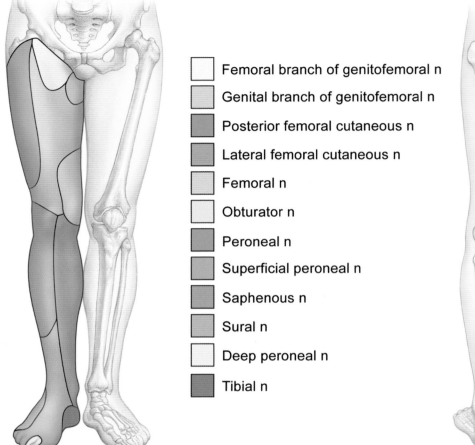
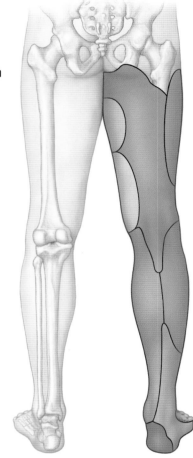

Femoral branch of genitofemoral n

Genital branch of genitofemoral n

Posterior femoral cutaneous n

Lateral femoral cutaneous n

Femoral n

Obturator n

Peroneal n

Superficial peroneal n

Saphenous n

Sural n

Deep peroneal n

Tibial n

Figure 2. Lower extremity cutaneous innervation.

the lateral border of the semimembranosus and semitendinosus muscles (Figure 6). These important anatomical landmarks can be accentuated by having the patient flex the leg against resistance while lying in the prone position.

Patient Position

The posterior approach to popliteal blockade is performed with the patient prone and the lower limb in a neutral position. The feet are extended beyond the edge of the bed to clearly discern the response to peripheral nerve stimulation (Figure 7). The proceduralist generally stands on the side of the patient to be blocked.

Technique

Neural Localization Techniques

The most common method of neural localization during popliteal blockade is peripheral nerve stimulation. An evoked motor response from the tibial component of the sciatic nerve produces plantar flexion at the ankle and foot inversion. Stimulation of the common peroneal component evokes ankle dorsiflexion and foot eversion. Ultrasound guidance may also be used for neural localization during the block technique. Although the sciatic nerve is a deeper anatomical structure than most peripheral nerves, ultrasound guidance

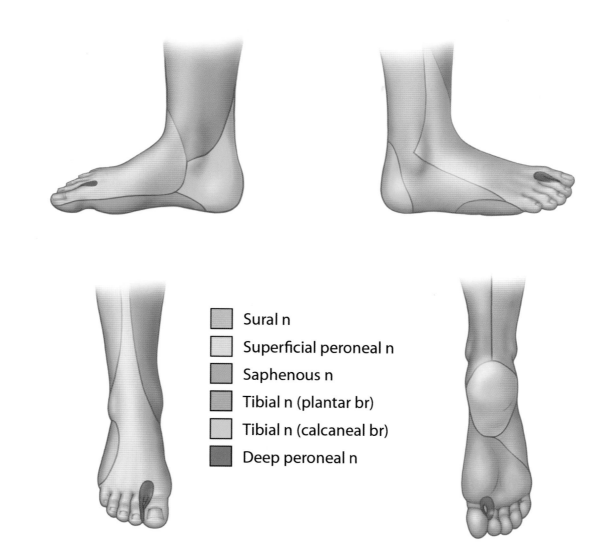

Figure 3. Cutaneous innervation of the foot and ankle.

may be used to identify important anatomical landmarks (e.g., popliteal artery and vein) and neural structures.

Needle Insertion Site

With the patient in the prone position, the borders of the popliteal fossa are identified and marked (Figure 6). The borders of the popliteal fossa include 1) the popliteal skin crease, 2) the medial border of the biceps femoris muscle (laterally), and 3) the lateral border of the semimembranosus and semitendinosus muscles

(medially). The borders of these muscles (i.e., the tendons) can be readily identified by having the patient flex the leg against resistance at the knee. This maneuver tightens the hamstring muscles and allows easy palpation of the associated tendons. The needle insertion site is a point 7 cm cephalad from the popliteal skin crease and 1 cm lateral to the midline of the triangle (Figure 6). A 21-gauge 4-inch (10-cm) insulated needle is inserted at an angle 45° to 60° from the skin and advanced in a cephalad direction (Figure 7).

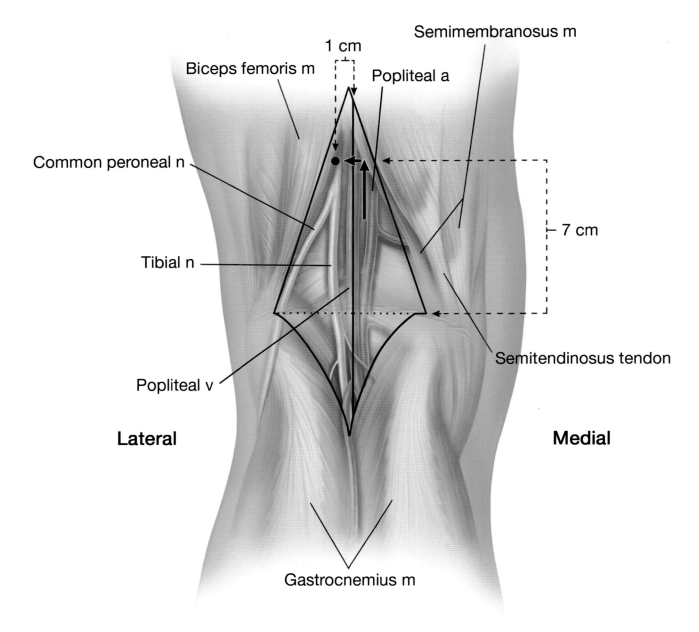

Figure 4. Neurovascular and muscular anatomy of the popliteal fossa.

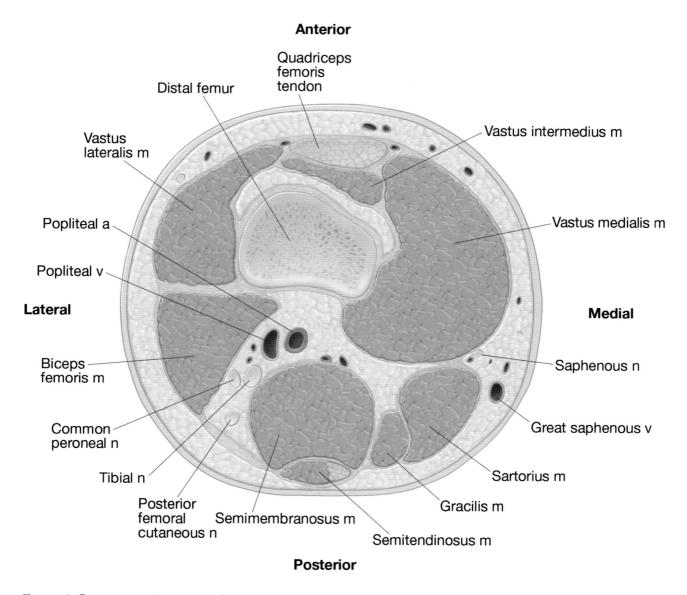

Figure 5. Cross-sectional anatomy of the popliteal fossa.

A tibial or common peroneal motor response is commonly elicited at a depth of 1.5 to 3 cm. After an appropriate motor response is elicited at a current of 0.5 mA or less, local anesthetic is slowly injected in 5-mL increments with intermittent aspiration to a total volume of 30 to 40 mL. A larger volume of local anesthetic is generally required during popliteal blockade to adequately anesthetize both the tibial and the common peroneal branches of the sciatic nerve. If a motor

response is unable to be elicited at a current of 0.5 mA or less, stimulation of the tibial nerve (at currents greater than 0.5 mA) may result in higher success rates.

Needle Redirection Cues
If an appropriate motor response is not elicited during the first needle pass, the needle is slightly withdrawn and redirected in a more lateral direction. Direct stimulation of the biceps femoris or semitendinosus muscle indicates

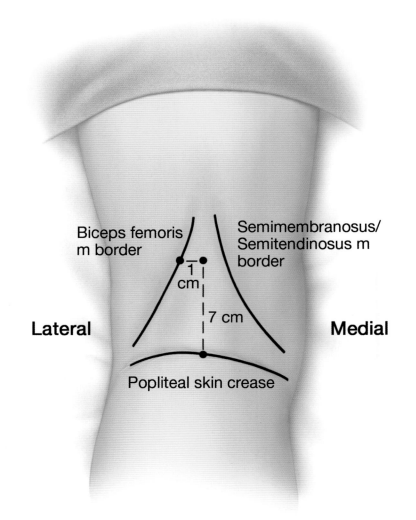

Biceps femoris
m border

Semimembranosus/
Semitendinosus m
border

1 cm

7 cm

Lateral

Medial

Popliteal skin crease

Figure 6. Surface landmarks for the posterior approach to popliteal blockade.

a needle trajectory that is either too lateral or too medial, respectively. If this occurs, appropriate redirection should be performed in small incremental maneuvers. If blood is aspirated during needle advancement, it is likely that either the popliteal artery or vein has been punctured. Under these circumstances, the needle is redirected to a more lateral and superficial (i.e., posterior) location. Finally, if bone (i.e., femur) is contacted, the needle has been advanced too deep (i.e., anterior), and the needle should be withdrawn to a more superficial location.

Alternative Techniques
The lateral approach to popliteal sciatic nerve blockade is a common alternative technique. Important surface landmarks for the lateral approach include the superior aspect of the patella and the muscular groove between the biceps femoris and vastus lateralis muscles. These important anatomical landmarks can be accentuated by having the patient flex the leg against resistance while lying in the supine position. Identification of the groove between the biceps femoris and vastus lateralis muscles may be difficult in obese patients.

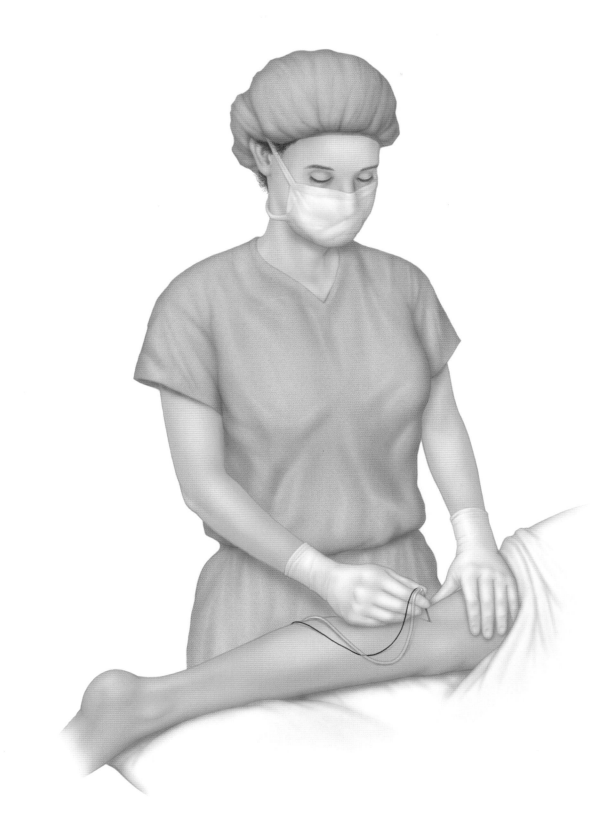

Figure 7. Patient-provider orientation during the posterior approach to popliteal blockade.

The lateral approach is performed with the patient supine and the lower limb in a neutral position (Figure 8). External rotation of the lower extremity may change the normal anatomical relationship of the sciatic nerve relative to the femur and biceps femoris muscle. The operative extremity may be elevated and the knee slightly flexed by placing a padded support or blanket under the knee or distal thigh. Similar to the posterior approach, the foot of the operative extremity should extend beyond the edge of the table to reliably discern subtle motor responses from peripheral nerve stimulation. The superior border of the patella is identified and a vertical line drawn laterally toward the table. The groove between the lateral border of the vastus lateralis muscle and the biceps femoris tendon is then identified and marked. The intersection of the two lines marks the site of needle insertion. A 21-gauge 4-inch (10-cm) insulated needle is inserted at an angle 30° from the coronal plane and advanced posteriorly until a tibial or common peroneal motor response is elicited (Figure 9). The common peroneal nerve is often stimulated first because of its lateral location relative to the tibial nerve. The tibial nerve is located deeper (i.e., more medial) and posterior to the common peroneal nerve. A motor response from *both* the common peroneal nerve and the tibial nerve should be identified to optimize block success. After an appropriate motor response is elicited at a current of

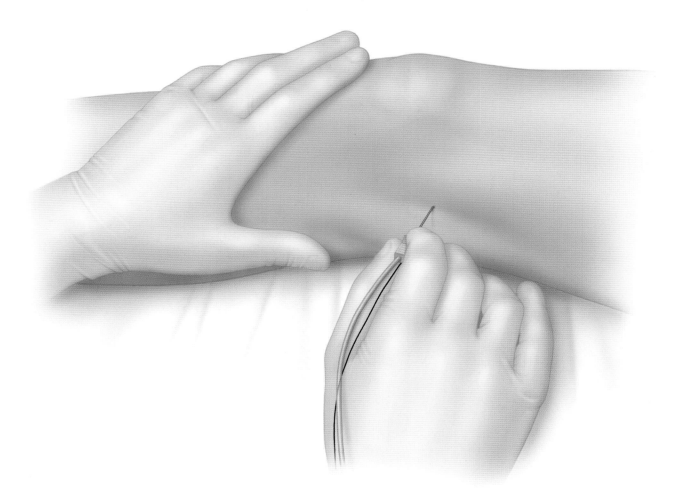

Figure 8. Needle insertion site for the lateral approach to popliteal blockade.

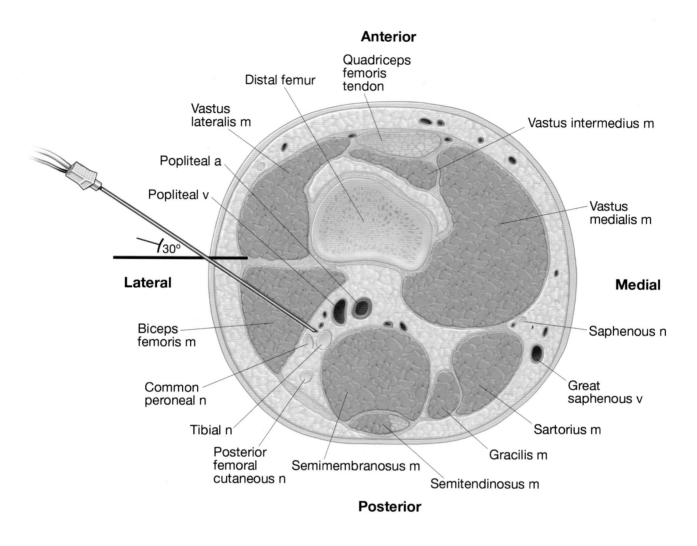

Figure 9. Cross-sectional anatomy of the popliteal fossa during needle advancement.

0.5 mA or less, local anesthetic is slowly injected in 5-mL increments with intermittent aspiration to a total volume of 15 to 20 mL onto both the tibial and the common peroneal nerves. If bone is contacted (i.e., femur), the needle is redirected more posteriorly in small incremental maneuvers until an appropriate motor response is elicited.

Several factors may increase the success rate of popliteal blockade. First, a double-stimulation technique (i.e., eliciting a motor response from both the tibial and the common peroneal nerve) is associated with higher success rates than single-injection techniques. Second, local anesthetic volume is important during single-injection techniques. For example, higher volumes of local anesthetic (e.g., 40 mL vs. 20 mL) will significantly increase the success rate of single-injection techniques. Finally, higher success rates have been reported with inversion and dorsiflexion motor responses. Inversion of the foot is due to stimulation of the tibialis posterior and tibialis anterior muscles. These two muscles are innervated by the tibial nerve and the deep peroneal nerve, respectively. Therefore, the elicitation of a strong inversion motor response during popliteal blockade suggests the needle tip is in proximity to both branches of the sciatic nerve—or to the sciatic nerve itself.

Ultrasound-Guided Popliteal Sciatic Nerve Blockade

Scanning Technique

Ultrasound-guided popliteal sciatic nerve blockade may be performed with the patient in either a supine or prone position. When the supine position is used, the extremity must be sufficiently elevated to allow adequate space under the leg for probe placement within the popliteal fossa. A more common approach is to have the patient prone with the leg in a neutral position. The ultrasound probe is placed within the popliteal region immediately proximal to the posterior skin crease and perpendicular to the long axis of the leg. This probe position allows providers to use either a posterior out-of-plane needle approach (Figure 10) or a lateral in-plane approach (Figure 11).

As the sciatic nerve descends the leg, it travels from a deep to superficial location within the extremity. Therefore, an ideal cross-sectional view of the sciatic nerve is difficult to obtain if the ultrasound probe is positioned perpendicular to the surface of the skin. To improve the angle of incidence—and therefore the image—the transducer should be angled cephalad 50° to 70° with the skin (i.e., directing the ultrasound beam caudad) to ensure a perpendicular intersection between the ultrasound beam and the neural target (Figure 10). Once the tibial and common peroneal nerves are identified, the ultrasound probe is moved in a cephalad direction to identify the point at which the two nerves converge to form the sciatic nerve (Figure 12). Ultrasound probes with mid- to high-range frequency (8-12 MHz) are most appropriate for imaging in this anatomical location.

Sonoanatomy

At the level of the popliteal skin crease, both the popliteal artery and the femur should be readily identifiable. The tibial and common peroneal nerves are located lateral and superficial (i.e., posterior) to both the popliteal artery and vein. Proximal to the skin crease, the sciatic nerve appears as a round hyperechoic structure with central honeycombing that is located superficial and slightly lateral to the popliteal artery (Figure 12). Scanning in a distal direction toward the skin crease will reveal the hyperechoic sciatic nerve separating into its tibial and common peroneal components (Figure 13). The tibial nerve is typically 2 to 4 cm from the skin surface and located medial and deep to the common peroneal nerve. In addition, the tibial nerve tends to be larger in diameter than the common peroneal nerve.

Ultrasound Approach

Ultrasound-guided popliteal sciatic nerve blockade may be performed using either a posterior out-of-plane needle approach (Figure 10) or a lateral in-plane approach (Figure 11). During the posterior out-of-plane approach, the probe is positioned so that the sciatic nerve is located near the center of the ultrasound image. A 21-gauge 4-inch (10-cm) stimulating needle is inserted 1 to 2 cm from the caudal edge of the transducer at an angle 45° to 60° from the skin (Figure 10). The needle is advanced to a position immediately lateral or medial to the sciatic nerve. Fine needle movements, tissue displacement, and hydrodissection are useful indicators of needle position and direction. Peripheral nerve stimulation can be used to confirm neural localization. After negative aspiration is confirmed, local anesthetic is injected circumferentially around the nerve in 5-mL increments with intermittent aspiration.

During the lateral in-plane approach, the needle insertion site is within the groove between the lateral border of the vastus lateralis muscle and the biceps femoris tendon. A 21-gauge 4-inch (10-cm) insulated needle is slowly advanced in a lateral to medial direction to a point immediately anterior or posterior to the sciatic nerve to minimize the risk of inadvertent needle trauma should the entire needle not be in view. If peripheral nerve stimulation is used to confirm neural identity, direct contact between the needle and the nerve may be necessary to elicit a motor response. Local anesthetic is then injected circumferentially around the nerves (Figure 14).

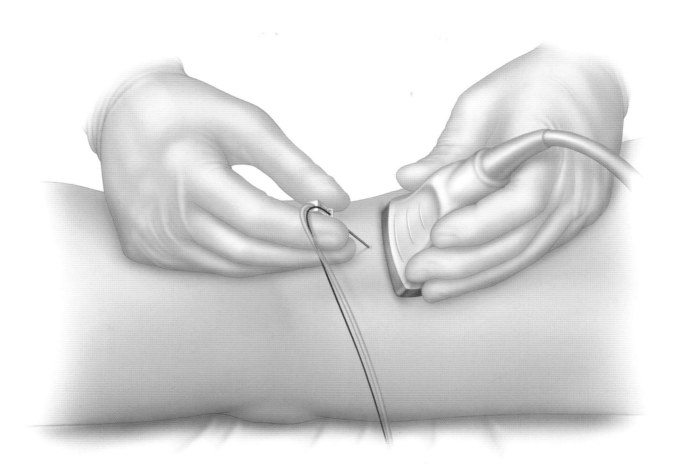

Figure 10. Popliteal ultrasound probe position, showing a posterior needle approach.

Continuous Peripheral Nerve Catheters

Continuous peripheral nerve catheters are commonly used as an adjunct to intraoperative anesthesia or for postoperative analgesia. Both stimulating and nonstimulating popliteal catheters have been used with success for patients undergoing inpatient and ambulatory surgical procedures. Although ultrasound technology can be used to accurately guide catheter placement, there is insufficient evidence to suggest that this technique is superior to more conventional methods of nerve stimulation.

Neural localization using peripheral nerve stimulation, including the site of needle insertion and needle redirection, is similar for both continuous and single-injection techniques. During popliteal catheter placement, an 18-gauge 4-inch (10-cm) insulated Tuohy needle is inserted using either the posterior or the lateral approach and advanced until a tibial or common peroneal motor response is elicited at a current of 0.5 mA or less. A 20-gauge catheter is then advanced 4 to 6 cm beyond the tip of the needle and secured with a sterile transparent dressing. Alternatively, the catheter may be tunneled subcutaneously to a location remote from the initial insertion site and covered with a protective dressing. The subcutaneous tunneling of catheters may decrease the risk of infectious complications or catheter dislodgement.

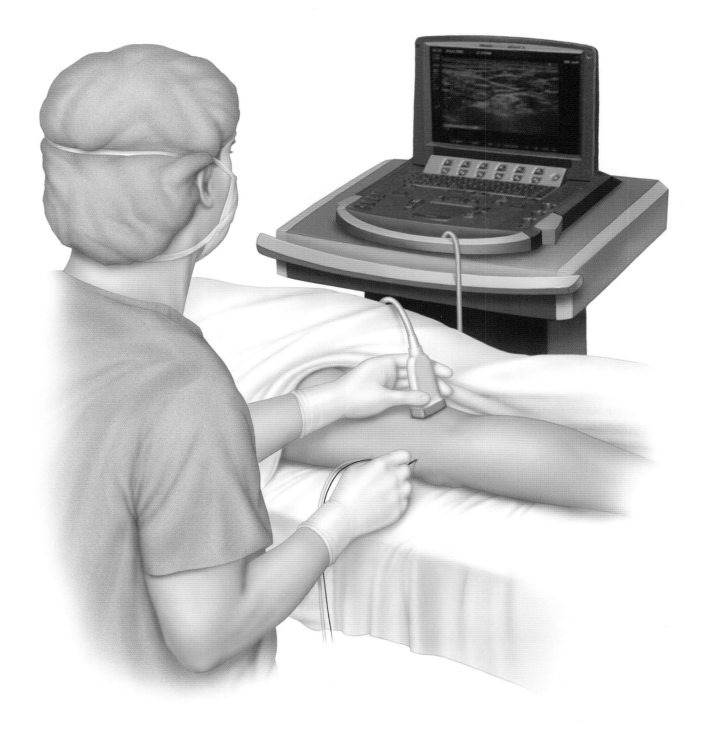

Figure 11. Popliteal ultrasound probe position, showing a lateral needle approach.

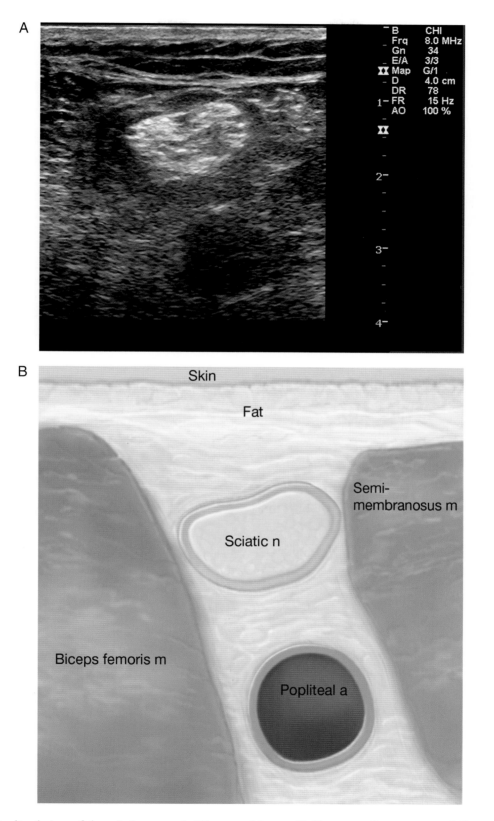

Figure 12. Popliteal view of the sciatic nerve. A, Ultrasound image. B, Corresponding anatomical illustration.

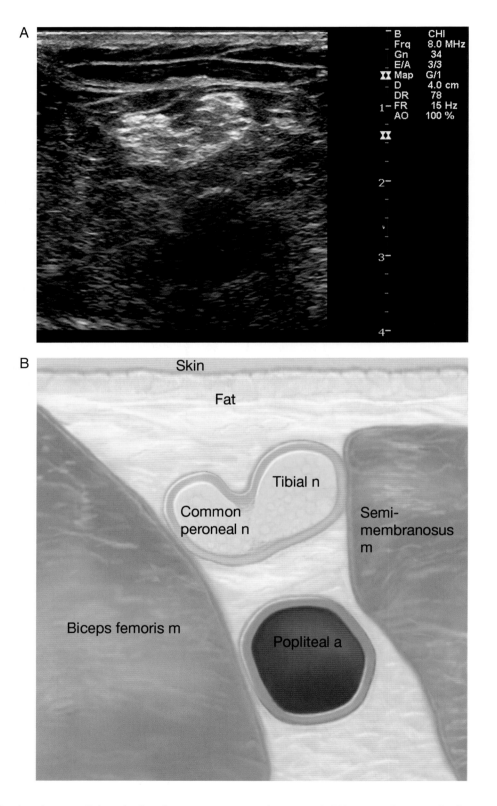

Figure 13. Popliteal view of the tibial and common peroneal nerves. A, Ultrasound image. B, Corresponding anatomical illustration.

Ultrasound-guided popliteal catheter placement is similar to that described for in-plane single-injection ultrasound techniques. Under direct visualization, an 18-gauge 4-inch (10-cm) insulated Tuohy needle is inserted using a lateral in-plane approach and slowly advanced in a medial direction. Location of the needle tip can be confirmed by injecting either saline or a dextrose-containing solution. After optimal needle placement (i.e., immediately adjacent to the sciatic nerve as it begins to diverge into the tibial and common peroneal components), a 20-gauge catheter is advanced 1 to 2 cm beyond the tip of the needle. The distribution of local anesthetic spread is confirmed using real-time ultrasound imaging. If circumferential spread of local anesthetic does not occur, catheter manipulation may be required with direct visualization. Once the catheter location has been optimized, the catheter is secured with a sterile transparent dressing.

Side Effects and Complications

Side effects and complications associated with popliteal sciatic nerve blockade are relatively uncommon. Localized bruising and tenderness may occur; however, true hematoma formation is quite rare. Inadvertent vascular puncture may also occur—particularly when using "blind" techniques. Serious complications due to systemic local anesthetic toxicity (e.g., seizures and cardiovascular collapse) have also been reported. However, these events are exceedingly rare. Finally, infectious complications remain a theoretical concern for both single-injection and continuous catheter techniques.

Postoperative sciatic nerve injury is one of the most feared complications of lower extremity regional blockade. The incidence of neural injury after sciatic nerve blockade is believed to be quite low—despite the fact that intraneural injection of local anesthetic during ultrasound-guided popliteal sciatic nerve blockade has been observed and documented within the literature. However, the precise role of neural blockade as a potential contributor to perioperative nerve injury remains undefined. Limited data suggest that the sciatic nerve may be more susceptible to mechanical, ischemic, or chemical injury than other peripheral nerves. Therefore, although definitive clinical evidence is lacking, it may be prudent to avoid sciatic nerve blockade in patients with multiple surgical or patient-related risk factors (e.g., prolonged tourniquet time, severe peripheral vascular disease, diabetes mellitus, new or progressive neurologic deficit) for peripheral nerve injury.

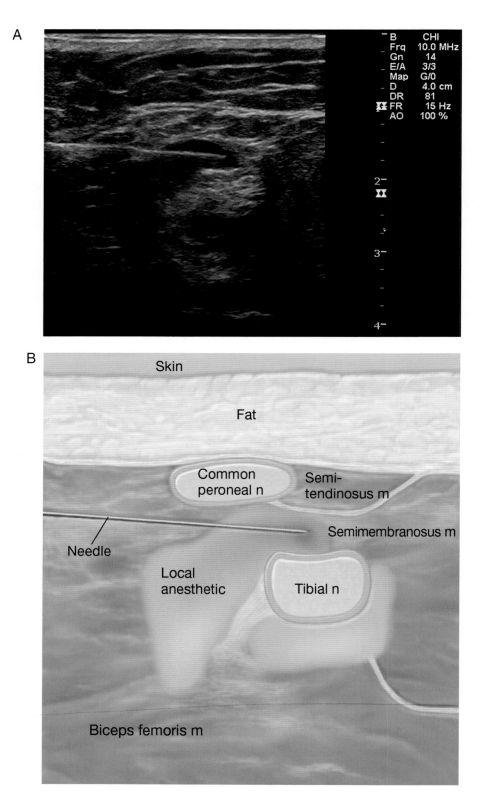

Figure 14. Ultrasound-guided popliteal sciatic nerve blockade. A, Ultrasound image. B, Corresponding anatomical illustration.

Suggested Reading

Benzon HT, Kim C, Benzon HP, Silverstein ME, Jericho B, Prillaman K, et al. Correlation between evoked motor response of the sciatic nerve and sensory blockade. Anesthesiology. 1997 Sep;87(3):547-52.

Borgeat A, Blumenthal S, Lambert M, Theodorou P, Vienne P. The feasibility and complications of the continuous popliteal nerve block: a 1001-case survey. Anesth Analg. 2006 Jul;103(1):229-33.

Chelly JE, Greger J, Casati A, Al-Samsam T, McGarvey W, Clanton T. Continuous lateral sciatic blocks for acute postoperative pain management after major ankle and foot surgery. Foot Ankle Int. 2002 Aug;23(8):749-52.

Enneking FK, Chan V, Greger J, Hadzić A, Lang SA, Horlocker TT. Lower-extremity peripheral nerve blockade: essentials of our current understanding. Reg Anesth Pain Med. 2005 Jan-Feb;30(1):4-35.

Feinglass NG, Clendenen SR, Torp KD, Wang RD, Castello R, Greengrass RA. Real-time three-dimensional ultrasound for continuous popliteal blockade: a case report and image description. Anesth Analg. 2007 Jul;105(1):272-4.

Grosser DM, Herr MJ, Claridge RJ, Barker LG. Preoperative lateral popliteal nerve block for intraoperative and postoperative pain control in elective foot and ankle surgery: a prospective analysis. Foot Ankle Int. 2007 Dec;28(12):1271-5.

Hadzić A, Vloka JD. A comparison of the posterior versus lateral approaches to the block of the sciatic nerve in the popliteal fossa. Anesthesiology. 1998 Jun;88(6):1480-6.

Ilfeld BM, Morey TE, Wand DR, Enneking FK. Continuous popliteal sciatic nerve block for postoperative pain control at home: a randomized, double-blinded, placebo-controlled study. Anesthesiology. 2002 Oct;97(4):959-65.

Paqueron X, Bouaziz H, Macalou D, Labaille T, Merle M, Laxenaire MC, et al. The lateral approach to the sciatic nerve at the popliteal fossa: one or two injections? Anesth Analg. 1999 Nov;89(5):1221-5.

Rorie DK, Byer DE, Nelson DO, Sittipong R, Johnson KA. Assessment of block of the sciatic nerve in the popliteal fossa. Anesth Analg. 1980 May;59(5):371-6.

Vloka JD, Hadzić A, April E, Thys DM. The division of the sciatic nerve in the popliteal fossa: anatomical implications for popliteal nerve blockade. Anesth Analg. 2001 Jan;92(1):215-7.

Zetlaoui PJ, Bouaziz H. Lateral approach to the sciatic nerve in the popliteal fossa. Anesth Analg. 1998 Jul;87(1):79-82.

CHAPTER

28

Ankle Blockade

Adam K. Jacob, M.D.

James R. Hebl, M.D.

Clinical Applications

Ankle blockade was first described in 1922 by Gaston Labat. In his textbook *Regional Anesthesia: Its Technic and Clinical Application*, Labat described local anesthesia blockade of the anterior and posterior tibial nerves for foot and ankle surgery. However, the technique was not popularized until 1976, when Schurman reintroduced the concept of ankle-block anesthesia. Since that time, ankle blockade has become a safe, efficacious, and well-tolerated anesthetic technique for foot and

ankle surgery. Although several variations in the technique have been described, conventional ankle blockade is generally performed at the level of the malleoli. The five terminal branches of the sciatic and femoral nerves are individually blocked to provide prolonged anesthesia and analgesia of the distal extremity. If a thigh or calf tourniquet is used during the surgical procedure, ankle blockade should be considered for only postoperative analgesia—because it will not prevent tourniquet-related pain or discomfort.

Relevant Anatomy

The five peripheral nerves of importance for complete ankle blockade include the terminal branches of the sciatic (i.e., tibial, sural, deep peroneal, and superficial peroneal) and femoral (i.e., saphenous) nerves. The tibial nerve and artery travel within the groove between the tibialis posterior and flexor digitorum longus muscles before passing posterior to the medial malleolus (Figure 1). At the level of the medial malleolus, the tibial nerve separates into the medial plantar, lateral plantar, and medial calcaneal nerves, which provide sensorimotor innervation to the plantar aspect of the foot (Figure 2).

The sural nerve is derived from the medial (i.e., derivative of the tibial nerve) and lateral (i.e., derivative of the common peroneal nerve) sural cutaneous nerves of the proximal leg. It descends the leg along the lateral border of the Achilles (i.e., calcaneal) tendon and passes posterior to the lateral malleolus. At the level of the lateral malleolus, the sural nerve branches into the lateral calcaneal and lateral dorsal cutaneous nerves, which provide sensory innervation to the lateral aspect of the foot and ankle (Figure 2).

The deep peroneal nerve travels within the anterior compartment of the leg with the anterior tibial artery between the tibialis anterior and extensor digitorum longus muscles. It crosses the ankle immediately lateral to the extensor hallucis longus tendon and medial to the extensor digitorum longus tendons (Figures 1 and 3). The deep peroneal nerve provides motor innervation to the tibialis anterior, extensor digitorum longus and brevis, and extensor hallucis longus and brevis muscles. It provides sensory innervation to the deep dorsal structures of the foot and the web space between the first and second toes (Figure 2).

The superficial peroneal nerve travels within the lateral compartment of the leg between the peroneus longus and extensor digitorum longus muscles and terminates in the foot anterior (i.e., superficial) and medial to the lateral malleolus (Figures 1 and 3). It provides motor innervation to the peroneus longus and brevis muscles and sensory innervation to the dorsal aspect of the foot (Figure 2).

The saphenous nerve is derived from the posterior division of the femoral nerve. It descends the leg along the medial border of the tibia within the subcutaneous tissue, immediately posterior to the great saphenous vein. At the level of the ankle, the saphenous nerve passes anterior to the medial malleolus (Figures 1 and 3), where it subdivides into an extensive network of smaller subcutaneous nerve fibers that provide sensory innervation to the medial aspect of the foot and ankle (Figure 2). Saphenous sensory innervation to the foot is variable, but it may extend as far as the base of the great toe.

Surface Anatomy

Important surface landmarks to identify prior to ankle blockade include the bony surfaces of the medial and lateral malleoli, the pulse of the posterior tibial artery, and the extensor hallucis longus tendon. The posterior tibial artery is palpated and marked in the fossa between the medial malleolus and the medial border of the Achilles tendon (Figures 1 and 4). The extensor hallucis longus tendon is identified at the level of the malleoli on the anterior aspect of the ankle (Figure 3). The tendon is accentuated when the patient extends the great toe against resistance. In some patients, the pulse of the anterior tibial artery can be palpated immediately adjacent to the extensor hallucis longus tendon.

Patient Position

The patient is positioned supine. The foot to be blocked is elevated using a padded support or blankets placed under the calf (Figure 5).

Technique

Neural Localization Techniques

Ankle blockade is typically performed using an infiltrative field block technique. The tibial nerve may also be located using peripheral nerve stimulation or ultrasonography.

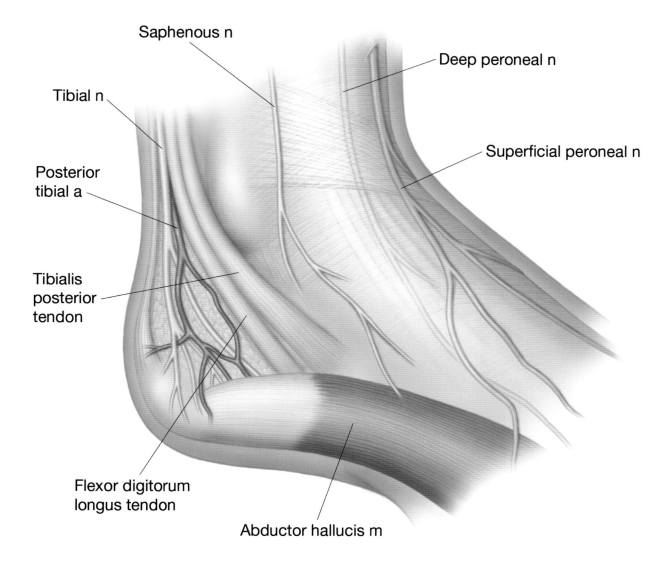

Figure 1. Neurovascular anatomy of the foot and ankle (medial view).

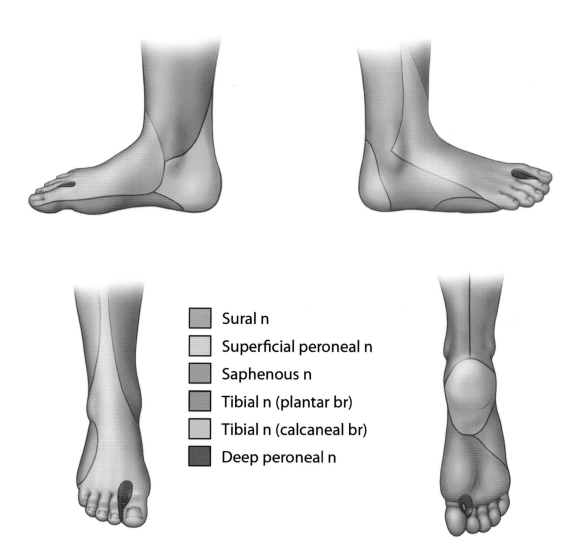

Figure 2. Cutaneous innervation of the foot and ankle.

Needle Insertion Site

Tibial Nerve

At the level of the medial malleolus, a 25-gauge 1.5-inch (3.8-cm) needle is inserted immediately posterior to the pulse of the posterior tibial artery and advanced toward the posterior border of the tibia (Figures 4 and 6). If the pulse cannot be palpated, the needle is inserted at the midpoint between the posterior border of the medial malleolus and the Achilles tendon. If the patient experiences a paresthesia during needle advancement, 8 to 10 mL of local anesthetic is slowly injected. If no paresthesia is elicited, the needle is advanced until the posterior border of the tibia is contacted. The needle is then slightly withdrawn, and, after negative aspiration, 8 to 10 mL of local anesthetic is injected.

Deep Peroneal Nerve

Before the deep peroneal nerve is blocked, the extensor hallucis longus tendon is identified by having the patient

Anterior

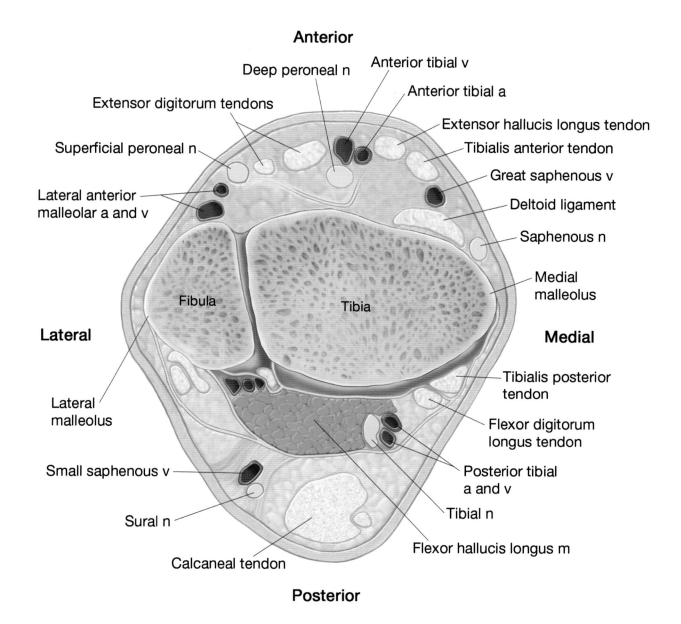

Deep peroneal n

Anterior tibial v

Anterior tibial a

Extensor digitorum tendons

Extensor hallucis longus tendon

Superficial peroneal n

Tibialis anterior tendon

Great saphenous v

Lateral anterior malleolar a and v

Deltoid ligament

Saphenous n

Fibula

Tibia

Medial malleolus

Lateral

Medial

Lateral malleolus

Tibialis posterior tendon

Flexor digitorum longus tendon

Small saphenous v

Posterior tibial a and v

Sural n

Tibial n

Calcaneal tendon

Flexor hallucis longus m

Posterior

Figure 3. Cross-sectional anatomy of the ankle.

extend the great toe against resistance. A 25-gauge 1.5-inch (3.8-cm) needle is then inserted perpendicular to the skin at the intramalleolar level, immediately lateral to the extensor hallucis longus tendon (Figures 6 and 7). The needle is advanced until the tibia is contacted. The needle is then slightly withdrawn, and 5 to 8 mL of local anesthetic is slowly injected.

Superficial Peroneal Nerve
A 25-gauge 1.5-inch (3.8-cm) needle is used to subcutaneously infiltrate 5 to 7 mL of local anesthetic from the needle insertion site used for deep peroneal nerve blockade to the *lateral* malleolus (Figure 6). Diffuse subcutaneous infiltration is required to ensure comprehensive blockade.

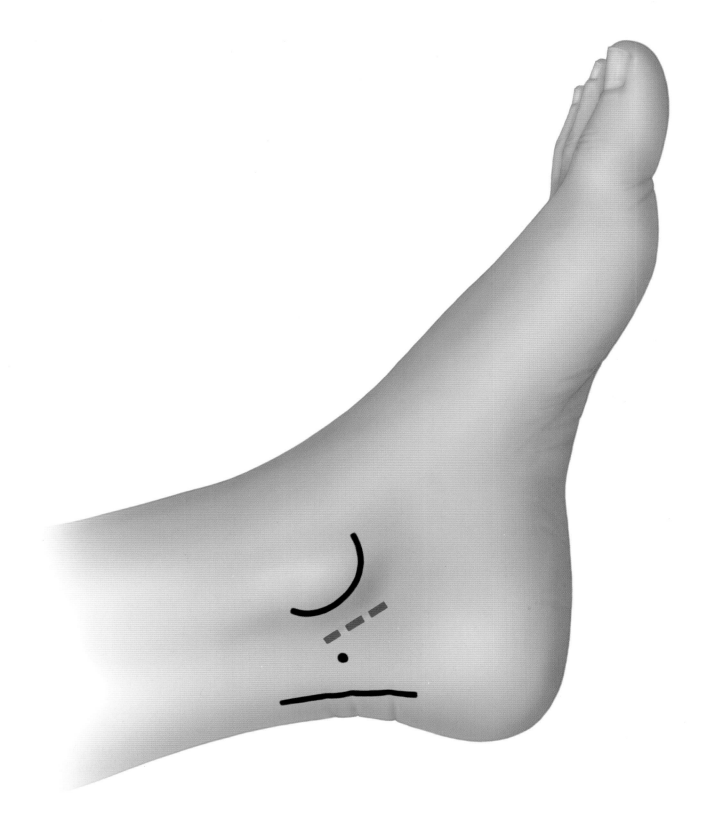

Figure 4. Surface landmarks for tibial nerve blockade.

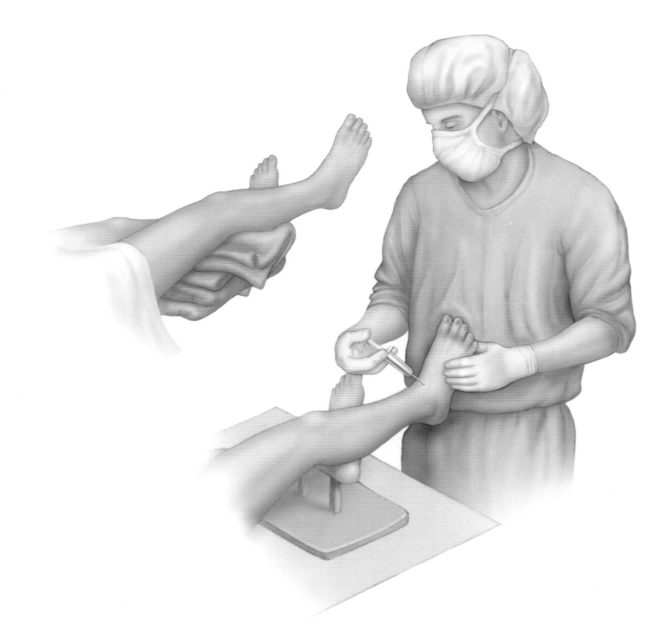

Figure 5. Patient-provider orientation during ankle blockade.

Saphenous Nerve

A 25-gauge 1.5-inch (3.8-cm) needle is used to sub-cutaneously infiltrate 5 to 7 mL of local anesthetic from the needle insertion site used for deep peroneal nerve blockade to the *medial* malleolus (Figure 6). Diffuse subcutaneous infiltration is required to ensure comprehensive blockade.

Sural Nerve

At the cephalic border of the lateral malleolus, a 25-gauge 1.5-inch (3.8-cm) needle is inserted along the lateral aspect of the Achilles tendon and advanced toward the posterior border of the fibula (Figure 6). Five to 8 mL of local anesthetic is injected from the subcutaneous tissue to the posterior border of the lateral malleolus.

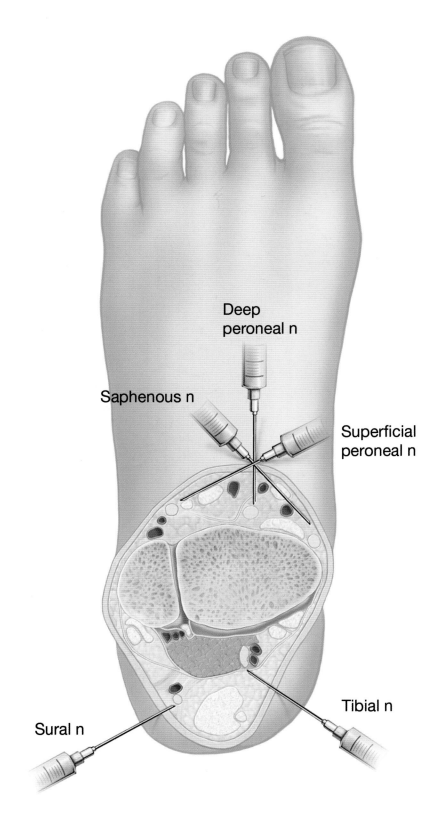

Figure 6. Needle insertion sites during ankle blockade.

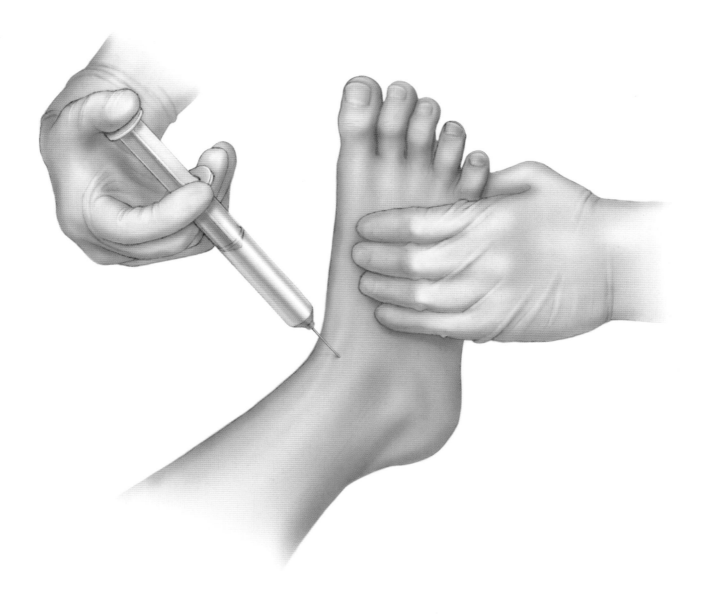

Figure 7. Deep peroneal nerve blockade.

Side Effects and Complications

Side effects and complications associated with ankle blockade are extremely rare. Persistent tingling and paresthesias have been reported in 2% to 25% of patients for a limited time during the postoperative period. However, it is unclear whether these symptoms are caused by prolonged neural blockade, surgical trauma, tourniquet ischemia, or neural injury. Localized bruising and tenderness may also occur after ankle blockade; however, true hematoma formation is quite rare. Other theoretical concerns include infection, bleeding, intravascular injection, and local anesthetic toxicity. Local anesthetic solutions containing epinephrine should *not* be used during ankle blockade—particularly if local anesthetic is injected circumferentially around the ankle. Small distal vessels may be susceptible to vasoconstriction, resulting in peripheral ischemia.

Suggested Reading

Brown DL. Atlas of regional anesthesia. 2nd ed. Philadelphia: W. B. Saunders; c1999.

Hebl JR. Peripheral nerve injury. In: Neal JM, Rathmell JP, editors. Complications in regional anesthesia and pain medicine. Philadelphia: W. B. Saunders; c2007. p. 125-40.

Labat G. Regional anesthesia: its technic and clinical application. Philadelphia: W. B. Saunders; c1922.

Schabort D, Boon JM, Becker PJ, Meiring JH. Easily identifiable bony landmarks as an aid in targeted regional ankle blockade. Clin Anat. 2005 Oct;18(7):518-26.

Schurman DJ. Ankle block anesthesia for foot surgery. Anesthesiology. 1976 Apr;44(4):348-52.

Turan I, Assareh H, Rolf C, Jakobsson J. Multi-modal-analgesia for pain management after Hallux Valgus surgery: a prospective randomised study on the effect of ankle block. J Orthop Surg Res. 2007 Dec 18;2:26.

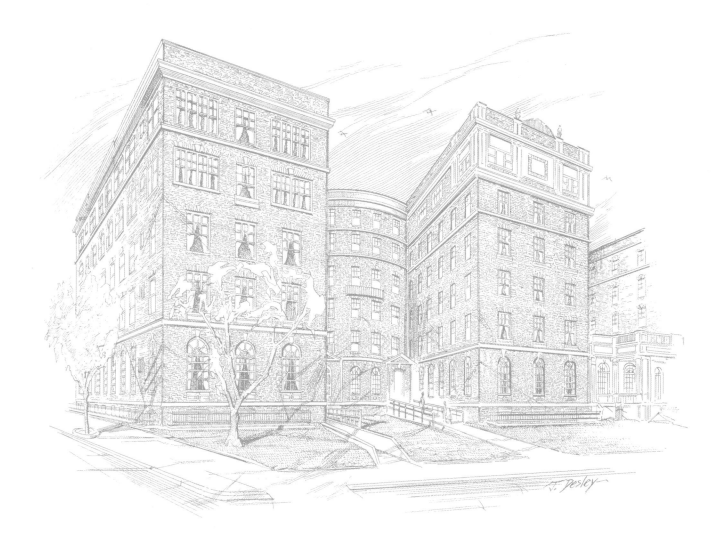

INDEX

Page references that contain *f* refer to figures; those containing *t* refer to tables.